ANTIBIOTIC ESSENTIALS

Burke A. Cunha, M.D.

Chief, Infectious Disease Division
Winthrop-University Hospital
Mineola, New York
Professor of Medicine
State University of New York
School of Medicine
Stony Brook, New York

PHYSICIANS' PRESS

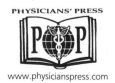

www.physicianspress.com

ABOUT THE EDITOR

Burke A. Cunha, M.D., is Chief, Infectious Disease Division at Winthrop-University Hospital, Mineola, New York, Professor of Medicine, State University of New York School of Medicine, Stony Brook, New York, and is one of the world's leading authorities on the treatment of infectious diseases. During his 30-year career, he has contributed more than 800 articles, 150 book chapters, and 10 books on infectious diseases to the medical literature. He has received numerous teaching awards, including the prestigious Aesculapius Award for outstanding teaching. He also serves on the editorial boards of more than two dozen medical journals, is Editor-in-Chief of *Infectious Disease Practice* and *Antibiotics for Clinicians*, and is Infectious Disease Editor-in-Chief for eMedicine on-line. Dr. Cunha is a Fellow of the Infectious Disease Society of America, American Academy of Microbiology, American College of Clinical Pharmacology, and American College of Chest Physicians. He has had a life-long interest in antimicrobial therapy in normal and compromised hosts, antibiotic pharmacokinetics/pharmacodynamics, pharmacoeconomics, and antibiotic resistance. Dr. Cunha is a Master of the American College of Physicians, awarded for achievements as a master clinician and teacher.

Be sure to visit www.physicianspress.com for a complete listing of medical titles, along with topical reviews, self-assessment questions, and other clinical information. Undetected errors/omissions in *Antibiotic Essentials* discovered after publication, if any, will also be posted. Feel free to contact us by e-mail with comments or suggestions.

Additional copies of *Antibiotic Essentials* may be obtained at medical bookstores, or you may contact us directly at:

Physicians' Press
620 Cherry Street
Royal Oak, Michigan, 48073
Tel: (248) 616-3023
Fax: (248) 616-3003
www.physicianspress.com

Printed in the United States of America   ISBN: 1-890114-34-0

TABLE OF CONTENTS

CONTRIBUTORS

BURKE A. CUNHA, M.D.
Chief, Infectious Disease Division
Winthrop–University Hospital
Mineola, New York
Professor of Medicine
State University of New York School of Medicine
Stony Brook, New York
Overview of Antimicrobial Therapy
Empiric Therapy Based on Clinical Syndrome
Initial Therapy Based on Isolates
Parasites, Fungi, Unusual Organisms
Antibiotic Prophylaxis and Immunization
Antimicrobial Drug Summaries

Paul Ambrose, Pharm.D.
Director, Infectious Diseases
Kendle International
Princeton, New Jersey
Antimicrobial Drug Interactions

Christy Owens, Pharm.D.
Department of Medical and Scientific Affairs
Novartis
South Freeport, Maine
Antimicrobial Drug Interactions

Robert C. Owens, Jr., Pharm.D.
Clinical Specialist, Infectious Diseases
Maine Medical Center
Clinical Instructor
University of Vermont College of Medicine
Burlington, Vermont
Antimicrobial Drug Interactions

Paul E. Sax, M.D.
Director, HIV Program
Brigham and Women's Hospital
Assistant Professor of Medicine
Harvard Medical School
Boston, Massachusetts
HIV Infection

Kenneth F. Wagner, D.O.
Attending Physician, Infectious Disease Consultant
National Naval Medical Center
Associate Professor of Medicine
Uniformed Services
University of the Health Sciences
F. Edward Hebert School of Medicine
Bethesda, Maryland
Parasites, Fungi, Unusual Organisms

REVIEWERS

Pierre Dorsainvil, M.D.
Mineola, New York
Parasites, Fungi, Unusual Organisms

Theodore C. Eickhoff, M.D.
Denver, Colorado
Prophylaxis and Immunization

Pierce Gardner, M.D.
Washington, D.C.
Prophylaxis and Immunization

Eric A. Hansen, D.O.
Cape May, New Jersey
Parasites, Fungi, Unusual Organisms

Diane H. Johnson, M.D.
Mineola, New York
Prophylaxis and Immunization

Mark H. Kaplan, M.D.
Manhasset, New York
HIV Drug Summaries

Mary Y. Ma, Pharm.D.
Los Angeles, California
Antimicrobial Drug Summaries

James H. Maguire, M.D.
Atlanta, Georgia
Parasites, Fungi, Unusual Organisms

Venkat R. Minnaganti, M.D.
Decatur, Illinois
Parasites, Fungi, Unusual Organisms

Kathleen E. Sartoris, Pharm.D.
Queens, New York
Antimicrobial Drug Summaries

David Schlossberg, M.D.
Philadelphia, Pennsylvania
Empiric Therapy

Paul E. Schoch, Ph.D.
Mineola, New York
Medical Microbiology

ACKNOWLEDGMENTS

To accomplish the task of presenting the data compiled in this reference, a small, dedicated team of professionals was assembled. This team focused their energy and discipline for many months into typing, revising, designing, illustrating, and formatting the many chapters that make up this text. I wish to acknowledge Monica Crowder-Kaufmann, Lisa Lusardi, Rebecca Smith, and Cindy Gillespie for their important contribution. I would also like to thank the many contributors and reviewers who graciously contributed their time and energy amidst busy professional lives, Mark Freed, M.D., President and Editor-in-Chief of Physicians' Press, for his vision, commitment, and guidance, Norman Lyle for cover design, and the staff at Dickinson Press for their printing expertise.

I am indebted to these individuals, and hope their efforts are well received.

Burke A. Cunha, M.D.

NOTICE

for
Marie

"Grace in her steps,
Heaven in her eye,
In every gesture, dignity and love"
Milton

ABBREVIATIONS

A-V	atrio-ventricular
AAC	antibiotic associated colitis
AAD	antibiotic associated diarrhea
ABE	acute bacterial endocarditis
ABM	acute bacterial meningitis
AFB	acid fast bacilli
ANA	antinuclear antibody
ARC	AIDS-related complex
ARDS	adult respiratory distress syndrome
ASD	atrial septal defect
AV	arteriovenous
β-lactams	penicillins, cephalosporins, cephamycins (not monobactams or carbapenems)
BAL	bronchoalveolar lavage
CAB	catheter associated bacteriuria
CABG	coronary artery bypass grafting
CAH	chronic active hepatitis
CAP	community acquired pneumonia
CCU	critical care unit
CD_4	CD_4 T-cell lymphocyte
CE	California encephalitis virus
CIE	counter-immunoelectrophoresis
CLL	chronic lymphocytic leukemia
CMV	Cytomegalovirus
CNS	central nervous system
CPH	chronic persistent hepatitis
CPK	creatine phosphokinase
CrCl	creatinine clearance
CSD	Cat Scratch Disease
CSF	cerebrospinal fluid
CT	computerized tomography
CVA	costovertebral angle
CXR	chest x-ray
D & C	dilatation and curettage
DFA	direct fluorescent antibody
DI	diabetes insipidus
DIC	disseminated intravascular coagulation
DM	diabetes mellitus
DNA	deoxyribonucleic acid
e.g.	for example
EBV	Ebstein-Barr virus
EEE	Eastern equine encephalitis virus
EEG	electroencephalogram
EIA	enzyme immunoassay
ELISA	enzyme-linked immunosorbent assay
EM	erythema migrans
EMB	ethambutol
ENT	ear, nose, throat
Enterobacteriaceae:	Citrobacter, Edwardsiella, Enterobacter, E. coli, Klebsiella, Proteus, Providencia, Salmonella, Serratia, Shigella
ESBLs	extended spectrum β-lactamases
esp	especially
ESR	erythrocyte sedimentation rate
ESRD	end-stage renal disease
ET	endotracheal
FTA-ABS	fluorescent treponemal antibody absorption test
FUO	fever of unknown origin
g	gram
G6PD	glucose-6-phosphate dehydrogenase
GC	gonococcus/gonorrhea
GI	gastrointestinal
gm	gram
GU	genitourinary
HAV	Hepatitis A virus
HBcAb	hepatitis B core antibody
HBsAg	hepatitis B surface antigen
HAV	Hepatitis A virus
HBV	Hepatitis B virus
HCV	Hepatitis C virus
HDCV	human diploid cell vaccine
HDV	Hepatitis D virus
HEENT	head, eyes, ears, nose, throat
HEV	Hepatitis E virus
HFV	Hepatitis F virus
HGE	human granulocytic ehrlichiosis
HHV-6	human Herpes virus 6
HLA	histocompatibility antigen
HME	human monocytic ehrlichiosis
HPV	human papilloma virus
HRIG	human rabies immune globulin
HSV	Herpes simplex virus
I & D	incision and drainage
IBD	inflammatory bowel disease
IFA	immunofluorescent antibody
IgA	immunoglobulin A
IgG	immunoglobulin G
IgM	immunoglobulin M
INH	isoniazid
IT	intrathecal
ITP	idiopathic thrombocytopenic purpura
IUD	intrauterine device
IV/PO	IV or PO

IV	intravenous	PO	oral
IVDA	intravenous drug abuser	PPNG	penicillinase-producing N. gonorrhoeae
kg	kilogram	PVD	peripheral vascular disease
L	liter	PVE	prosthetic valve endocarditis
LCM	lymphocytic choriomeningitis	PZA	pyrazinamide
LDH	lactate dehydrogenase	q__h	every __ hours
LFT	liver function test	q__d	every __ days
LGV	lymphogranuloma venereum	qmonth	once a month
LLQ	left lower quadrant	qweek	once a week
LUQ	left upper quadrant	RBC	red blood cells
MAI	Mycobacterium avium-intracellulare	RLQ	right lower quadrant
mcg	microgram	RMSF	Rocky Mountain spotted fever
mcL	microliter	RNA	ribonucleic acid
mg	milligram	RUQ	right upper quadrant
mL	milliliter	RVA	rabies vaccine absorbed
MIC	minimum inhibitory concentration	SBE	subacute bacterial endocarditis
min	minute	SGOT/SGPT	liver function test
MMR	measles, mumps, rubella	SLE	systemic lupus erythematosus
MRI	magnetic resonance imaging	sp.	species
MRSA	methicillin-resistant S. aureus	SPEP	serum protein electrophoresis
MRSE	methicillin-resistant S. epidermidis	SQ	subcutaneous
MSSA	methicillin-sensitive S. aureus	STD	sexually transmitted diseases
MSSE	methicillin-sensitive S. epidermidis	TAH/BSO	total abdominal hysterectomy/bilateral salpingoopherectomy
MTT	methlytetrathiazolethiol		
MVP	mitral valve prolapse	TB	tuberculosis
NNRTI	non-nucleoside reverse transcriptase inhibitor	TEE	transesophageal echocardiogram
		TID	three times per day
NP	nosocomial pneumonia	TMP	trimethoprim
NRTI	nucleoside reverse transcriptase inhibitor	TMP-SMX	trimethoprim-sulfamethoxazole
		TRNG	tetracycline-resistant N. gonorrhoeae
NS	neurosurgical	TST	tuberculin skin test
NSAIDS	nonsteroidal anti-inflammatory drugs	TTE	transthoracic echocardiogram
OI	opportunistic infection	TURP	transurethral resection of prostate
PBS	protected brush specimen	UTI	urinary tract infection
PCEC	purified chick embryo cells	VA	ventriculoatrial
PCN	penicillin	VP	ventriculoperitoneal
PCP	Pneumocystis carinii pneumonia	VAP	ventilator-associated pneumonia
PCR	polymerase chain reaction	VCA	viral capsid antigen
PDA	patent ductus arteriosus	VEE	Venezuelan equine encephalitis virus
PEP	post-exposure prophylaxis	VRE	vancomycin-resistant enterococci
PI	protease inhibitor	VZV	Varicella zoster virus
PML	progressive multifocal leukoencephalopathy	WBC	white blood cells
		WNE	Western Nile encephalitis virus
PMN	polymorphonuclear leucocytes	yrs	years

Chapter 1
Overview of Antimicrobial Therapy
Burke A. Cunha, M.D.

Overview of Antimicrobial Therapy

Infectious diseases are the leading cause of morbidity and mortality worldwide. The ability of bacteria, viruses, mycobacteria, fungi, protozoa, chlamydiae, mycoplasmas, spirochetes, rickettsia, and helminths to cause infection is a balance between inoculum size, virulence, and the adequacy of host defenses. Despite the ability of antimicrobial therapy to augment normal host defenses and prevent/control infection, prescribing errors are common, including treatment of colonization, suboptimal empiric therapy, inappropriate combination therapy, dosing and duration errors, and mismanagement of apparent antibiotic failure. Inadequate consideration of antibiotic resistance potential, tissue penetration, drug interactions, side effects, and cost also limits the effectiveness of antimicrobial therapy. *Antibiotic Essentials* is a concise, practical, and authoritative guide to the treatment and prevention of infectious diseases commonly encountered in clinical practice.

FACTORS IN ANTIBIOTIC SELECTION

A. **Spectrum.** Antibiotic spectrum refers to the range of microorganisms an antibiotic is usually effective against, and is the basis for empiric antibiotic therapy (Chapter 2).

B. **Tissue Penetration**. Antibiotics that are effective against a microorganism in-vitro but unable to reach the site of infection are of little or no benefit to the host. Antibiotic tissue penetration depends on properties of the antibiotic (e.g., lipid solubility, molecular size) and tissue (e.g, adequacy of blood supply, presence of inflammation). Antibiotic tissue penetration is rarely problematic in acute infections due to increased microvascular permeability from local release of chemical inflammatory mediators. In contrast, chronic infections (e.g., chronic pyelonephritis, chronic prostatitis, chronic osteomyelitis) and infections caused by intracellular pathogens often rely on chemical properties of an antibiotic (e.g., high lipid solubility, small molecular size) for adequate tissue penetration. Antibiotics cannot be expected to eradicate organisms from areas that are difficult to penetrate or have impaired blood supply, such as abscesses, which usually require surgical drainage for cure. In addition, implanted foreign materials associated with infection usually need to be removed for cure, since microbes causing infections associated with prosthetic joints, shunts, and intravenous lines produce a slime/glycocalyx on plastic/metal surfaces that permits organisms to survive despite antimicrobial therapy. Antimicrobial penetration into cerebrospinal fluid (CSF) is shown in Table 1.

C. **Antibiotic Resistance.** Bacterial resistance to antimicrobial therapy can be natural or acquired, and relative or absolute. Pathogens not covered by the usual spectrum of an antibiotic are *naturally* resistant (e.g., 25% of S. pneumoniae are naturally resistant to macrolides), while *acquired* resistance occurs when a previously sensitive pathogen is no longer as sensitive to an antibiotic (e.g., ampicillin-resistant H. influenzae). Organisms with *intermediate level (relative)* resistance manifest increases in minimum inhibitory

Table 1. Antimicrobial Penetration Into Cerebrospinal Fluid

Class	Excellent Penetration	Good Penetration	Poor Penetration

Antibiotics	TMP-SMX
	Chloramphenicol
	Cycloserine
	Pyrazinamide
	INH
	Rifampin
	Minocycline
	Linezolid
		Meropenem
		Doxycycline
		3rd generation
		  cephalosporins
		Cefepime
		Aztreonam
		Nafcillin
		Tetracycline
			Most penicillins
			$1^{st}, 2^{nd}$ generation
			  cephalosporins
			Aminoglycosides
			Quinolones
			Quinupristin/dalfopristin
			Macrolides
			Vancomycin
			Imipenem
			Polymyxin B
			Clindamycin

Antivirals	Zidovudine Vidarabine	Acyclovir Stavudine Saquinavir Didanosine Ritonavir Indinavir Valacyclovir Famciclovir	Other antivirals
Antifungals	Flucytosine Fluconazole Voriconazole	Itraconazole	Amphotericin B Caspofungin

concentrations (MICs) to an antibiotic over time, but remain susceptible to the antibiotic at achievable serum/tissue concentrations (e.g., penicillin-resistant S. pneumoniae). In contrast, organisms with *high level (absolute)* resistance manifest a sudden increase in MICs during therapy, and cannot be overcome by higher-than-usual antibiotic doses (e.g., gentamicin-resistant P. aeruginosa).

Antibiotic resistance is *agent-specific*, not a class phenomenon (e.g, ciprofloxacin-resistant S. pneumoniae are not resistant to other quinolones), and is *not* related to volume or duration of use: Antibiotics with low resistance potential (e.g., levofloxacin) manifest little or no resistance even when used in high volume, while other antibiotics (e.g., ciprofloxacin) can develop resistance with minimal use. Successful antibiotic resistance control strategies include eliminating antibiotics from animal feeds, microbial surveillance to detect resistance problems early, infection control precautions to limit/contain spread of clonal resistance, restricted hospital formulary (i.e., controlled use of high resistance potential antibiotics), and preferential use of low resistance potential antibiotics by clinicians. Unsuccessful strategies include rotating formularies, restricted use of certain antibiotic classes (e.g., 3rd generation cephalosporins, fluoroquinolones), and use of combination therapy. In choosing between similar antibiotics, always select an antibiotic with a low resistance potential. In addition to usual resistance problems (Table 2), imipenem, ceftazidime, and ciprofloxacin are associated with increased prevalence of methicillin-resistant S. aureus (MRSA), and vancomycin is associated with increased prevalence of vancomycin-resistant enterococci (VRE).

D. Safety Profile. Whenever possible, avoid antibiotics with serious/frequent side effects.

E. Cost. Switching early from IV to PO antibiotics is the single most important cost saving strategy in hospitalized patients, as the institutional cost of IV administration (~$10/dose) may exceed the cost of the antibiotic itself. Antibiotic costs can also be minimized by using antibiotics with long half-lives, and by choosing monotherapy over combination therapy. Other factors adding to the cost of antimicrobial therapy include the need for an obligatory second antimicrobial agent, antibiotic side effects (e.g., diarrhea, cutaneous reactions, seizures, phlebitis), and outbreaks of resistant organisms, which require cohorting and prolonged hospitalization.

Table 2. Resistance Potential of Commonly Used Antibiotics

Antibiotics with High Resistance Potential	
Antibiotic	**Usual Resistance Problems**
Ampicillin	H. influenzae, E. coli, S. aureus
Tetracycline	S. aureus, S. pneumoniae, N. gonorrhoeae
TMP-SMX	S. pneumoniae, H. influenzae
Cefamandole	H. influenzae, Enterobacter
Ceftazidime[1]	P. aeruginosa, Enterobacter, Klebsiella
Gentamicin	P. aeruginosa
Tobramycin	P. aeruginosa
Imipenem[1]	P. aeruginosa
Ciprofloxacin[1]	P. aeruginosa, S. pneumoniae
Rifampin[2]	Enterobacteriaceae

Antibiotics with Low Resistance Potential[3]			
Amikacin	Doxycycline	Ofloxacin	Cefotetan
Clindamycin	Minocycline	Gatifloxacin	Cefoxitin
Chloramphenicol	Aztreonam	Gemifloxacin	Cefprozil
Azithromycin	Ertapenem	Grepafloxacin	Cefuroxime
Telithromycin	Meropenem	Levofloxacin	3rd generation cephalosporins[5]
Vancomycin[4]	Polymyxin B	Moxifloxacin	Cefepime
Quinupristin/	Nitrofurantoin	Sparfloxacin	Ampicillin/sulbactam
dalfopristin	Metronidazole	Trovafloxacin	Piperacillin/tazobactam
Linezolid	Nafcillin	Fosfomycin	Antipseudomonal penicillins[6]

1. Use associated with increased prevalence of methicillin-resistant S. aureus (MRSA)
2. Increased resistance if used alone, but not in combination
3. Antibiotics not associated with widespread resistance problems, even with prolonged/unrestricted use
4. Vancomycin does not increase E. faecalis resistance, but increases the prevalence of vancomycin-resistant E. faecium (VRE)
5. Except ceftazidime
6. Except carbenicillin

FACTORS IN ANTIBIOTIC DOSING

Usual antibiotic dosing assumes normal renal and hepatic function. Patients with significant renal insufficiency and/or hepatic dysfunction may require dosage reduction in antibiotics metabolized/eliminated by these organs (Table 3). Specific dosing recommendations based on the degree of renal and hepatic insufficiency are detailed in Chapter 7.

A. **Renal Insufficiency.** Since most antibiotics eliminated by the kidneys have a wide "toxic-to-therapeutic ratio," dosing strategies are frequently based on formula-derived estimates of creatinine clearance (Table 3), rather than precise quantitation of glomerular filtration rates. Dosage adjustments are especially important for antibiotics with narrow toxic-to-therapeutic ratios (e.g., aminoglycosides), and for patients who are receiving other nephrotoxic medications or have preexisting renal disease.

  1. **Loading and Maintenance Dosing in Renal Insufficiency.** For drugs eliminated by the kidneys, the loading dose (if required) is left unchanged, and the maintenance dose and dosing interval are modified in proportion to the degree of renal insufficiency. For moderate renal insufficiency (CrCl ~ 40-60 mL/min), the maintenance dose is usually cut in half and the dosing interval is left unchanged. For severe renal insufficiency (CrCl ~ 10-40 mL/min), the maintenance dose is usually cut in half and the dosing interval is doubled. Dosing adjustment problems in renal insufficiency can be circumvented by selecting an antibiotic with a similar spectrum that is eliminated by the hepatic route.

  2. **Aminoglycoside Dosing.** Aminoglycosides have a narrow toxic-to-therapeutic ratio and high nephrotoxic potential, and are of particular concern for patients with renal insufficiency. Single daily dosing—adjusted for the degree of renal insufficiency after the loading dose is administered—has virtually eliminated the nephrotoxic potential of aminoglycosides, and is recommended for all patients, including the critically ill. (A possible exception is enterococcal endocarditis, where gentamicin dosing every 8 hours may be preferable.) Aminoglycoside-induced tubular dysfunction is best assessed by quantitative renal tubular cast counts in urine, which more accurately reflect aminoglycoside nephrotoxicity than serum creatinine.

B. **Hepatic Insufficiency.** Antibiotic dosing for patients with hepatic dysfunction is problematic, since there is no hepatic counterpart to the serum creatinine to accurately assess liver function. In practice, antibiotic dosing is based on clinical assessment of the severity of liver disease. For practical purposes, dosing adjustments are usually not required for mild or moderate hepatic insufficiency. For severe hepatic insufficiency, dosing adjustments are usually made for antibiotics with hepatotoxic potential (Chapter 7). Relatively few antibiotics depend solely on hepatic inactivation/elimination, and dosing adjustment problems in these cases can be circumvented by selecting an appropriate antibiotic eliminated by the renal route.

Table 3. Dosing Strategies in Hepatic/Renal Insufficiency*

Hepatic Insufficiency
- Decrease total daily dose of hepatically-eliminated antibiotic by 50% in presence of clinically severe liver disease
- Alternative: Use antibiotic eliminated/inactivated by the renal route in usual dose

Renal Insufficiency
- If creatinine clearance ~ 40-60 mL/min, decrease dose of renally-eliminated antibiotic by 50% and maintain the usual dosing interval
- If creatinine clearance ~10-40 mL/min, decrease dose of renally-eliminated antibiotic by 50% and double the dosing interval
- Alternative: Use antibiotic eliminated/inactivated by the hepatic route in usual dose

Major Route of Elimination			
Hepatobiliary		**Renal**	
Chloramphenicol	Quinupristin/dalfopristin	Most β-lactams	Vancomycin
Cefoperazone	Nafcillin	Aminoglycosides	Most quinolones
Doxycycline	Linezolid	TMP-SMX	Nitrofurantoin
Minocycline	INH	Monobactams	Fluconazole
Sparfloxacin	Pyrazinamide	Carbapenems	Acyclovir
Trovafloxacin	Rifampin	Polymyxin B	Valacyclovir
Grepafloxacin	Clindamycin	Tetracycline	Famciclovir
Gemifloxacin	Metronidazole		
Moxifloxacin	Itraconazole		
Macrolides	Caspofungin		
Ketolides	Voriconazole		

* See individual drug summaries in Chapter 7 for specific dosing recommendations
Creatinine clearance (CrCl) is used to assess renal function, and can be estimated by the following formula:
CrCl (mL/min) = [(140 − age) x weight (kg)] / [72 x serum creatinine (mg/dL)]. Multiply by 0.85 if female. It is important to recognize that due to age-dependent declines in renal function, elderly patients with "normal" serum creatinines may have CrCls requiring dosage adjustment. For example, a 70-year-old, 50-kg female with a serum creatinine of 1.2 mg/dL has an estimated CrCl of 34 mL/min

C. **Combined Renal and Hepatic Insufficiency.**   There are no good dosing adjustment guidelines for patients with hepatorenal insufficiency. If renal insufficiency is worse than hepatic insufficiency, antibiotics eliminated by the liver are often administered at half the total daily dose. If hepatic insufficiency is worse than renal insufficiency, antibiotics eliminated by the kidneys are usually administered and dosed in proportion to renal function.

OTHER CONSIDERATIONS IN ANTIMICROBIAL THERAPY

A. **Bactericidal vs. Bacteriostatic Therapy.** For most infections, bacteriostatic and bactericidal antibiotics inhibit/kill organisms at the same rate, and should not be a factor in antibiotic selection. Bactericidal antibiotics have an advantage in certain infections, such endocarditis, meningitis, and febrile leukopenia, but there are exceptions even in these cases.

B. **Monotherapy vs. Combination Therapy**. Monotherapy is preferred to combination therapy, and is possible for most infections. In addition to cost savings, monotherapy results in less chance of medication error and fewer missed doses/drug interactions. Combination therapy may be useful for drug synergy or for extending spectrum beyond what can be obtained with a single drug. However, since drug synergy is difficult to assess and the possibility of antagonism always exists, antibiotics should be combined for synergy only if synergy is likely based on experience or actual testing. Combination therapy is not effective in preventing antibiotic resistance, except in very few situations (Table 4).

C. **Intravenous vs. Oral Switch Therapy.** Patients admitted to the hospital are usually started on IV antibiotic therapy, then switched to equivalent oral therapy after clinical improvement/defervescence (usually within 72 hours). Advantages of early IV-to-PO switch programs include reduced cost, early hospital discharge, less need for home IV therapy, and virtual elimination of IV line infections. Drugs well-suited for IV-to-PO switch or for treatment entirely by the oral route include doxycycline, minocycline, clindamycin, metronidazole, chloramphenicol, amoxicillin, trimethoprim-sulfamethoxazole, levofloxacin, and linezolid. Only some penicillins and cephalosporins are useful for IV-to-PO switch programs, due to limited bioavailability.

Table 4. Combination Therapy and Antibiotic Resistance

Antibiotic Combinations That Prevent Resistance
Anti-pseudomonal penicillin (carbenicillin) + aminoglycoside (gentamicin, tobramycin, amikacin)
Rifampin + other TB drugs (INH, ethambutol, pyrazinamide)
5-flucytosine + amphotericin B

Frequently Used Antibiotic Combinations That Do Not Prevent Resistance*
TMP-SMX
Ceftazidime in combination with any other antibiotic
Ciprofloxacin in combination with any other antibiotic
Imipenem in combination with any other antibiotic
Most other antibiotic combinations

* These combinations are often prescribed to prevent resistance when, in actuality, they do not

Most infectious diseases should be treated orally, unless the patient is critically ill, cannot take antibiotics by mouth, or there is no equivalent oral antibiotic. If the patient is able to take/absorb oral antibiotics, there is no difference in clinical outcome using equivalent IV or PO antibiotics. It is more important to think in terms of antibiotic spectrum, bioavailability and tissue penetration, rather than route of administration. Nearly all non-critically ill patients should be treated in part or entirely with oral antibiotics. When switching from IV to PO therapy, the oral antibiotic chosen ideally should achieve the same blood and tissue levels as the equivalent IV antibiotic (Table 5).

D. Duration of Therapy. Most bacterial infections in normal hosts are treated with antibiotics for 1-2 weeks. The duration of therapy may need to be extended in patients with impaired immunity (e.g., diabetes, SLE, alcoholic liver disease, neutropenia, diminished splenic function, etc.), chronic bacterial infections (e.g., endocarditis, osteomyelitis), chronic viral and fungal infections, or certain bacterial intracellular pathogens (Table 6). Infections such as HIV and CMV in compromised hosts usually require life-long suppressive therapy. Antibiotic therapy should ordinarily not be continued for more than 2 weeks, even if low-grade fevers persist. Prolonged therapy offers no benefit, and increases the risk of adverse side effects, drug interactions, and superinfections.

Table 5. Bioavailability of Oral Antimicrobials

Bioavailability	Antimicrobials		
Excellent[1]	Amoxicillin	TMP	Minocycline
	Clindamycin	TMP-SMX	Linezolid
	Most quinolones	Doxycycline	Fluconazole
	5-Flucytosine	Chloramphenicol	Voriconazole
	Rifampin	Metronidazole	
Good[2]	Most beta-lactams	Acyclovir	
	Most 1st,2nd,3rd gen.	Valacyclovir	
	oral cephalosporins	Famciclovir	
	Macrolides		
	Itraconazole		
Inadequate[3]	Vancomycin		

1. Oral administration results in equivalent blood/tissue levels as the same dose given IV (PO = IV)
2. Oral administration results in lower blood/tissue levels than the same dose given IV (PO < IV)
3. Oral administration results in inadequate blood/tissue levels

Table 6. Infectious Diseases Requiring Prolonged Antimicrobial Therapy

Duration of Therapy	Infectious Diseases
3 weeks	Lymphogranuloma venereum (LGV), syphilis (late latent)
4 weeks	Chronic otitis media, chronic sinusitis, acute osteomyelitis, chronic pyelonephritis, brain abscess, SBE (viridans streptococci), Legionella
6 weeks	Acute bacterial endocarditis (S. aureus, enterococcal), H. pylori
3 months	Chronic prostatitis, lung abscess[1]
6 months	Pulmonary TB, extrapulmonary TB, Actinomycosis[2], Nocardia[3], chronic osteomyelitis[4]
12 months	Whipple's disease
> 12 months	Bartonella, chronic suppressive therapy for Pneumocystis carinii pneumonia (PCP), cytomegalovirus (CMV), HIV, prosthetic-related infections[5]

1. Treat until resolved or until chest x-ray is normal/nearly normal and remains unchanged
2. May require longer treatment; treat until resolved
3. May require longer treatment in compromised hosts
4   Adequate surgical debridement is required for cure
5. Implanted foreign materials associated with infection (prosthetic valves, vascular grafts, joint replacements, hemodialysis shunts) should be removed as soon as possible after diagnosis. If removal is not feasible, then chronic suppressive therapy may be attempted, although clinical failure is the rule

---

EMPIRIC ANTIBIOTIC THERAPY

Microbiology susceptibility data are not ordinarily available prior to initial treatment with antibiotics. Empiric therapy is based on directing coverage against the most likely pathogens, and takes into consideration drug allergy history, hepatic/renal function, possible antibiotic side effects, resistance potential, and cost. If a patient is moderately or severely ill, empiric therapy is usually initiated intravenously. Patients who are mildly ill, whether hospitalized or ambulatory, may be started on oral antibiotics with high bioavailability. Cultures of appropriate clinical specimens (e.g., sputum, urine) should be obtained prior to starting empiric therapy to provide bacterial isolates for in-vitro susceptibility testing. Empiric therapy for common infectious diseases is described in Chapter 2.

MICROBIOLOGY AND SUSCEPTIBILITY TESTING

A. **Overview.** In-vitro susceptibility testing provides information about microbial sensitivities to various antibiotics, and is useful in guiding therapy. Proper application of microbiology and susceptibility data requires careful assessment of the in-vitro results to determine if they are consistent with the clinical context; if not, the clinical impression usually should take precedence.

B. **Limitations of Microbiology Susceptibility Testing**
   1. **In-vitro data do not differentiate between colonizers and pathogens.** Before treating a culture report from the microbiology laboratory, it is important to determine whether the organism is a pathogen or a colonizer in the clinical context. As a rule, colonization should not be treated.

   2. **In-vitro data do not necessarily translate into in-vivo efficacy.** Reports which indicate an organism is "sensitive" or "resistant" to a given antibiotic in-vitro do not necessarily reflect in-vivo activity. Table 7 lists antibiotic-microorganism combinations for which susceptibility testing is usually unreliable.

   3. **In-vitro susceptibility testing is dependent on the microbe, methodology, and antibiotic concentration.** In-vitro susceptibility testing by the microbiology laboratory *assumes* the isolate was recovered from *blood*, and is being exposed to *serum* concentrations of an antibiotic given in the *usual* dose. Since some body sites (e.g., bladder, urine) contain higher antibiotic concentrations than found in serum, and other body sites (e.g., CSF) contain lower antibiotic concentrations than found in serum, in-vitro data may be misleading for non-bloodstream infections. For example, a Klebsiella pneumoniae isolate obtained from the CSF may be reported as "sensitive" to cefazolin even though cefazolin does not penetrate the CSF. Likewise, E. coli and Klebsiella urinary isolates are often reported as "resistant" to ampicillin/sulbactam despite in-vivo efficacy, due to high antibiotic concentrations in the urinary tract. Because microbial susceptibility is *concentration-dependent*, antibiotics should be prescribed at the usual recommended doses. Attempts to lower cost by reducing dosage may decrease antibiotic efficacy (e.g., cefoxitin 2 gm IV inhibits ~ 85% of B. fragilis isolates, whereas 1 gm IV inhibits only ~ 20% of strains).

C. **Summary.** In-vitro susceptibility testing is useful in most situations, but should not be followed blindly. Many factors need to be considered when interpreting in-vitro microbiologic data, and infectious disease consultation is recommended for all but the most straightforward susceptibility interpretation problems. Since susceptibility is concentration-dependent, IV-to-PO switch changes using antibiotics of the same class is

Table 7.   Antibiotic-Organism Combinations for Which In-Vitro Susceptibility Testing Is Unreliable[1]

Antibiotic	"Sensitive" Organism
Penicillin	H. influenzae, Yersinia pestis
TMP-SMX	Klebsiella, Enterococci, Bartonella
Polymyxin B	Proteus, Salmonella
Imipenem	Stenotrophomonas maltophilia[2]
Gentamicin	Mycobacterium tuberculosis
Vancomycin	Erysipelothrix rhusiopathiae
Aminoglycosides	Streptococci, Salmonella, Shigella
Clindamycin	Fusobacteria, Clostridia, enterococci, Listeria
Macrolides	P. multocida
1st,2nd generation cephalosporins	Salmonella, Shigella, Bartonella
3rd,4th generation cephalosporins[4]	Enterococci, Listeria, Bartonella
All antibiotics except vancomycin, minocycline, quinupristin/dalfopristin, linezolid	MRSA[3]

1. In-vitro susceptibility *does not* predict in-vivo activity; susceptibility data cannot be relied upon to guide therapy for antibiotic-organism combinations in this table
2. Formerly Pseudomonas
3. In spite of apparent in-vitro susceptibility of many antibiotics against MRSA, only vancomycin, quinupristin/dalfopristin, linezolid, and minocycline are effective in-vivo
4. Cefoperazone is the only cephalosporin with clinically useful anti-enterococcal activity (E. faecalis, not E. faecium [VRE])

best made when the oral antibiotic can achieve similar blood/tissue levels as the IV antibiotic. For example, IV-to-PO switch from cefazolin 1 gm (IV) to cephalexin 500 mg (PO) may not be effective against all pathogens at all sites, since cephalexin 500 mg (PO) achieves much lower serum concentrations compared to cefazolin 1 gm (IV) (16 mcg/mL vs. 200 mcg/mL).

ANTIBIOTIC FAILURE

There are many possible causes of *apparent* antibiotic failure, including drug fever, antibiotic-unresponsive infections, and febrile non-infectious diseases. The most common error in the management of apparent antibiotic failure is changing/adding additional antibiotics instead of determining the cause (Tables 8, 9).

Table 8. Causes of Apparent/Actual Antibiotic Failure

In-vitro susceptibility but inactive in-vivo
Antibiotic tolerance with gram-positive cocci
Inadequate coverage/spectrum
Inadequate antibiotic blood levels
Inadequate antibiotic tissue levels
    Undrained abscess
    Foreign body-related infection
    Protected focus (e.g., cerebrospinal fluid)
    Organ hypoperfusion/diminished blood supply (e.g., chronic osteomyelitis in diabetics)
Drug-induced interactions
    Antibiotic inactivation
    Antibiotic antagonism
Decreased antibiotic activity in tissue
Fungal superinfection
Treating colonization, not infection
Non-infectious diseases
    Medical disorders mimicking infection (e.g., SLE)
    Drug fever (Table 9)
Antibiotic-unresponsive infectious diseases
    Most viral infections

Table 9. Clinical Features of Drug Fever

History
    Many but not all individuals are atopic
    Patients have been on a sensitizing medication for days or years "without a problem"
Physical exam
    Fevers may be low- or high-grade, but usually range between 102°-104°F, and may exceed 106°F
    Relative bradycardia*
    Patient appears "inappropriately well" for degree of fever
Laboratory tests
    Elevated WBC count (usually with left shift)
    Eosinophils almost always present, but eosinophilia is uncommon
    Elevated erythrocyte sedimentation rate in majority of cases
    Early, transient, mild elevations of serum transaminases (common)
    Negative blood cultures (excluding contaminants)

* Relative bradycardia refers to heart rates that are inappropriately slow relative to body temperature (pulse must be taken simultaneously with temperature elevation). Applies to adult patients with temperature ≥ 102°F; does not apply to patients with second/third-degree heart block, pacemaker-induced rhythms, or those taking beta-blockers.
Appropriate Temperature-Pulse Relationships

Pulse (beats/min)	Temperature
150	41.1°C (106°F)
140	40.6°C (105°F)
130	40.7°C (104°F)
120	39.4°C (103°F)
110	38.9°C (102°F)

PITFALLS IN ANTIBIOTIC PRESCRIBING

- Use of antibiotics to treat non-infectious or antibiotic-unresponsive infectious diseases (e.g., viral infections)

- Use of antibiotics to treat colonization

- Overuse of combination therapy. Monotherapy is preferred over combination therapy unless compelling reasons prevail, such as drug synergy or extended spectrum beyond what can be obtained with a single drug. Monotherapy reduces the risk of drug interactions and side effects, and is usually less expensive

- Use of antibiotics for persistent fevers. For patients with persistent fevers on an antimicrobial regimens that appears to be failing, it is important to reassess the patient rather than add additional antibiotics. Causes of prolonged fevers include undrained septic foci, non-infectious medical disorders, and drug fevers. Undiagnosed causes of leukocytosis/low-grade fevers should not be treated with prolonged courses of antibiotics

- Inadequate surgical therapy. Infections involving infected prosthetic materials or fluid collections (e.g., abscesses) often require surgical therapy for cure. For infections such as chronic osteomyelitis, surgery is the only way to cure the infection; antibiotics are useful only for suppression or to prevent local infectious complications

- Home IV therapy. There is less need to use home IV therapy given the vast array of excellent oral antibiotics (e.g., linezolid)

Chapter 2

Empiric Therapy Based on Clinical Syndrome

Burke A. Cunha, M.D.

This chapter is organized by clinical syndrome, patient subset, and in some cases, specific organism. Clinical summaries immediately follow each treatment grid.

Therapeutic recommendations are based on antimicrobial effectiveness, reliability, cost, safety, and resistance potential. Switching to a more specific/narrow spectrum antimicrobial is not more effective than well-chosen empiric/initial therapy, and usually results in increased cost and more side effects/drug interactions. The antimicrobial dosages in this section represent the usual dosages for normal renal and hepatic function. Dosage adjustments, side effects, drug interactions, and other important prescribing information is described in the individual drug summaries in Chapter 7.

"IV-to-PO Switch" in the last column of the shaded title bar in each treatment grid indicates the clinical syndrome should be treated either by IV therapy alone or IV followed by PO therapy, but *not* by PO therapy alone. "PO Therapy or IV-to-PO Switch" indicates the clinical syndrome can be treated by IV therapy alone, PO therapy alone, or IV followed by PO therapy (unless otherwise indicated in the footnotes under each treatment grid).

Most patients on IV therapy able to take PO medications should be switched to PO equivalent therapy after clinical improvement.

Empiric Therapy of CNS Infections

Acute Bacterial Meningitis (ABM)

Subset	Usual Pathogens	Preferred IV Therapy	Alternate IV Therapy	IV-to-PO Switch
Normal host	N. meningitidis H. influenzae S. pneumoniae	Ceftriaxone 2 gm (IV) q12h x 2 weeks	Cefotaxime 3 gm (IV) q6h x 2 weeks **or** Ceftizoxime 3 gm (IV) q6h x 2 weeks	Chloramphenicol 500 mg (PO) q6h x 2 weeks
Elderly or malignancy	Listeria monocytogenes plus usual meningeal pathogens in normal hosts	<u>Before culture results</u> Ceftriaxone 2 gm (IV) q12h x 2 weeks **plus** Ampicillin 2 gm (IV) q4h x 2 weeks <u>After culture results</u> <u>*Listeria present*</u> Ampicillin 2 gm (IV) q4h x 2 weeks <u>*Listeria not present*</u> Treat as normal host	<u>After culture results</u> <u>*Listeria present*</u> TMP-SMX 5 mg/kg (IV) q6h x 2 weeks **or** Chloramphenicol 500 mg (IV) q6h x 2 weeks <u>*Listeria not present*</u> Treat as for normal host, above	<u>For Listeria meningitis only</u> TMP-SMX 5 mg/kg (PO) q6h x 2 weeks **or** Chloramphenicol 500 mg (PO) q6h x 2 weeks <u>For usual meningeal pathogens</u> Chloramphenicol 500 mg (PO) q6h x 2 weeks
CNS shunt infections (VA shunts) (Treat initially for MSSA; if later identified as MSRA, MSSE, or MSRE, treat accordingly)	S. aureus S. epidermidis (coagulase-negative staphylococci)	<u>MSSA/MSSE</u> Cefotaxime 3 gm (IV) q6h x 1 week after shunt removal **or** Ceftizoxime 3 gm (IV) q6h x 1 week after shunt removal <u>MRSA/MRSE</u> Linezolid 600 mg (IV) q12h x 1 week after shunt removal	<u>MSSA/MSSE</u> Cefepime 2 gm (IV) q8h x 1 week after shunt removal **or** Meropenem 2 gm (IV) q8h x 1 week after shunt removal <u>MRSA/MRSE</u> Vancomycin 1 gm (IV) q12h x 1 week after shunt removal plus 20 mg (IT) q24h until shunt removal	<u>MSSE/MRSE</u> Linezolid 600 mg (PO) q12h x 1 week after shunt removal <u>MSSA/MRSA</u> Minocycline 100 mg (PO) q12h x 1 week after shunt removal **or** Linezolid 600 mg (PO) q12h x 1 week after shunt removal

Acute Bacterial Meningitis (ABM) (cont'd)

Subset	Usual Pathogens	Preferred IV Therapy	Alternate IV Therapy	IV-to-PO Switch
CNS shunt infections (VP shunts)	E. coli K. pneumoniae Enterobacter S. marcescens	Cefotaxime 3 gm (IV) q6h x 2 weeks after shunt removal **or** Ceftizoxime 3 gm (IV) q6h x 2 weeks after shunt removal	Ceftriaxone 2 gm (IV) q12h x 2 weeks after shunt removal **or** TMP-SMX 5 mg/kg (IV) q6h x 2 weeks after shunt removal	TMP-SMX 5 mg/kg (PO) q6h x 2 weeks after shunt removal

MSSA/MRSA = methicillin-sensitive/resistant S. aureus; MSSE/MRSE = methicillin-sensitive/resistant S. epidermidis.
Duration of therapy represents total time IV or IV + PO. Most patients on IV therapy able to take PO meds should be switched to PO therapy after clinical improvement

Clinical Presentation: Abrupt onset of fever, headache, stiff neck
Diagnosis: CSF gram stain/culture

Acute Bacterial Meningitis (Normal Hosts)

Diagnostic Considerations: Gram stain of centrifugated CSF is still the best diagnositic test. CSF antigen/CIE are unhelpful in establishing the diagnosis (many false-negatives). Blood cultures are positive for ABM pathogen in 80-90%. Typical CSF findings include a WBC count of 100-5000 cells/mm^3, elevated opening pressure, elevated protein and lactic acid levels (> 4-6 mmol/L), and a positive CSF gram stain. If the WBC is extremely high (> 20,000 cells/mm^3), suspect brain abscess with rupture into the ventricular system, and obtain a CT/MRI to confirm. S. pneumoniae meningitis is associated with cranial nerves abnormalities, mental status changes, and neurologic sequelae. With H. influenzae or S. pneumoniae meningitis, obtain a head CT/MRI to rule out other CNS pathology
Pitfalls: If ABM is suspected, always perform lumbar puncture (LP) *before* obtaining a CT scan, since early antibiotic therapy is critical to prognosis. A CT/MRI should be obtained before LP *only* if a mass lesion/suppurative intracranial process is of primary concern, after blood cultures have been drawn. A stiff neck on physical examination has limited diagnostic value in the elderly, since nuchal rigidity may occur without meningitis (e.g., cervical arthritis) and meningitis may occur without nuchal rigidity. Recurrence of fever during the first week of H. influenzae meningitis is commonly due to subdural effusion, which usually resolves spontaneously over several days. Meningococcal meningitis may occur with or without meningococcemia. On gram stain, S. pneumoniae may be mistaken for H. influenzae, and Listeria may be mistaken for S. pneumoniae
Therapeutic Considerations: Do not reduce meningeal antibiotic dosing as the patient improves. Repeat LP only if the patient is not responding to antibiotics after 48 hours; lack of response may be due to therapeutic failure, relapse, or a non-infectious CNS disorder. For S. pneumoniae meningitis, obtain penicillin MICs on all CSF isolates; nearly all penicillin-resistant strains have relatively low MICs (2-5 mcg/mL) and are susceptible to meningeal doses of beta-lactam antibiotics (e.g., ceftriaxone). All but the most highly penicillin-resistant pneumococci are still effectively treated with meningeal doses of beta-lactams. Highly resistant pneumococcal strains (rare in the CSF) may be treated for 2 weeks with meropenem 2 gm (IV) q8h, cefepime 2 gm (IV) q8h, linezolid 600 mg (IV) q12h, or vancomycin (IV/IT). Dexamethasone 0.15 mg/kg (IV) q6h x 4 days may be given to children with ABM to reduce the incidence/severity of neurologic sequelae, although the value of steroids in adult ABM is unclear; if used, give dexamethasone 30 minutes before the initial antibiotic dose
Prognosis: Uniformly fatal without treatment. Case-fatality rates in treated adults are 10-20%. Neurological deficits on presentation are associated with a poor prognosis. Permanent neurological

deficits are more frequent with S. pneumoniae than H. influenzae, even with prompt therapy. In meningococcal meningitis with meningococcemia, prognosis is related to the number of petechiae, with few or no neurological deficits in survivors

Acute Bacterial Meningitis (Elderly Patients/Malignancy)

Diagnostic Considerations: Diagnosis by CSF gram stain/culture. ABM pathogens include usual pathogens in normal hosts plus Listeria monocytogenes, a gram-positive, aerobic, bacillus. Listeria is the most common ABM pathogen in patients with malignancies, and is a common pathogen in the elderly. With Listeria meningitis, CSF cultures are positive in 100%, but CSF gram stain is negative in 50%. Meningeal carcinomatosis is suggested by multiple cranial nerve abnormalities

Pitfalls: "Diphtheroids" isolated from CSF should be speciated to rule out Listeria. Listeria are motile and hemolytic on blood agar plate, diphtheroids are not

Therapeutic Considerations: Elderly patients and cancer patients with ABM require empiric coverage of Listeria plus other common pathogens in normal hosts (N. meningitidis, H. influenzae, S. pneumoniae). Specific monotherapy can be administered once the organism is known. Third-generation cephalosporins are not active against Listeria

Prognosis: Related to underlying health of host

Acute Bacterial Meningitis (CNS Shunt Infections)

Diagnostic Considerations: Diagnosis by CSF gram stain/culture. S. epidermidis meningitis usually occurs only with infected prosthetic implant material (e.g., CNS shunt/plate)

Pitfalls: Blood cultures are usually negative for shunt pathogens

Therapeutic Considerations: 15% of S. epidermidis strains are resistant to nafcillin/clindamycin. In addition to systemic antibiotics in meningeal doses, adjunctive intraventricular/intrathecal antibiotics are sometimes given to control shunt infections before shunt removal

Prognosis: Good if prosthetic material is removed

Acute Non-Bacterial Meningitis/Chronic Meningitis

Subset	Usual Pathogens	IV Therapy	IV-to-PO Switch
Viral (aseptic)	EBV VZV LCM Enteroviruses WNE	Not applicable	Not applicable
	HSV-1 HSV-2	Acyclovir 10 mg/kg (IV) q8h x 14-21 days	Acyclovir 400 mg (PO) 5x/day x 14-21 days **or** Valacyclovir 500 mg (PO) q8h x 14-21 days **or** Famciclovir 500 mg (PO) q8h x 14-21 days
Primary amebic meningo-encephalitis (PAM)	Naegleria fowleri	Amphotericin B 1 mg/kg (IV) q24h until cured **plus** Amphotericin B 1 mg into ventricles via Ommaya reservoir q24h until cured	Not applicable

Acute Non-Bacterial Meningitis/Chronic Meningitis (cont'd)

Subset	Usual Pathogens	Preferred IV Therapy	Alternate IV Therapy	PO Therapy or IV-to-PO Switch
Granuloma-tous amebic meningo-encephalitis	Acanthamoeba	No proven treatment*		
TB	M. tuberculosis	IV Therapy Not applicable	PO Therapy INH 300 mg (PO) q24h x 6-9 months **plus** Rifampin 600 mg (PO) q24h x 6-9 months If multiresistant TB strain likely, also add: EMB 15 mg/kg (PO) q24h x 6-9 months **plus** PZA 25 mg/kg (PO) q24h x 6-9 months	
Fungal *Non-HIV*	Cryptococcus neoformans	Amphotericin B 1 mg/kg (IV) q24h x 6 weeks **plus** 5-FC 1 mg/kg (PO) q6h x 6 weeks, **followed by** Fluconazole 800 mg (IV or PO) x 1 dose, then 400 mg (PO) q24h x 10 weeks	Amphotericin B lipid formulation 5 mg/kg (IV) q24h x 6 weeks, then 3x/week x 4 weeks **plus** Fluconazole 800 mg (IV or PO) x 1 dose, then 400 mg (PO) q24h x 10 weeks	PO therapy alone Not applicable
HIV	Cryptococcus neoformans	See p. 217		
Chronic meningitis	M. tuberculosis, Brucella, Leptospirosis, Listeria, T. pallidum, Cryptococcus, Coccidioidomycosis, Histoplasmosis, Toxoplasmosis, Toxocariasis, CMV, Neurocysticercosis, Neuroborreliosis, Enteroviruses	Treat specific pathogen after confirming diagnosis. Do not treat empirically		

Duration of therapy represents total time PO (for TB), IV, or IV + PO. Most patients on IV therapy able to take PO meds should be switched to PO therapy after clinical improvement

* *Amphotericin B, fluconazole, ketoconazole, itraconazole, flucytosine, rifampin, isoniazid, aminoglycosides, sulfonamides, pentamidine mostly with little success. Success reported in transplant recipient with IV pentamidine followed by itraconazole, and in AIDS patient with ketoconazole plus flucytosine*

Viral (Aseptic) Meningitis

Clinical Presentation: Headache, low-grade fever, mild meningismus, photophobia

Diagnostic Considerations: Diagnosis by specific serological tests/viral culture. HSV-2 genital infections are often accompanied by mild CNS symptoms, which usually do not require anti-viral therapy. HSV-1 causes a variety of CNS infections, including meningitis, meningoencephalitis, and encephalitis (most common; see pp. 22-23). HSV meningitis is indistinguishable clinically from other causes of viral meningitis. EBV meningitis is usually associated with clinical/laboratory features of EBV infectious mononucleosis; suspect the diagnosis in a patient with a positive monospot and unexplained meningoencephalitis. VZV meningitis is typically associated with cutaneous vesicular lesions (H. zoster), and usually does not require additional therapy beyond that given for shingles. LCM meningitis begins as a "flu-like" illness usually in the fall after hamster contact, and may have low CSF glucose. Enterovirus meningitis is often associated with a maculopapular rash, non-exudative pharyngitis, diarrhea, and rarely low CSF glucose

Pitfalls: Consider NSAIDs and IV immunoglobulin as non-infectious causes of aseptic meningitis

Therapeutic Considerations: Treat specific pathogen

Prognosis: Without neurological deficits, full recovery is the rule

Primary Amebic Meningoencephalitis (PAM) (Naegleria fowleri)

Clinical Presentation: Acquired by freshwater exposure containing the protozoa, often by jumping into a lake/pool. Affects healthy children/young adults. Organism penetrates cribiform plate and enters CSF. Symptoms occur within 7 days of exposure and are indistinguishable from fulminant bacterial meningitis, including headache, fever, anorexia, vomiting, signs of meningeal inflammation, altered mental status, coma. May complain of unusual smell/taste sensations early in infection. CSF has RBCs and very low glucose

Diagnostic Considerations: Diagnosis by demonstrating organism in CSF. Worldwide distribution. Free-living fresh water amoeba flourish in warmer climates. Key to diagnosis rests on clinical suspicion based on history of freshwater exposure in previous 1-2 weeks

Pitfalls: CSF findings resemble bacterial meningitis, but RBCs present

Therapeutic Considerations: Often fatal despite early treatment

Prognosis: Almost always fatal

Granulomatous Amebic Meningoencephalitis (Acanthamoeba)

Clinical Presentation: Insidious onset with focal neurologic deficits ± mental status changes, seizures, fever, headache, hemiparesis, meningismus, ataxia, visual disturbances. May be associated with Acanthamoeba keratoconjunctivitis, skin ulcers, or disseminated disease. Usually seen only in immunocompromised/debilitated patients

Diagnostic Considerations: Diagnosis by demonstrating organism in brain biopsy specimen. CT/MRI shows mass lesions. "Stellate cysts" characteristic of Acanthamoeba vs. "round cysts" of Naegleria. Worldwide distribution. Strong association with extended wear of contact lenses

Pitfalls: Not associated with freshwater exposure, unlike primary amebic meningoencephalitis (Naegleria fowleri). Resembles subacute/chronic meningitis. No trophozoites in CSF. Skin lesions may be present for months before onset of CNS symptoms

Therapeutic Considerations: No proven treatment. Often fatal despite early treatment

Prognosis: Usually fatal

TB Meningitis (Mycobacterium tuberculosis)

Clinical Presentation: Subacute onset of non-specific symptoms. Fever usually present ± headache, nausea, vomiting. Acute presentation and cranial nerve palsies uncommon

Diagnostic Considerations: Diagnosis by CSF AFB smear/culture. PCR of CSF is sensitive/specific. CSF may be normal, but often shows low glucose, increased protein, RBCs, and increased lactic acid. May find characteristic "pellicle" in CSF after 12 hours. Look for TB elsewhere

Pitfalls: CSF may have PMN predominance early, before developing typical lymphocytic predominance. Eosinophils in CSF is not a feature of TB, and should suggest another diagnosis

Therapeutic Considerations: Dexamethasone 4 mg (IV or PO) q6h x 2-4 weeks is useful to reduce CSF inflammation if given early

Prognosis: Poor prognostic factors include delay in treatment, neurologic deficits, or hydrocephalus. Proteinaceous TB exudates may obstruct ventricles and cause hydrocephalus, which is diagnosed by CT/MRI and may require shunt

Fungal (Cryptococcal) Meningitis (Cryptococcus neoformans)

Clinical Presentation: Insidious onset of non-specific symptoms. Headache most common. Chronic cases may have CNS symptoms for weeks to months with intervening asymptomatic periods. Acute manifestations are more common in AIDS, chronic steroid therapy, lymphoreticular malignancies. 50-80% of patients are abnormal hosts

Diagnostic Considerations: C. neoformans is the most common cause of fungal meningitis, and the only encapsulated yeast in the CSF to cause meningitis. Diagnosis by CSF India ink cryptococcal latex antigen/culture. Rule out HIV and other underlying immunosuppressive diseases

Pitfalls: CSF latex antigen titer may not return to zero in HIV/AIDS patients. Continue treatment until titers decline/do not decrease further, and until CSF culture is negative for cryptococci. India ink smears of CSF are useful for initial infection, but should not be relied on to diagnose recurrent episodes, since smears may be positive despite negative CSF cultures (dead cryptococci may remain in CSF for years). Diagnosis of recurrences rests on CSF culture

Therapeutic Considerations: Treat until CSF is sterile or initial CSF latex antigen titer is zero or remains near zero on serial lumbar punctures. After patient defervesces on amphotericin B/5FC, switch to oral fluconazole x 10 weeks. Amphotericin B lipid formulations may be used if amphotericin B cannot be tolerated. HIV patients require life-long suppressive therapy with fluconazole 200 mg (PO) q24h

Prognosis: Good. Poor prognostic factors include no CSF pleocytosis, many organisms in CSF, and altered consciousness on admission

Chronic Meningitis

Clinical Presentation: Same as acute meningitis, but signs/symptoms less prominent and clinical presentation is subacute (> 1 month)

Diagnostic Considerations: Differential diagnosis is too broad for empiric treatment. Subacute/chronic clinical presentation allows time for complete diagnostic work-up. Culture CSF and obtain CSF/serum tests to identify a specific pathogen, then treat

Pitfalls: If infectious etiology is not found, consider NSAIDs, SLE, meningeal carcinomatosis, sarcoidosis, etc. Chronic CMV or enterococcal meningitis should prompt search for underlying host defense defects/immunosuppression

Therapeutic Considerations: If suspicion of TB meningitis is high, empiric anti-TB treatment is warranted. Otherwise, treat only after diagnosing specific infection

Prognosis: Related to underlying health of host

Encephalitis

Subset	Usual Pathogens	IV-to-PO Switch
Herpes	HSV-1	Acyclovir 10 mg/kg (IV) q8h x 7 days, then if able to take oral medications, complete 14-21 days of total therapy with acyclovir 400 mg (PO) 5x/day or valacyclovir 1 gm (PO) q8h or famciclovir 500 mg (PO) q8h
Arbovirus	Usual Pathogens California encephalitis (CE), Western equine encephalitis (WEE), Venezuelan equine encephalitis (VEE), Eastern equine encephalitis (EEE), St. Louis encephalitis (SLE), Japanese encephalitis (JE), West Nile encephalitis (WNE) IV/PO Therapy Not applicable	

Encephalitis (cont'd)

Subset	Usual Pathogens	Preferred IV Therapy	Alternate IV Therapy	IV-to-PO Switch
Mycoplasma	M. pneumoniae	Doxycycline 200 mg (IV) q12h x 3 days, then 100 mg (IV) q12h x 2-4 weeks	Minocycline 100 mg (IV) q12h x 2-4 weeks	Doxycycline 200 mg (PO) q12h x 3 days, then 100 mg (PO) q12h x 2-4 weeks* **or** Minocycline 100 mg (PO) q12h x 2-4 weeks
Solid organ transplants, HIV/AIDS	CMV T. gondii	See p. 217		

Duration of therapy represents total time IV or IV + PO. Most patients on IV therapy able to take PO meds should be switched to PO therapy after clinical improvement
* Loading dose is not needed PO if given IV with the same drug

Herpes Encephalitis (HSV-1)
Clinical Presentation: Acute onset of fever and change in mental status without nuchal rigidity
Diagnostic Considerations: EEG is best early (< 72 hours) presumptive test, showing unilateral temporal lobe abnormalities. Brain MRI is abnormal before CT scan, which may require several days before a temporal lobe focus is seen. Definitive diagnosis is by CSF PCR for HSV-1 DNA. Usually presents as encephalitis or meningoencephalitis, presentation as meningitis alone is uncommon. Profound decrease in sensorium is characteristic of HSV meningoencephalitis. CSF may have PMN predominance and low glucose levels, unlike other viral causes of meningitis
Pitfalls: Rule out non-infectious causes of encephalopathy
Therapeutic Considerations: HSV is the only treatable common cause of viral encephalitis in normal hosts. Treat as soon as possible, since neurological deficits may be mild and reversible early on, but severe and irreversible later
Prognosis: Related to extent of brain injury and early antiviral therapy

Arboviral Encephalitis
Clinical Presentation: Acute onset of fever, headache, change in mental status days to weeks after inoculation of virus through the bite of an infected insect (e.g., mosquito/tick). May progress over several days to stupor/coma
Diagnostic Considerations: Diagnosis by specific arboviral serology
Pitfalls: Usually occurs in summer/fall. Diagnosis suggested by arboviral contact/travel history. Electrolyte abnormalities due to syndrome of inappropriate antidiuretic hormone (SiADH) may occur
Therapeutic Considerations: Only supportive therapy is available at present
Prognosis: Permanent neurological deficits are common, but not predictable. May be fatal

Mycoplasma Encephalitis
Clinical Presentation: Acute onset of fever and change in mental status without nuchal rigidity
Diagnostic Considerations: Diagnosis suggested by CNS and extra-pulmonary manifestations—sore throat, otitis, E. multiforme, soft stools/diarrhea—in a patient with community-acquired pneumonia, elevated IgM Mycoplasma titers, and very high (≥ 1:1024) cold agglutinin titers. CSF shows mild mononucleosis/pleocytosis and normal/low glucose
Pitfall: CNS findings may overshadow pulmonary findings

Therapeutic Considerations: Macrolides will treat pulmonary infection, but not CNS infection (due to poor CNS penetration)
Prognosis: With early treatment, prognosis is good without neurologic sequelae

CMV Encephalitis (see p. 223)

Toxoplasma Encephalitis (see p. 222)

Brain Abscess/Subdural Empyema/Cavernous Vein Thrombosis/Intracranial Suppurative Thrombophlebitis

Subset	Usual Pathogens	Preferred IV Therapy	Alternate IV Therapy	IV-to-PO Switch
Brain Abscess (Single Mass Lesion)				
Open trauma	S. aureus Entero-bacteriaceae P. aeruginosa	Cefepime 2 gm (IV) q8h x 2 weeks	Meropenem 2 gm (IV) q8h x 2 weeks	Not applicable
Neurosurgical procedure (Treat initially for MSSA; if later identified as MRSA, MSSE or MRSE, treat accordingly)	S. aureus S. epidermidis	<u>MSSA/MSSE</u> Nafcillin 2 gm (IV) q4h x 2 weeks **or** Ceftizoxime 3 gm (IV) q6h x 2 weeks **or** Cefepime 2 gm (IV) q8h x 2 weeks <u>MRSA/MRSE</u> Linezolid 600 mg (IV) q12h x 2 weeks	<u>MSSA/MRSA</u> Linezolid 600 mg (PO) q12h x 2 weeks	
Mastoid/ otitic source	Enterobacter Proteus	Cefepime 2 gm (IV) q8h x 2 weeks	Meropenem 2 gm (IV) q8h x 2 weeks	Not applicable
Dental source	Oral anaerobes Actinomyces	Ceftizoxime 3 gm (IV) q6h x 2 weeks	Ceftriaxone 2 gm (IV) q12h x 2 weeks **plus** Metronidazole 1 gm (IV) q24h x 2 weeks	Not applicable
Subdural empyema/ sinus source	Oral anaerobes H. influenzae	Ceftizoxime 3 gm (IV) q6h x 2 weeks	Ceftriaxone 2 gm (IV) q12h x 2 weeks **plus** Metronidazole 1 gm (IV) q24h x 2 weeks	Not applicable

Pitfalls: Do not overlook underlying sinus infection, which may need surgical drainage
Therapeutic Considerations: Obtain ENT consult for possible surgical debridement of sinuses
Prognosis: Good prognosis if sinus is drained

Brain Abscess (Cardiac Source; Acute Bacterial Endocarditis)

Diagnostic Considerations: Diagnosis by blood cultures positive for acute bacterial endocarditis (ABE) pathogen and multiple brain lesions on head CT/MRI
Pitfalls: Do not overlook right-to-left cardiac shunt (e.g., patent foramen ovale, atrial septal defect) as source of brain abscess. Cerebral embolization results in aseptic meningitis in SBE, but septic meningitis/brain abscess in ABE (due to high virulence of pathogens)
Therapeutic Considerations: Multiple lesions suggest hematogenous spread. Use sensitivity of blood culture isolates to determine coverage. Meningeal doses are the same as endocarditis doses
Prognosis: Related to location/size of CNS lesions and extent of cardiac valvular involvement

Brain Abscess (Pulmonary Source)

Diagnostic Considerations: Diagnosis suggested by underlying bronchiectasis, empyema, cystic fibrosis, or lung abscess in a patient with a brain abscess
Pitfalls: Brain abscesses are associated with chronic suppurative lung disease (e.g., bronchiectasis, lung abscess/empyema), not chronic bronchitis
Therapeutic Considerations: Lung abscess may need surgical drainage
Prognosis: Related to extent/location of CNS lesions, drainage of lung abscess/empyema, and control of lung infection

Empiric Therapy of HEENT Infections

Facial/Periorbital Cellulitis

Subset	Usual Pathogens	Preferred IV Therapy	Alternate IV Therapy	PO Therapy or IV-to-PO Switch
Facial cellulitis	Group A streptococci H. influenzae	Cefotaxime 2 gm (IV) q6h x 2 weeks **or** Ceftriaxone 1 gm (IV) q24h x 2 weeks	Ceftizoxime 2 gm (IV) q8h x 2 weeks	Any oral 2nd or 3rd gen. cephalosporin x 2 weeks **or** Levofloxacin 500 mg (PO) q24h x 2 weeks **or** Gatifloxacin 400 mg (PO) q24h x 2 weeks

Duration of therapy represents total time IV, PO, or IV + PO. Most patients on IV therapy able to take PO meds should be switched to PO therapy soon after clinical improvement (usually < 72 hours)

Clinical Presentation: Acute onset of warm, painful, facial rash without discharge, swelling, pruritus
Diagnostic Considerations: Diagnosis by clinical appearance. May spread rapidly across face. Purplish hue suggests H. influenzae
Pitfalls: If periorbital cellulitis, obtain head CT/MRI to rule out underlying sinusitis/CNS involvement
Therapeutic Considerations: May need to treat x 3 weeks in compromised hosts (chronic steroids,

Brain Abscess/Subdural Empyema/Cavernous Vein Thrombosis/Intracranial Suppurative Thrombophlebitis (cont'd)

Subset	Usual Pathogens	Preferred IV Therapy	Alternate IV Therapy	IV-to-PO Switch
Brain Abscess (Multiple Mass Lesions)				
Cardiac source (ABE; right-to-left shunt)	S. aureus S. pneumoniae H. influenzae	Cefepime 2 gm (IV) q8h x 2 weeks	Cefotaxime 3 gm (IV) q6h x 2 weeks **or** Meropenem 1 gm (IV) q8h x 2 weeks	Not applicable
Pulmonary source	Oral anaerobes Actinomyces	Ceftizoxime 3 gm (IV) q6h x 2 weeks	Ceftriaxone 2 gm (IV) q12h x 2 weeks **plus** Metronidazole 1 gm (IV) q24h x 2 weeks	Not applicable

*MSSA/MRSA = methicillin-sensitive/resistant S. aureus; MSSE/MRSE = methicillin-sensitive/resistant S. epidermidis.
Duration of therapy represents total time IV or IV + PO. Most patients on IV therapy able to take PO meds should be switched to PO therapy after clinical improvement*

Clinical Presentation: Variable presentation, with fever, change in mental status, cranial nerve abnormalities ± headache

Diagnostic Considerations: Diagnosis by CSF gram stain/culture. If brain abscess is suspected, obtain head CT/MRI. Lumbar puncture may induce herniation

Pitfalls: CSF analysis is negative for bacterial meningitis unless abscess ruptures into ventricular system

Therapeutic Considerations: Treatment with meningeal doses of antibiotics is required. Large single abscesses may be surgically drained; multiple small abscesses are best treated medically

Prognosis: Related to underlying source and health of host

Brain Abscess (Mastoid/Otitic Source)

Diagnostic Considerations: Diagnosis by head CT/MRI demonstrating focus of infection in mastoid

Pitfalls: Rule out associated subdural empyema

Therapeutic Considerations: ENT consult for possible surgical debridement of mastoid

Prognosis: Good. May require mastoid debridement for cure

Brain Abscess (Dental Source)

Diagnostic Considerations: Diagnosis by panorex x-rays/gallium scan of jaw demonstrating focus in mandible/erosion into sinuses

Pitfalls: Apical root abscess may not be apparent clinically

Therapeutic Considerations: Large single abscess may be surgically drained. Multiple small abscesses are best treated medically. Treat until lesions on CT/MRI resolve or do not become smaller on therapy

Prognosis: Good if dental focus is removed

Brain Abscess (Subdural Empyema/Sinus Source)

Diagnostic Considerations: Diagnosis by sinus films/CT/MRI to confirm presence of sinusitis/bone erosion (cranial osteomyelitis/epidural abscess). Usually from paranasal sinusitis

diabetics, SLE, etc.)
Prognosis: Good with early treatment; worse if underlying sinusitis/CNS involvement

Sinusitis

Subset	Usual Pathogens	Preferred IV Therapy	Alternate IV Therapy	PO Therapy or IV-to-PO Switch
Acute	S. pneumoniae H. influenzae M. catarrhalis	Levofloxacin 500 mg (IV) q24h x 2 weeks	Ceftriaxone 1 gm (IV) q24h x 2 weeks **or** Gatifloxacin 400 mg (IV) q24h x 2 weeks **or** Moxifloxacin 400 mg (IV) q24h x 2 weeks	Levofloxacin 500 mg (PO) q24h x 2 weeks **or** Gatifloxacin 400 mg (PO) q24h x 2 weeks **or** Moxifloxacin 400 mg (PO) q24h x 2 weeks **or** Doxycycline 200 mg (IV or PO) q12h x 3 days, then 100 mg (PO) q12h x 11 days*
Chronic	H. influenzae S. pneumoniae M. catarrhalis Oral anaerobes	Not applicable	Levofloxacin 500 mg (PO) q24h x 4 weeks **or** Gatifloxacin 400 mg (PO) q24h x 4 weeks **or** Moxifloxacin 400 mg (PO) q24h x 4 weeks **or** Doxycycline 100 mg (PO) q12h x 4 weeks	

Duration of therapy represents total time IV, PO, or IV + PO. Most patients on IV therapy able to take PO meds should be switched to PO therapy soon after clinical improvement (usually < 72 hours)
* *Loading dose is not needed PO if given IV with the same drug*

Acute Sinusitis
Clinical Presentation: Headache and percussion tenderness over infected sinus
Diagnostic Considerations: Diagnosis by sinus films or head CT/MRI showing air/fluid level(s) and/or sinus mucosal thickening
Pitfalls: May present as periorbital cellulitis. Obtain head CT/MRI to rule out underlying sinusitis. If CT/MRI demonstrates "post-septal" involvement, treat as acute bacterial meningitis
Therapeutic Considerations: Treat for full 2 weeks, not 7-10 days. Avoid macrolides and TMP-SMX (predispose to resistant S. pneumoniae); macrolides miss 25% of S. pneumoniae
Prognosis: Good if treated for full 2 weeks. Relapses may occur with suboptimal treatment

Chronic Sinusitis
Clinical Presentation: Generalized headache with low-grade fevers and little/no sinus tenderness by percussion in a patient with a history of acute sinusitis
Diagnostic Considerations: Diagnosis by sinus films or head CT/MRI showing air/fluid level(s) and/or sinus mucosal thickening

Pitfalls: Clinical presentation is variable/non-specific. Head CT/MRI is needed to confirm the diagnosis and rule out sinus tumor
Therapeutic Considerations: Therapeutic failure/relapse is usually due to inadequate antibiotic duration, dose, or tissue penetration. Treat for a full 4 weeks (2-3 weeks is usually inadequate). If symptoms persist after 4 weeks of therapy, refer to ENT for surgical drainage procedure
Prognosis: Good

Keratitis

Subset	Usual Pathogens	Topical Therapy
Bacterial	S. aureus M. catarrhalis P. aeruginosa	Antibacterial eyedrops (ciprofloxacin, ofloxacin, or tobramycin/bacitracin/polymyxin B) hourly while awake x 2 weeks
Viral	HSV-1	Trifluridine 1% solution 1 drop hourly while awake x 2 days, then 1 drop q6h x 14-21 days **or** Viral ophthalmic topical ointment (e.g., vidarabine) at bedtime x 14-21 days
Amebic	Acanthamoeba	Propamidine (0.1%), neomycin, gramicidin, or polymyxin B eyedrops hourly while awake x 1-2 weeks **or** Polyhexamethylene biguanide (0.02%) eyedrops hourly while awake x 1-2 weeks **or** Chlorhexidine (0.02%) eyedrops hourly while awake x 1-2 weeks

Clinical Presentation: Corneal haziness, infiltrates, or ulcers
Diagnosis: Appearance of corneal lesions/culture

Bacterial Keratitis
Diagnostic Considerations: Usually secondary to eye trauma. Always obtain ophthalmology consult
Pitfalls: Be sure to culture ulcer. Unusual organisms are common in eye trauma
Therapeutic Considerations: Treat until lesions resolve. Ointment easier/lasts longer than solutions. Avoid topical steroids
Prognosis: Related to extent of trauma/organism. S. aureus, P. aeruginosa have a worse prognosis

Viral Keratitis (HSV-1)
Diagnostic Considerations: "Dendritic" corneal ulcers characteristic. Obtain ophthalmology consult
Pitfalls: Small corneal ulcers may be missed without fluorescein staining
Therapeutic Considerations: Treat until lesions resolve. Oral acyclovir is not needed. Avoid ophthalmic steroid ointment
Prognosis: Good if treated early (before eye damage is extensive)

Amebic Keratitis (Acanthamoeba)
Diagnostic Considerations: Usually associated with extended use of soft contact lenses. Corneal scrapings are positive with calcofluor staining. Acanthamoeba keratitis is painful with typical circular, hazy, corneal infiltrate. Always obtain ophthalmology consult
Pitfalls: Do not confuse with HSV-1 dendritic ulcers. Avoid topical steroids

Therapeutic Considerations: If secondary bacterial infection, treat as bacterial keratitis
Prognosis: No good treatment. Poor prognosis

Conjunctivitis

Subset	Usual Pathogens	IV Therapy	PO/Topical Therapy
Bacterial	M. catarrhalis H. influenzae S. pneumoniae	Not applicable	Antibacterial eyedrops (ciprofloxacin, ofloxacin, or tobramycin/bacitracin/polymyxin B) q12h x 1 week plus antibacterial ointment (same antibiotic) at bedtime x 1 week
Viral	Adenovirus	Not applicable	Not applicable
	VZV	Not applicable	Famciclovir 500 mg (PO) q8h x 10-14 days **or** Valacyclovir 1 gm (PO) q8h x 10-14 days
Chlamydial	C. trachomatis C. psittaci	Not applicable	Doxycycline 100 mg (PO) q12h x 1-2 weeks **or** Azithromycin 1 gm (PO) x 1 dose

Bacterial Conjunctivitis
Clinical Presentation: Profuse, purulent exudate from conjunctiva
Diagnostic Considerations: Reddened conjunctiva; culture for specific pathogen
Pitfalls: Do not confuse with allergic conjunctivitis, which itches and has a clear discharge
Therapeutic Considerations: Obtain ophthalmology consult. Ointment lasts longer in eye than solution. Do not use topical steroids without an antibacterial
Prognosis: Excellent when treated early, with no residual visual impairment

Viral Conjunctivitis
Adenovirus
Clinical Presentation: Reddened conjunctiva, watery discharge, negative bacterial culture
Diagnostic Considerations: Diagnosis by cloudy/steamy cornea with negative bacterial cultures. Clue is punctate infiltrates with a cloudy cornea. Extremely contagious; careful handwashing is essential. Obtain viral culture of conjunctiva for diagnosis
Pitfalls: Pharyngitis a clue to adenoviral etiology (pharyngoconjunctival fever)
Therapeutic Considerations: No treatment available. Usually resolves in 1-2 weeks
Prognosis: Related to degree of corneal haziness. Severe cases may take weeks to clear

VZV Ophthalmicus
Diagnostic Considerations: Vesicles on tip of nose predict eye involvement
Pitfalls: Do not miss vesicular lesions in external auditory canal in patients with facial palsy (Ramsey-Hunt Syndrome)
Therapeutic Considerations: Obtain ophthalmology consult. Topical steroids may be used if given with anti-VZV therapy
Prognosis: Good if treated early with systemic antivirals

Chlamydial Conjunctivitis
Diagnostic Considerations: Diagnosis by direct fluorescent antibody (DFA)/culture of conjunctiva
Pitfalls: Do not confuse bilateral, upper lid, granular conjunctivitis of Chlamydia with viral/bacterial

conjunctivitis, which involves both upper and lower eyelids
Therapeutic Considerations: Ophthalmic erythromycin treatment is useful for neonates
Prognosis: Excellent with early treatment

Chorioretinitis

Subset	Usual Pathogens	Preferred IV Therapy	Alternate IV Therapy	PO Therapy or IV-to-PO Switch
Viral	CMV	See p. 221		
Fungal†	Candida albicans	Fluconazole 800 mg (IV) x 1 dose, then 400 mg (IV) q24h x 2 weeks **or** Caspofungin 70 mg (IV) x 1 dose, then 50 mg (IV) q24h x 2 weeks **or** Voriconazole 400 mg (IV) x 1 dose, then 200 mg (IV) q12h x 2 weeks	Amphotericin B 0.6 mg/kg (IV) q24h for total dose of 1 gm **or** Amphotericin B lipid formulation 5 mg/kg (IV) q24h x 3 weeks	Fluconazole 800 mg (PO) x 1 dose, then 400 mg (PO) q24h x 2 weeks* **or** Voriconazole 400 mg (PO) x 1 dose, then 200 mg (PO) q12h x 2 weeks*
Protozoal	Toxoplasma gondii	IV Therapy Not applicable	PO Therapy Pyrimethamine 75 mg (PO) x 1 dose, then 25 mg (PO) q24h x 6 weeks **plus either** Sulfadiazine 1 gm (PO) q6h x 6 weeks **or** Clindamycin 300 mg (PO) q8h x 6 weeks	

Duration of therapy represents total time IV, PO, or IV + PO. Most patients on IV therapy able to take PO meds should be switched to PO therapy after clinical improvement
† *Treat only IV or IV-to-PO switch*
* *Loading dose is not needed PO if given IV with the same drug*

CMV Chorioretinitis (see p. 227)

Candida Chorioretinitis
Clinical Presentation: Small, raised, white, circular lesions on retina
Diagnostic Considerations: Fundus findings similar to white, raised colonies on blood agar plates
Pitfalls: Candida endophthalmitis signifies invasive/disseminated candidiasis
Therapeutic Considerations: Treat as disseminated candidiasis
Prognosis: Good with early treatment

Toxoplasma Chorioretinitis
Clinical Presentation: Grey/black pigmentation of macula
Diagnostic Considerations: Diagnosis by IgM IFA toxoplasmosis titers
Pitfalls: Unilateral endophthalmitis usually indicates acquired toxoplasmosis; congenital toxoplasmosis is usually bilateral
Therapeutic Considerations: Obtain ophthalmology consult. Treat only acute/active toxoplasmosis with visual symptoms; do not treat chronic chorioretinitis. Add folinic acid 10 mg (PO) q24h to prevent folic acid deficiency
Prognosis: Related to degree of immunosuppression

Benign External Otitis (Pseudomonas aeruginosa)

Clinical Presentation: Acute external ear canal drainage without perforation of tympanic membrane or bone involvement

Diagnostic Considerations: Diagnosis suggested by external ear drainage after water exposure. Usually acquired from swimming pools ("swimmers ear"). Not an invasive infection

Pitfalls: Be sure external otitis is not associated with perforated tympanic membrane, which requires ENT consultation and systemic antibiotics

Therapeutic Considerations: Treat topically until symptoms/infection resolve

Prognosis: Excellent with topical therapy

Malignant External Otitis (Pseudomonas aeruginosa)

Clinical Presentation: External ear canal drainage with bone involvement

Diagnostic Considerations: Diagnosis by demonstrating P. aeruginosa in soft tissue culture from ear canal plus bone/cartilage involvement on x-ray. Usually affects diabetics. CT/MRI of head shows bony involvement of external auditory canal

Pitfalls: Rare in non-diabetics

Therapeutic Considerations: Requires surgical debridement plus antibiotic therapy for cure

Prognosis: Related to control of diabetes mellitus

Otitis Media

Subset	Usual Pathogens	IV Therapy	PO Therapy
Acute	S. pneumoniae H. influenzae M. catarrhalis	Ceftriaxone 1 gm (IV) q24h x 1 dose	Amoxicillin 1 gm (PO) q8h x 2 weeks **or** Levofloxacin 500 mg (PO) q24h x 2 weeks **or** Gatifloxacin 400 mg (PO) q24h x 2 weeks **or** Cefprozil 500 mg (PO) q12h x 2 weeks **or** Doxycycline 100 mg (PO) q12h x 2 weeks
Chronic	H. influenzae S. pneumoniae M. catarrhalis	Not applicable	Levofloxacin 500 mg (PO) q24h x 4-6 weeks **or** Gatifloxacin 400 mg (PO) q24h x 4-6 weeks **or** Cefprozil 500 mg (PO) q12h x 4-6 weeks **or** Moxifloxacin 400 mg (PO) q24h x 4-6 weeks

Acute Otitis Media

Clinical Presentation: Acute unilateral ear pain with fever and reddened tympanic membrane

Diagnostic Considerations: Diagnosis is clinical with reddened tympanic membrane

Pitfalls: Use antibiotics with good penetration into middle ear fluid. Uncommon in adults

Therapeutic Considerations: Treat empirically for all pathogens, since culture of middle ear fluid is usually not possible. Treat for full 2 weeks or relapse is common

Prognosis: Tends to recur in children; patency/angularity of eustachian tube determines risk

Chronic Otitis Media

Clinical Presentation: Earache with minimally reddened tympanic membrane and a history of acute otitis media

Diagnostic Considerations: Diagnosis is clinical, with mildly reddened tympanic membrane. H influenzae is more common than S. pneumoniae

Pitfalls: Usual cause of chronic otitis media is improperly/inadequately treated acute otitis media. Use antibiotics in full dose for full course

Therapeutic Considerations: Short courses of antibiotic therapy may fail. Treatment with macrolides, TMP-SMX, and oral cephalosporins (except cefprozil) predisposes to resistant S. pneumoniae

Prognosis: Good if tympanic membrane is not perforated. Tends to relapse with short (< 4 week) antibiotic courses

Mastoiditis

Subset	Usual Pathogens	Preferred IV Therapy	Alternate IV Therapy	PO Therapy or IV-to-PO Switch
Acute	S. pneumoniae H. influenzae S. aureus	Cefotaxime 2 gm (IV) q6h x 2 weeks **or** Cefepime 2 gm (IV) q12h x 2 weeks **or** Levofloxacin 500 mg (IV) q24h x 2 weeks	Meropenem 1 gm (IV) q8h x 2 weeks **or** Imipenem 1 gm (IV) q6h x 2 weeks	Clindamycin 300 mg (PO) q8h x 2 weeks **plus** Levofloxacin 500 mg (PO) q24 x 2 weeks
Chronic	S. pneumoniae H. influenzae S. aureus Oral anaerobes P. aeruginosa	Cefepime 2 gm (IV) q12h x 4-6 weeks **or** Levofloxacin 750 mg (IV) q24h x 4-6 weeks	Meropenem 1 gm (IV) q8h x 4-6 weeks **or** Imipenem 1 gm (IV) q6h x 4-6 weeks	Levofloxacin 750 mg (PO) q24h x 4-6 weeks

Duration of therapy represents total time IV, PO, or IV + PO. Most patients on IV therapy able to take PO meds should be switched to PO therapy soon after clinical improvement (usually < 72 hours)

Acute Mastoiditis

Clinical Presentation: Pain/tenderness over mastoid with fever

Diagnostic Considerations: Diagnosis by CT/MRI showing mastoid involvement

Pitfalls: Obtain head CT/MRI to rule out extension into CNS presenting as acute bacterial meningitis

Prognosis: Good if treated early

Chronic Mastoiditis

Clinical Presentation: Subacute pain/tenderness over mastoid with low-grade fever

Diagnostic Considerations: Diagnosis by CT/MRI showing mastoid involvement

Pitfalls: Obtain head CT/MRI to rule out CNS extension

Therapeutic Considerations: Usually requires surgical debridement for cure. Should be viewed as chronic osteomyelitis

Prognosis: Progressive without surgery. Poor prognosis with associated meningitis/brain abscess

Suppurative Parotitis

Subset	Usual Pathogens	Preferred IV Therapy	Alternate IV Therapy	PO Therapy or IV-to-PO Switch
Parotitis	S. aureus Entero-bacteriaceae Oral anaerobes	Meropenem 1 gm (IV) q8h x 2 weeks **or** Imipenem 1 gm (IV) q6h x 2 weeks **or** Ceftizoxime 2 gm (IV) q8h x 2 weeks	Clindamycin 600 mg (IV) q8h x 2 weeks **plus** Levofloxacin 500 mg (IV) q24h x 2 weeks	Clindamycin 300 mg (PO) q8h x 2 weeks **plus** Levofloxacin 500 mg (PO) q24h x 2 weeks

Duration of therapy represents total time IV, PO, or IV + PO. Most patients on IV therapy able to take PO meds should be switched to PO therapy soon after clinical improvement (usually < 72 hours)

Clinical Presentation: Unilateral parotid pain/swelling with discharge from Stensen's duct ± fever
Diagnostic Considerations: Diagnosis by clinical presentation, ↑ amylase, CT/MRI demonstrating stone in parotid duct/gland involvement
Pitfalls: Differentiate from unilateral mumps by purulent discharge from Stensen's duct
Therapeutic Considerations: If duct is obstructed, remove stone
Prognosis: Good with early therapy/hydration

Pharyngitis/Chronic Fatigue Syndrome (CFS)

Subset	Usual Pathogens	IV Therapy	PO Therapy
Bacterial	Group A streptococci	Not applicable	Amoxicillin 1 gm (PO) q8h x 7-10 days **or** Cefprozil 500 mg (PO) q12h x 7-10 days **or** Clindamycin 300 mg (PO) q8h x 7-10 days **or** Azithromycin 500 mg (PO) x 1 dose, then 250 mg (PO) q24h x 4 days
Viral	Respiratory viruses EBV, CMV, HHV-6	Not applicable	Not applicable
Other	M. pneumoniae C. pneumoniae	Not applicable	Levofloxacin 500 mg (PO) q24h x 2 weeks **or** Gatifloxacin 400 mg (PO) q24h x 2 weeks **or** Doxycycline 100 mg (PO) q12h x 2 weeks **or** Azithromycin 500 mg (PO) x 1 dose, then 250 mg (PO) q24h x 4 days
Chronic fatigue syndrome	Not known (not EBV)	Not applicable	See therapeutic considerations (p. 37)

Bacterial Pharyngitis
Clinical Presentation: Acute sore throat with fever, bilateral anterior cervical adenopathy, and elevated ASO titer. No hoarseness
Diagnostic Considerations: Diagnosis of Group A streptococcal pharyngitis by elevated ASO titer after initial sore throat and positive throat culture. Rapid strep tests unnecessary, since delay in culture results (~1 week) still allows adequate time to initiate therapy and prevent acute rheumatic fever. Group A streptococcal pharyngitis is rare in adults > 30 years
Pitfalls: Gram stain of throat exudate differentiates Group A streptococcal colonization (few or no PMNs) from infection (many PMNs) in patients with a positive throat culture or rapid strep test. Neither throat culture nor rapid strep test alone differentiates colonization from infection
Therapeutic Considerations: Benzathine penicillin 1.2 mu (IM) x 1 dose can be used as an alternative to oral therapy. Penicillin, erythromycin, and ampicillin fail in 15% of cases due to poor penetration into oral secretions or beta-lactamase producing oral organisms
Prognosis: Excellent. Treat within 10 days to prevent acute rheumatic fever

Viral Pharyngitis
Clinical Presentation: Acute sore throat. Other features depend on specific pathogen
Diagnostic Considerations: Most cases of viral pharyngitis are caused by respiratory viruses, and are frequently accompanied by hoarseness, but not high fever, pharyngeal exudates, palatal petechiae, or posterior cervical adenopathy. Other causes of viral pharyngitis (EBV, CMV, HHV-6) are usually associated with posterior cervical adenopathy and ↑ SGOT/SGPT. EBV mono may present with exudative or non-exudative pharyngitis, and is diagnosed by negative ASO titer with a positive mono spot test or elevated EBV IgM viral capsid antigen (VCA) titer. Before mono spot test turns positive (may take up to 8 weeks), a presumptive diagnosis of EBV mono can be made by ESR and SGOT, which are elevated in EBV and normal in Group A streptococcal pharyngitis. If EBV mono spot is negative, retest weekly x 8 weeks; if still negative, obtain IgM CMV/toxoplasmosis titers to diagnose the cause of "mono spot negative" pharyngitis
Pitfalls: 30% of patients with viral pharyngitis have Group A streptococcal colonization. Look for viral features to suggest the correct diagnosis (leukopenia, lymphocytosis, atypical lymphocytes)
Therapeutic Considerations: Symptomatic care only. Short-term steroids should only be used in EBV infection if airway obstruction is present/imminent. Since 30% of patients with viral pharyngitis are colonized with Group A streptococci, do not treat throat cultures positive for Group A streptococci if non-streptococcal pharyngitis features are present (e.g., bilateral posterior cervical adenopathy)
Prognosis: Related to extent of systemic infection. Post-viral fatigue is common. CMV may remain active in liver for 6-12 months with mildly elevated serum transaminases

Mycoplasma/Chlamydia Pharyngitis
Clinical Presentation: Acute sore throat ± laryngitis. Usually non-exudative
Diagnostic Considerations: Diagnosis by elevated IgM M. pneumoniae or C. pneumoniae titers. Consider diagnosis in patients with non-exudative pharyngitis without viral or streptococcal pharyngitis. Mycoplasma pharyngitis is often accompanied by otitis/bullous myringitis
Pitfalls: Patients with C. pneumoniae frequently have laryngitis, which is not a feature of EBV, CMV, Group A streptococcal, or M. pneumoniae pharyngitis
Therapeutic Considerations: Treatment of C. pneumoniae laryngitis results in rapid (~ 3 days) return of normal voice, which does not occur with viral pharyngitis
Prognosis: Excellent

Chronic Fatigue Syndrome (CFS)
Clinical Presentation: Fatigue > 1 year with cognitive impairment ± mild pharyngitis
Diagnostic Considerations: Rule out other causes of chronic fatigue (cancer, adrenal/thyroid disease, etc.) before diagnosing CFS. HHV-6/Coxsackie B titers are usually elevated. Some have ↓ natural kill

(NK) cells/activity. ESR ~ 0. Crimson crescents in the posterior pharynx are common
Pitfalls: ↑ VCA IgG EBV titers is common in CFS, but EBV does not cause CFS. Do not confuse CFS with fibromyalgia, which has muscular "trigger points" and no cognitive impairment. CFS and fibromyalgia may coexist
Therapeutic Considerations: No specific therapy is available. Patients with ↓ NK cells may benefit from beta-carotene 50,000 U (PO) q24h x 3 weeks. Patients with ↑ C. pneumoniae titers may benefit from doxycycline 100 mg (PO) q24h x 2 weeks or azithromycin 250 mg (PO) q24h x 2 weeks
Prognosis: Cyclical illness with remissions and flares (precipitated by exertion). Avoid exercise

Mouth Ulcers/Vesicles

Subset	Usual Pathogens	Preferred IV Therapy	Alternate IV Therapy	PO Therapy or IV-to-PO Switch
Vincent's angina	Borrelia Fusobacterium	Clindamycin 600 mg (IV) q8h x 2 weeks	Ceftizoxime 2 gm (IV) q8h x 2 weeks **or** Any beta-lactam (IV) x 2 weeks	Clindamycin 300 mg (PO) q8h x 2 weeks **or** Amoxicillin 1 gm (PO) q8h x 2 weeks
Ludwig's angina	Group A streptococci	Clindamycin 600 mg (IV) q8h x 2 weeks	Ceftizoxime 2 gm (IV) q8h x 2 weeks **or** Any beta-lactam (IV) x 2 weeks	Clindamycin 300 mg (PO) q8h x 2 weeks **or** Amoxicillin 1 gm (PO) q8h x 2 weeks
Stomatitis	Normal mouth flora	Not applicable	Not applicable	
Herpangina	Coxsackie A virus	Not applicable	Not applicable	
Herpes gingivo-stomatitis	HSV-1	Not applicable	Acyclovir 400 mg (PO) 5x/day x 1 week **or** Valacyclovir 500 mg (PO) q12h x 1 week **or** Famciclovir 500 mg (PO) q12h x 1 week	
Aphthous ulcers	Normal mouth flora	Not applicable	Not applicable	

Duration of therapy represents total time IV, PO, or IV + PO. Most patients on IV therapy able to take PO meds should be switched to PO therapy soon after clinical improvement (usually < 72 hours)

Clinical Presentation: Painful mouth ulcers/vesicles without fever

Vincent's Angina (Borrelia/Fusobacterium)
Diagnostic Considerations: Foul breath, poor dental hygiene/pyorrhea
Pitfalls: Do not attribute foul breath to poor dental hygiene without considering other serious causes (e.g., lung abscess, renal failure)
Therapeutic Considerations: After control of acute infection, refer to dentist
Prognosis: Excellent with early treatment

Ludwig's Angina (Group A streptococci)
Diagnostic Considerations: Fever with elevated floor of mouth is diagnostic. Massive neck swelling may be evident
Pitfalls: C_{1q} deficiency has perioral/tongue swelling, but no fever or floor of mouth elevation
Therapeutic Considerations: Surgical drainage is not necessary. May need airway emergently; have tracheotomy set at bedside
Prognosis: Early airway obstruction has adverse impact on prognosis

Stomatitis (normal mouth flora)
Diagnostic Considerations: Diagnosis based on clinical appearance
Pitfalls: Do not miss a systemic cause (e.g., acute leukemia)
Therapeutic Considerations: Painful; treat symptomatically
Prognosis: Related to severity of underlying systemic disease

Herpangina (Coxsackie A virus)
Diagnostic Considerations: Ulcers located posteriorly in pharynx. No gum involvement or halitosis
Pitfalls: Do not confuse with anterior vesicular lesions of HSV
Therapeutic Considerations: No good treatment available. Usually resolves spontaneously in 2 weeks
Prognosis: Good, but may be recurrent

Herpes Gingivostomatitis (HSV-1)
Diagnostic Considerations: Anterior ulcers in pharynx. Associated with bleeding gums, not halitosis
Pitfalls: Do not miss a systemic disease associated with bleeding gums (e.g., acute myelogenous leukemia). Periodontal disease is not usually associated with oral ulcers
Therapeutic Considerations: Oral analgesic solutions may help in swallowing
Prognosis: Excellent with early treatment

Aphthous Ulcers (normal mouth flora)
Diagnostic Considerations: Usually an isolated finding. Ulcers are painful
Pitfalls: May be a clue to systemic disorder (e.g., Behcet's syndrome). Mouth ulcers in SLE are painless
Therapeutic Considerations: Usually refractory to all treatment and often recurrent. Steroid ointment (Kenalog in orabase) may be helpful
Prognosis: Good, but tends to recur

Deep Neck Infections, Lemierre's Syndrome, Severe Dental Infections

Subset	Usual Pathogens	Preferred IV Therapy	Alternate IV Therapy	IV-to-PO Switch
Deep neck infections (lateral pharyngeal, retro-pharyngeal, prevertebral space)	Oral anaerobes Oral streptococci	Meropenem 1 gm (IV) q8h x 2 weeks **or** Imipenem 1 gm (IV) q6h x 2 weeks	Clindamycin 600 mg (IV) q8h x 2 weeks **or** Ceftizoxime 2 gm (IV) q8h x 2 weeks	Clindamycin 300 mg (PO) q8h x 2 weeks **or** Doxycycline 200 mg (PO) q12h x 3 days, then 100 mg (PO) q12h x 11 days*
Lemierre's Syndrome	Fusobacterium necrophorum	Treat as deep neck infection, above		
Severe dental infections	Oral anaerobes Oral streptococci	Clindamycin 600 mg (IV) q8h x 2 weeks **or** Piperacillin/ tazobactam 4.5 gm (IV) q8h x 2 weeks	Meropenem 1 gm (IV) q8h x 2 weeks **or** Imipenem 1 gm (IV) q6h x 2 weeks	Clindamycin 300 mg (PO) q8h x 2 weeks **or** Doxycycline 200 mg (PO) q12h x 3 days, then 100 mg (PO) q12h x 11 days*

Duration of therapy represents total time IV or IV + PO. Most patients on IV therapy able to take PO meds should be switched to PO therapy after clinical improvement
* Loading dose is not needed PO if given IV with the same drug

Clinical Presentation: Neck pain and fever
Diagnosis: Clinical presentation plus confirmatory CT/MRI scan

Deep Neck Infections
(lateral pharyngeal, retropharyngeal, prevertebral space)
Diagnostic Considerations: Patients are usually toxemic with unilateral posterior pharyngeal soft tissue mass on oral exam. Neck stiffness may be present with retropharyngeal space infection/abscess
Pitfalls: Retropharyngeal "danger space" infection may extend to mediastinum and present as mediastinitis
Therapeutic Considerations: Obtain ENT consult for surgical drainage
Prognosis: Poor without surgical drainage

Lemierre's Syndrome
Clinical Presentation: Jugular vein septic thrombophlebitis with fever, toxemic appearance, and tenderness over angle of jaw/jugular vein
Diagnostic Considerations: May present as multiple septic pulmonary emboli. Usually follows recent dental infection
Pitfalls: Suspect Lemierre's syndrome in patients with sore throat and shock
Therapeutic Considerations: If unresponsive to antibiotic therapy, may need venotomy
Prognosis: Poor with septic pulmonary emboli/shock

Severe Dental Infections
Diagnostic Considerations: Obtain CT/MRI of jaws to rule out osteomyelitis or abscess
Pitfalls: Chronic drainage in a patient with an implant is diagnostic of chronic osteomyelitis/abscess until proven otherwise
Therapeutic Considerations: Abscesses must be drained for cure
Prognosis: Poor prognosis and recurrent without adequate surgical drainage

Epiglottitis

Subset	Usual Pathogens	Preferred IV Therapy	Alternate IV Therapy	IV-to-PO Switch
Epiglottitis	S. pneumoniae H. influenzae Respiratory viruses	Ceftriaxone 1 gm (IV) q24h x 2 weeks **or** Ceftizoxime 2 gm (IV) q8h x 2 weeks	Meropenem 1 gm (IV) q8h x 2 weeks **or** Imipenem 1 gm (IV) q6h x 2 weeks	Levofloxacin 500 mg (PO) q24h x 2 weeks **or** Cefprozil 500 mg (PO) q12h x 2 weeks

Duration of therapy represents total time IV or IV + PO. Most patients on IV therapy able to take PO meds should be switched to PO therapy after clinical improvement

Clinical Presentation: Stridor with upper respiratory infection
Diagnostic Considerations: Lateral film of neck shows epiglottic edema. Neck CT/MRI may help if neck films are nondiagnostic
Pitfalls: Do not attempt to culture the epiglottis (may precipitate acute upper airway obstruction)
Therapeutic Considerations: Treat empirically as soon as possible. Obtain ENT consult
Prognosis: Early airway obstruction is associated with an adverse prognosis

Empiric Therapy of Lower Respiratory Tract Infections

Acute Exacerbation of Chronic Bronchitis (AECB)

Subset	Usual Pathogens	IV Therapy	PO Therapy
AECB	S. pneumoniae H. influenzae M. catarrhalis C. pneumoniae	Not applicable	Levofloxacin 500 mg (PO) q24h x 5 days **or** Gatifloxacin 400 mg (PO) q24h x 5 days **or** Moxifloxacin 400 mg (PO) q24h x 5 days **or** Doxycycline 100 mg (PO) q12h x 5 days

Clinical Presentation: Productive cough and negative chest x-ray in a patient with chronic bronchitis
Diagnostic Considerations: Diagnosis by productive cough, purulent sputum, and chest x-ray negative for pneumonia. H. influenzae is relatively more common than other pathogens
Pitfalls: Do not obtain sputum cultures in chronic bronchitis; cultures usually reported as normal/mixed flora and should not be used to guide therapy
Therapeutic Considerations: Treat as community-acquired pneumonia, since pathogens are the same (even though H. influenzae is relatively more frequent). Bronchodilators helpful for bronchospasm
Prognosis: Related to underlying cardiopulmonary status

Mediastinitis

Subset	Usual Pathogens	Preferred IV Therapy	Alternate IV Therapy	IV-to-PO Switch
Following esophageal perforation or thoracic surgery	Oral anaerobes	Piperacillin/ tazobactam 4.5 gm (IV) q8h x 2 weeks **or** Ampicillin/ sulbactam 3 gm (IV) q6h x 2 weeks	Meropenem 1 gm (IV) q8h x 2 weeks **or** Imipenem 1 gm (IV) q6h x 2 weeks **or** Ertapenem 1 gm (IV) q24h x 2 weeks	Amoxicillin 1 gm (PO) q8h x 2 weeks **or** Levofloxacin 500 mg (PO) q24h x 2 weeks

Duration of therapy represents total time IV or IV + PO. Most patients on IV therapy able to take PO meds should be switched to PO therapy after clinical improvement

Diagnostic Considerations: Chest x-ray usually shows perihilar infiltrate in mediastinitis. Pleural effusions from esophageal tears have elevated amylase levels
Pitfalls: Do not overlook esophageal tear in mediastinitis with pleural effusions

Therapeutic Considerations: Obtain surgical consult if esophageal perforation is suspected
Prognosis: Related to extent, location, and duration of esophageal tear/mediastinal infection

Community-Acquired Pneumonia (CAP)

Subset	Usual Pathogens*	Preferred IV Therapy	Alternate IV Therapy	PO Therapy or IV-to-PO Switch
Typical bacterial pathogens	S. pneumoniae H. influenzae M. catarrhalis	Levofloxacin 500 mg (IV) q24h x 2 weeks **or** Gatifloxacin 400 mg (IV) q24h x 2 weeks **or** Moxifloxacin 400 mg (IV) q24h x 2 weeks	Doxycycline 200 mg (IV) q12h x 3 days, then 100 mg (IV) q12h x 11 days **or** Azithromycin 500 mg (IV) x 1 dose, then 250 mg (IV) q24h x 2 weeks	Levofloxacin 500 mg (PO) q24h x 2 weeks **or** Gatifloxacin 400 mg (PO) q24h x 2 weeks **or** Moxifloxacin 400 mg (PO) q24h x 2 weeks **or** Doxycycline 200 mg (PO) q12h x 3 days, then 100 mg (PO) q12h x 11 days** **or** Azithromycin 500 mg (PO) x 1 dose, then 250 mg (PO) q24h x 2 weeks**
Atypical pathogens *Zoonotic*	Chlamydia psittaci (psittacosis) Coxiella burnetii (Q fever) Francisella tularensis (tularemia)	Doxycycline 200 mg (IV) q12h x 3 days, then 100 mg (IV) q12h x 2-4 weeks	Levofloxacin 500 mg (IV) q24h x 2-4 weeks	Doxycycline 200 mg (PO) q12h x 3 days, then 100 mg (PO) q12h x 2-4 weeks** **or** Levofloxacin 500 mg (PO) q24h x 2-4 weeks

Community-Acquired Pneumonia (CAP) (cont'd)

Subset	Usual Pathogens*	Preferred IV Therapy	Alternate IV Therapy	PO Therapy or IV-to-PO Switch
Atypical pathogens *Non-zoonotic*	Legionella sp. Mycoplasma pneumoniae Chlamydia pneumoniae	Levofloxacin 500 mg (IV) q24h x 2-4 weeks **or** Gatifloxacin 400 mg (IV) q24h x 2-4 weeks **or** Moxifloxacin 400 mg (IV) q24h x 2-4 weeks	Doxycycline 200 mg (IV) q12h x 3 days, then 100 mg (IV) q12h x 2-4 weeks **or** Azithromycin 500 mg (IV) x 1 dose, then 250 mg (IV) q24h x 4 days. Follow in 2 weeks with azithromycin 500 mg (PO) x 1 dose, then 250 mg (PO) q24h x 4 days	Levofloxacin 500 mg (PO) q24h x 2-4 weeks **or** Gatifloxacin 400 mg (PO) q24h x 2-4 weeks **or** Moxifloxacin 400 mg (PO) q24h x 2-4 weeks **or** Doxycycline 200 mg (PO) q12h x 3 days, then 100 mg (PO) q12h x 2-4 weeks** **or** Azithromycin** 500 mg (PO) x 1 dose, then 250 mg (PO) q24h x 4 days. Repeat in 2 weeks
Aspiration	Oral anaerobes S. pneumoniae H. influenzae M. catarrhalis	Levofloxacin 500 mg (IV) q24h x 2 weeks **or** Gatifloxacin 400 mg (IV) q24h x 2 weeks **or** Moxifloxacin 400 mg (IV) q24h x 2 weeks	Ceftriaxone 1 gm (IV) q24h x 2 weeks	Levofloxacin 500 mg (PO) q24h x 2 weeks **or** Gatifloxacin 400 mg (PO) q24h x 2 weeks **or** Moxifloxacin 400 mg (PO) q24h x 2 weeks
HIV *PCP*	P. carinii	See p. 216		
Sputum (+) for AFB	M. tuberculosis MAI	See p. 216		
Sputum (–) for AFB	S. pneumoniae H. influenzae Salmonella Legionella C. pneumoniae	Levofloxacin 500 mg (IV) q24h x 2 weeks **or** Gatifloxacin 400 mg (IV) q24h x 2 weeks	Ceftriaxone 1 gm (IV) q24h x 2 weeks **plus** Azithromycin 500 mg (IV) q24h x 1 week	Levofloxacin 500 mg (PO) q24h x 2 weeks **or** Gatifloxacin 400 mg (PO) q24h x 2 weeks

Community-Acquired Pneumonia (CAP) (cont'd)

Subset	Usual Pathogens*	Preferred IV Therapy	Alternate IV Therapy	PO Therapy or IV-to-PO Switch
Atypical tuberculosis	Mycobacterium avium-intracellulare (MAI)	Not applicable	<u>Treat for 3-6 months/until CD4 ↑:</u> Ethambutol 15 mg/kg (PO) q24h **plus either** Clarithromycin 500 mg (PO) q12h **or** Azithromycin 500 mg (PO) q24h <u>May also choose to add:</u> Ciprofloxacin 750 mg (PO) q12h **or** Ofloxacin 400 mg (PO) q12h or Levofloxacin 500 mg (PO) q24h	
Tuberculosis (TB)	M. tuberculosis	Not applicable	INH 300 mg (PO) q24h x 6-12 months **plus** Rifampin 600 mg (PO) q24h x 6-12 months <u>If multiresistant TB strain likely, also add:</u> EMB 15 mg/kg (PO) q24h x 6-12 months **plus** PZA 25 mg/kg (PO) q24h x 6-12 months	
Chronic alcoholics	K. pneumoniae S. pneumoniae H. influenzae M. catarrhalis	Ceftriaxone 1 gm (IV) q24h x 2 weeks	Levofloxacin 500 mg (IV) q24h x 2 weeks **or** Gatifloxacin 400 mg (IV) q24h x 2 weeks **or** Moxifloxacin 400 mg (IV) q24h x 2 weeks	Levofloxacin 500 mg (PO) q24h x 2 weeks **or** Gatifloxacin 400 mg (PO) q24h x 2 weeks **or** Moxifloxacin 400 mg (PO) q24h x 2 weeks
Post-viral influenza	S. aureus S. pneumoniae H. influenzae	Levofloxacin 500 mg (IV) q24h x 2 weeks **plus either** Nafcillin 2 gm (IV) q4h x 2 weeks **or** Clindamycin 600 mg (IV) q8h x 2 weeks	Ceftriaxone 1 gm (IV) q24h x 2 weeks **plus either** Vancomycin 1 gm (IV) q12h x 2 weeks **or** Linezolid 600 mg (IV) q12h x 2 weeks	Levofloxacin 500 mg (PO) q24h x 2 weeks **plus** Clindamycin 300 mg (PO) q8h x 2 weeks
Bronchiectasis, cystic fibrosis	P. aeruginosa	Treat as nosocomial pneumonia (p. 50)		

Community-Acquired Pneumonia (CAP) (cont'd)

Subset	Usual Pathogens*	Preferred IV Therapy	Alternate IV Therapy	PO Therapy or IV-to-PO Switch
Nursing home-acquired pneumonia (NHAP)	H. influenzae S. pneumoniae M. catarrhalis C. pneumoniae	Levofloxacin 500 mg (IV) q24h x 2 weeks **or** Gatifloxacin 400 mg (IV) q24h x 2 weeks **or** Moxifloxacin 400 mg (IV) q24h x 2 weeks	Doxycycline 200 mg (IV) q12h x 3 days, then 100 mg (IV) q12h x 11 days	Levofloxacin 500 mg (PO) q24h x 2 weeks **or** Gatifloxacin 400 mg (PO) q24h x 2 weeks **or** Doxycycline 200 mg (PO) q12h x 3 days, then 100 mg (PO) q12h x 11 days** **or** Moxifloxacin 400 mg (PO) q24h x 2 weeks
Chronic steroid therapy† (If perihilar infiltrates/hypoxemia, treat as PCP until lung biopsy)	Aspergillus	Amphotericin B 1 mg/kg (IV) q24h until 1-2 grams **or** Caspofungin 70 mg (IV) x 1 dose, then 50 mg (IV) q24h x 4 weeks **or** Voriconazole 400 mg (IV) x 1 dose, then 200 mg (IV) q12h x 4 weeks	Amphotericin B lipid formulation 5 mg/kg (IV) x 4-8 weeks **or** Itraconazole 200 mg (IV) q12h x 2 days, then 200 mg (IV) q24h for total of 4 weeks	Itraconazole 200 mg (IV) q12h x 2 days, then 200 mg (PO) q12h for total of 4 weeks** **or** Voriconazole 400 mg (PO) x 1 dose, then 200 mg (PO) q12h x 4 weeks**
	P. carinii (PCP)	TMP-SMX 5 mg/kg (IV) q6h x 3 weeks	Pentamidine 4 mg/kg (IV) q24h x 3 weeks	TMP-SMX 5 mg/kg (PO) q6h x 3 weeks
Organ transplants†	CMV	Ganciclovir 2.5 mg/kg (IV) q8h x 21 days, then 5 mg/kg (IV) 3-5x/week x 20 doses **plus** IVIG 500 mg/kg (IV) q48h x 10 doses, then 500 mg/kg (IV) 2x/wk x 8 doses	Not applicable	Valganciclovir 900 mg (PO) q12h x 3 weeks, then 900 mg (PO) q24h life-long
	P. carinii (PCP)	TMP-SMX 5 mg/kg (IV) q6h x 3 weeks	Pentamidine 4 mg/kg (IV) q24h x 3 weeks	TMP-SMX 5 mg/kg (PO) q6h x 3 weeks

Community-Acquired Pneumonia (CAP) (cont'd)

Subset	Usual Pathogens*	Preferred Therapy
Other pathogens	Blastomyces, Histoplasma, Coccidioides, Paracoccidioides, Actinomyces, Nocardia, Pseudallescheria boydii, Sporothrix, Mucor	See pp. 168-169

Duration of therapy represents total time IV, PO, or IV + PO. Most patients on IV therapy able to take PO meds should be switched to PO therapy soon after clinical improvement
* Compromised hosts are predisposed to organisms listed, but may be infected by usual pathogens in normal hosts
** Loading dose is not needed PO if given IV with the same drug
† Treat only IV or IV-to-PO switch

Clinical Presentation: Fever, cough, respiratory symptoms, chest x-ray consistent with pneumonia
Diagnosis: Identification of organism on sputum gram stain/culture. Same organism is found in blood if blood cultures are positive

Community-Acquired Pneumonia (Typical Bacterial Pathogens)
Diagnostic Considerations: Sputum is useful if a single organism predominates and is not contaminated by saliva. Purulent sputum, pleuritic chest pain, pleural effusion favor typical pathogens
Pitfalls: Obtain a chest x-ray to verify the diagnosis and rule out non-infectious mimics (e.g., heart failure). Treat COPD/chronic bronchitis patients empirically (sputum is unhelpful; usually shows "mixed/normal flora")
Therapeutic Considerations: Do not switch to narrow-spectrum antibiotic after organism is identified on gram stain/blood culture. Pathogen identification is important for prognostic and public health reasons, not for therapy. Severity of CAP is related to the degree of cardiopulmonary/immune dysfunction and impacts the length of hospital stay, not the therapeutic approach or antibiotic choice
Prognosis: Related to cardiopulmonary status and splenic function

Community-Acquired Pneumonia (Atypical Pathogens)
Clinical Presentation: CAP with extra-pulmonary symptoms, signs, or laboratory abnormalities
Diagnosis: Confirm by specific serological tests

Zoonotic Infections (Psittacosis, Q fever, Tularemia)
Diagnostic Considerations: Zoonotic contact history is key to presumptive diagnosis: psittacosis (parrots and relatives); Q fever (sheep, parturient cats); tularemia (rabbit, deer, deer fly bite)
Pitfalls: Organisms are difficult/dangerous to grow. Do not culture. Use serological tests for diagnosis
Therapeutic Considerations: Q fever endocarditis requires prolonged therapy
Prognosis: Good except for Q fever with complications (e.g., SBE)

Non-Zoonotic Infections (Legionella sp., M. pneumoniae, C. pneumoniae)
Diagnostic Considerations: Each atypical pathogen has a different and characteristic pattern of extra-pulmonary organ involvement. Legionnaire's disease is suggested by relative bradycardia, ↓ PO_4^-, ↑ SGOT, microscopic hematuria, abdominal pain, diarrhea
Pitfalls: Failure to respond to beta-lactams should suggest diagnosis of atypical CAP
Therapeutic Considerations: Treat Legionella x 4 weeks. Treat Mycoplasma or Chlamydia x 2 weeks
Prognosis: Related to severity of underlying cardiopulmonary disease

Aspiration Pneumonia
Diagnostic Considerations: Sputum not diagnostic. No need for transtracheal aspirate culture

Pitfalls: Lobar location varies with patient position during aspiration
Therapeutic Considerations: Oral anaerobes are sensitive to all beta-lactams and most antibiotics used to treat CAP. Additional anaerobic (B. fragilis) coverage is not needed
Prognosis: Related to severity of CNS/esophageal disease

Pneumonia in HIV
Pneumocystis carinii Pneumonia (PCP) (see p. 221)

Sputum Positive for AFB (TB/MAI) (see pp. 222, 225)

Sputum Negative for AFB
Clinical Presentation: CAP in HIV patient with focal infiltrate(s) and normal/slightly depressed CD_4
Diagnostic Considerations: Diagnosis by sputum gram stain/culture ± positive blood cultures (bacterial pathogens) or Legionella/Chlamydia serology (atypical pathogens). Blood cultures are most often positive for S. pneumoniae or H. influenzae. Only cover S. aureus in IV drug abusers with pre-terminal disease
Pitfalls: Atypical chest x-ray appearance is not uncommon. Treat syndrome of CAP, not chest x-ray. CAP in HIV does not resemble PCP, which presents with profound hypoxemia without focal infiltrates
Therapeutic Considerations: Treat the same as CAP in normal hosts
Prognosis: Clinically resolves the same as CAP in normal hosts

Mycobacterium avium-intracellulare (MAI) Pneumonia
Clinical Presentation: Community-acquired pneumonia in immunosuppressed/HIV patient with focal single/multiple infiltrates
Diagnostic Considerations: Diagnosis by AFB smear/culture
Pitfalls: Must differentiate TB and MAI by AFB culture
Therapeutic Considerations: MAI requires life-long suppressive therapy after initial treatment
Prognosis: Related to degree of immunosuppression/CD_4 count

Tuberculous (TB) Pneumonia
Clinical Presentation: Community-acquired pneumonia with single/multiple infiltrates
Diagnostic Considerations: Diagnosis by sputum AFB smear/culture. Respiratory isolation important. Lower lobe effusion common in lower lobe primary TB. Reactivation TB is usually bilateral/apical ± old, healed Ghon complex; cavitation/fibrosis are common, but pleural effusion is absent
Pitfalls: Primary TB may present as CAP; reactivation TB presents as chronic pneumonia
Therapeutic Considerations: 1-2 weeks of therapy is usually required to eliminate AFBs from sputum
Prognosis: Related to underlying health status

Pneumonia in Chronic Alcoholics
Diagnostic Considerations: Klebsiella pneumoniae usually occurs only in chronic alcoholics, and is characterized by blood-flecked "currant jelly" sputum and cavitation (typically in 3-5 days)
Pitfalls: Suspect Klebsiella in "pneumococcal" pneumonia that cavitates. Empyema is more common than pleural effusion
Therapeutic Considerations: Monotherapy with newer anti-Klebsiella agents is as effective or superior to "double-drug" therapy with older agents
Prognosis: Related to degree of hepatic/splenic dysfunction

Post-Viral Influenza Pneumonia
Diagnostic Considerations: S. aureus pneumonia usually only affects patients with viral influenza pneumonia, and is characterized by cyanosis and rapid cavitation on chest x-ray. Do not diagnose

staphylococcal pneumonia without these signs
Pitfalls: Bacterial pneumonia may be superimposed or follow viral influenza pneumonia
Therapeutic Considerations: Usually no need to cover MRSA
Prognosis: Related to severity of influenza pneumonia and type of superinfection

Bronchiectasis/Cystic Fibrosis (P. aeruginosa)
Diagnostic Considerations: Cystic fibrosis/bronchiectasis is characterized by viscous secretions ± low grade fevers; less commonly may present as lung abscess. Onset of pneumonia/lung abscess heralded by cough/decrease in pulmonary function
Pitfalls: Sputum colonization is common (e.g., S. maltophilia, B. cepacia) and may not reflect lung pathogens
Therapeutic Considerations: Important to select antibiotics with low resistance potential and good penetration into respiratory secretions (e.g., quinolones, meropenem). Treated the same as nosocomial pneumonia
Prognosis: Related to extent of underlying lung disease/severity of infection

Nursing Home-Acquired Pneumonia (NHAP)
Diagnostic Considerations: Difficult to obtain sputum in elderly/debilitated patients. H. influenzae is common; K. pneumoniae is uncommon in non-alcoholics, even in this population
Pitfalls: Resembles community-acquired pneumonia in terms of pathogens and length of hospital stay, not nosocomial pneumoni
Therapeutic Considerations: Treat as community-acquired pneumonia, not nosocomial pneumonia. No need to cover P. aeruginosa
Prognosis: Related to underlying cardiopulmonary status

Pneumonia in Chronic Steroid Therapy
If fungal infection is suspected, obtain lung biopsy to confirm diagnosis/identify causative organism. Non-responsiveness to appropriate antibiotics should suggest fungal infection. Do not empirically treat fungi; confirm diagnosis by lung biopsy first. Prognosis related to degree of immunosuppression

Acute Aspergillus Pneumonia
Clinical Presentation: Chest x-ray shows progressive necrotizing pneumonia unresponsive to antibiotic therapy. No characteristic appearance on chest x-ray. Usually seen only in compromised hosts
Diagnostic Considerations: Diagnosis by lung biopsy (not broncho-alveolar lavage) demonstrating hyphae invading lung parenchyma/blood vessels. Usually occurs only in patients receiving chronic steroids or cancer chemotherapy, organ transplants, leukopenic compromised hosts, or patients with chronic granulomatous disease
Pitfalls: Aspergillus pneumonia does not occur in normal hosts
Prognosis: Almost always fatal despite appropriate therapy

Pneumonia in Organ Transplants
Clinical Presentation: CAP with perihilar infiltrates and hypoxemia
Diagnostic Considerations: CMV is diagnosed by stain/culture of lung biopsy
Therapeutic Considerations: Treat as CMV pneumonia if CMV is predominant pathogen on lung biopsy. CMV may progress despite ganciclovir therapy
Prognosis: Related to degree of immunosuppression

Other Pneumonias (Blastomyces, Histoplasma, Coccidioides, Paracoccidioides, Actinomyces, Nocardia, Pseudallescheria boydii, Sporothrix, Mucor) (see pp. 169-172)

Lung Abscess/Empyema

Subset	Usual Pathogens	Preferred IV Therapy	Alternate IV Therapy	PO Therapy or IV-to-PO Switch
Lung abscess/ empyema	Oral anaerobes S. aureus S. pneumoniae K. pneumoniae	Clindamycin 600 mg (IV) q8h until resolved **plus** Levofloxacin 500 mg (IV) q24h until resolved	Meropenem 1 gm (IV) q8h until resolved **or** Imipenem 1 gm (IV) q6h until resolved **or** Ertapenem 1 gm (IV) q24h until resolved **or** Piperacillin/ tazobactam 4.5 gm (IV) q8h until resolved	Clindamycin 300 mg (PO) q8h until resolved **plus** Levofloxacin 500 mg (PO) q24h until resolved
Bronchiectasis, cystic fibrosis	P. aeruginosa	Treat as nosocomial pneumonia (p. 50)		

Duration of therapy represents total time IV, PO, or IV + PO. Most patients on IV therapy able to take PO meds should be switched to PO therapy soon after clinical improvement (usually < 72 hours)

Clinical Presentation: Lung abscess presents as single/multiple cavitary lung lesion(s) with fever. Empyema presents as persistent fever with pleural effusion that does not layer out on lateral decubitus chest x-ray

Diagnostic Considerations: In lung abscess, plain film/CT scan demonstrates cavitary lung lesions appearing > 1 week after pneumonia. Most CAPs are not associated with pleural effusion, and few develop empyema. In empyema, pleural fluid pH is ≤ 7.2; culture purulent exudate for pathogen

Pitfalls: Pleural effusions secondary to CAP usually resolve rapidly with treatment. Suspect empyema in patients with persistent pleural effusions with fever

Therapeutic Considerations: Chest tube/surgical drainage needed for empyema. Treat lung abscess until it resolves (usually 3-12 months)

Prognosis: Good if adequately drained

Nosocomial Pneumonia (NP)

Subset	Usual Pathogens	Preferred IV Therapy	Alternate IV Therapy	IV-to-PO Switch
Nosocomial pneumonia	P. aeruginosa* E. coli K. pneumoniae S. marcescens	Cefepime 2 gm (IV) q12h x 2 weeks **or** Meropenem 1 gm (IV) q8h x 2 weeks **or** Imipenem 1 gm (IV) q6h x 2 weeks **or** Piperacillin 4 gm (IV) q8h x 2 weeks **or** Levofloxacin 750 mg (IV) q24h x 2 weeks	**One "A" drug + one "B" drug:** **"A" Drugs** Cefepime 2 gm (IV) q12h x 2 weeks **or** Meropenem 1 gm (IV) q8h x 2 weeks **"B" Drugs** Levofloxacin 500 mg (IV) q24h x 2 weeks **or** Gentamicin 120 mg (IV) q24h x 2 weeks **or** Aztreonam 2 gm (IV) q8h x 2 weeks	<u>P. aeruginosa</u> Levofloxacin 750 mg (PO) q24h x 2 weeks **or** Ciprofloxacin 750 mg (PO) q12h x 2 weeks <u>Non-P. aeruginosa</u> Levofloxacin 750 mg (PO) q24h x 2 weeks

Duration of therapy represents total time IV or IV + PO. Most patients on IV therapy able to take PO meds should be switched to PO therapy after clinical improvement
* *For confirmed P. aeruginosa NP, preferred IV therapy consists of combination drug therapy with [meropenem or imipenem] plus [cefepime or piperacillin or levofloxacin]*

Clinical Presentation: Pulmonary infiltrate compatible with a bacterial pneumonia occurring ≥ 1 week in-hospital ± fever/leukocytosis

Diagnostic Considerations: Definitive diagnosis by culture of lung biopsy. P. aeruginosa and S. aureus are common colonizers in CCU-ventilated patients. Proven P. aeruginosa NP is a necrotizing pneumonia with rapid cavitation (< 72 hours), microabscesses, and blood vessel invasion. S. aureus (MSSA/MRSA) rarely cause NP despite being cultured from 25% of ET tubes. Acinetobacter NP occurs usually in outbreak situations. Leukocytosis and fever are nonspecific/nondiagnostic of NP

Pitfalls: Do not cover non-pulmonary pathogens cultured from respiratory secretions in ventilated patients (Enterobacter, P. cepacia, P. maltophilia, Citrobacter, Flavobacterium, Enterococci); these organisms rarely if ever cause NP. S. aureus (MSSA/MRSA) cultured by bronchogenic techniques is not diagnostic for S. aureus NP. Semi-quantitative protected brush specimens (PBS) reflect airway colonization, not lung pathogens

Therapeutic Considerations: Monotherapy is as effective as combination therapy for non-P. aeruginosa NP, but 2-drug therapy is recommended for confirmed P. aeruginosa NP. After 2 weeks of appropriate antibiotic therapy, non-progressive/stable pulmonary infiltrates with fever and leukocytosis are usually due to a non-infectious cause, rather than persistent infection. Do not add anti-MSSA/MRSA coverage if S. aureus (MSSA/MRSA) is cultured from respiratory secretions of intubated patients

Prognosis: Related to underlying cardiopulmonary status

Empiric Therapy of Cardiovascular Infections

Subacute Bacterial Endocarditis (SBE)

Subset	Usual Pathogens	Preferred IV Therapy	Alternate IV Therapy	PO Therapy or IV-to-PO Switch
No obvious source	S. viridans Group B,C,G streptococci Nutritionally-variant streptococci	Ceftriaxone 2 gm (IV) q24h x 2 weeks **plus** Gentamicin 120 mg (IV) q24h x 2 weeks **or monotherapy with** Ceftriaxone 2 gm (IV) q24h x 2 weeks	Penicillin G 3 mu (IV) q4h x 2 weeks **plus** Gentamicin 180 mg (IV) q24h x 2 weeks **or monotherapy with** Vancomycin 1 gm (IV) q12h x 2 weeks **or** Linezolid 600 mg (IV) q12h x 2 weeks	Amoxicillin 1 gm (PO) q8h x 2 weeks **or** Linezolid 600 mg (PO) q12h x 2 weeks
GI/GU source likely (Treat initially for E. faecalis; if later identified as E. faecium, treat accordingly)	E. faecalis	Vancomycin 1 gm (IV) q12h x 4-6 weeks **plus** Gentamicin 80 mg (IV) q8h x 4-6 weeks **or monotherapy with** Ampicillin 2 gm (IV) q4h x 4-6 weeks	Meropenem 1 gm (IV) q8h x 4-6 weeks **or** Imipenem 1 gm (IV) q6h x 4-6 weeks **or** Linezolid 600 mg (IV) q12h x 4-6 weeks	Amoxicillin 1 gm (PO) q8h x 4-6 weeks **or** Linezolid 600 mg (PO) q12h x 4-6 weeks
	E. faecium (VRE)	Linezolid 600 mg (IV) q12h x 4-6 weeks	Quinupristin/ dalfopristin 7.5 mg/kg (IV) q8h x 4-6 weeks	Linezolid 600 mg (PO) q12h x 4-6 weeks
	S. bovis	Treat the same as "no obvious source" subset, above		

Subacute Bacterial Endocarditis (SBE) (cont'd)

Subset	Usual Pathogens	Preferred IV Therapy	Alternate IV Therapy	PO Therapy or IV-to-PO Switch
Apparent "culture negative" SBE*	Hemophilus sp. Actinobacillus actinomycetem-comitans Cardiobacterium hominis Eikenella corrodens Kingella kingae	Ceftriaxone 2 gm (IV) q24h x 4 weeks **or** Any 3rd generation cephalosporin (IV) x 4 weeks **or** Cefepime 2 gm (IV) q12h x 4 weeks	Ampicillin 2 gm (IV) q4h x 4 weeks **plus either** Gentamicin 120 mg (IV) q24h x 4 weeks **or** Levofloxacin 500 mg (IV) q24h x 4-6 weeks	Levofloxacin 500 mg (PO) q24h x 4 weeks **or** Ciprofloxacin 500 mg (PO) q12h x 4 weeks
True "culture negative" SBE*	Legionella Coxiella burnetii (Q fever) Chlamydia psittaci Brucella	Levofloxacin 500 mg (IV) q24h x 4-6 weeks	Doxycycline 200 mg (IV) q12h x 3 days, then 100 mg (IV) q12h x 4-6 weeks	Doxycycline 200 mg (PO) q12h x 3 days, then 100 mg (PO) q12h x 4-6 weeks** **or** Levofloxacin 500 mg (PO) q24h x 4-6 weeks

VRE = vancomycin-resistant enterococci. Duration of therapy represents total time IV, PO, or IV + PO. Most patients on IV therapy able to take PO meds should be switched to PO therapy soon after clinical improvement
*   Treat only IV or IV-to-PO switch
**   Loading dose is not needed PO if given IV with the same drug

Clinical Presentation: Subacute febrile illness ± localizing symptoms/signs in a patient with a heart murmur. Peripheral manifestations are commonly absent with early diagnosis/treatment
Diagnosis: Positive blood cultures plus vegetation on transthoracic/transesophageal echo

SBE (No Obvious Source)

Diagnostic Considerations: Most common pathogen is S. viridans. Source is usually from the mouth, although oral/dental infection is usually inapparent clinically
Pitfalls: Vegetations without positive blood cultures or peripheral manifestations of SBE are not diagnostic of endocarditis. SBE vegetations may persist after antibiotic therapy, but are sterile
Therapeutic Considerations: In penicillin-allergic (anaphylactic) patients, vancomycin may be used alone or in combination with gentamicin. Follow ESR weekly to monitor antibiotic response. No need to repeat blood cultures unless patient has persistent fever or is not responding clinically. Two-week treatment is acceptable for uncomplicated S. viridans SBE. Treat nutritionally-variant streptococci (B₆/pyridoxal deficient streptococci) the same as for S. viridans SBE
Prognosis: Related to extent of embolization/severity of heart failure

SBE (GI/GU Source Likely)

Diagnostic Considerations: Commonest pathogens from GI/GU source are Enterococci (especially E. faecalis). If S. bovis, look for GI polyp, tumor. Enterococcal SBE commonly follows GI/GU instrumentation
Therapeutic Considerations: E. faecalis SBE may be treated with ampicillin alone; gentamicin may be added if synergy testing is positive (e.g., isolate sensitive to < 500 mcg/mL of gentamicin). Do not

add gentamicin if MIC > 500 mcg/mL. For penicillin-allergic patients, use vancomycin plus gentamicin; vancomycin alone is inadequate for enterococcal (E. faecalis) SBE. Treat enterococcal PVE the same as for native valve enterococcal SBE. Treat S. bovis SBE the same as S. viridans SBE. Non-enterococcal Group D streptococci (S. bovis) is penicllin sensitive, unlike Group D enterococci (E. faecalis)

Prognosis: Related to extent of embolization/severity of heart failure

Apparent "Culture Negative" SBE

Diagnostic Considerations: Culture of HACEK organisms requires enhanced CO_2/special media (Castaneda vented bottles) and prolonged incubation (2-4 weeks). True "culture negative" SBE is rare, and is characterized by peripheral signs of SBE with a murmur, vegetation, and negative blood cultures

Pitfalls: Most cases of "culture negative" SBE are not really culture negative, but due to fastidious organisms (HACEK group) requiring prolonged incubation with enhanced CO_2 atmosphere for growth. Sterile vegetations may persist after antibiotic therapy

Therapeutic Considerations: Follow clinical improvement with serial ESRs, which should return to pretreatment levels with therapy. Verification of cure by blood culture is not needed if patient is afebrile and clinically well

Prognosis: Related to extent of embolization/severity of heart failure

True "Culture Negative" SBE

Diagnostic Considerations: Diagnosis by specific serology. Large vessel emboli suggests culture negative SBE in patients with negative blood cultures but signs of SBE

Pitfalls: Do not diagnose culture negative SBE in patients with a heart murmur and negative blood cultures if peripheral SBE manifestations are absent

Therapeutic Considerations: Treatment is based on specific organism identified by diagnostic tests

Prognosis: Related to extent of embolization/severity of heart failure

Acute Bacterial Endocarditis (ABE)

Subset	Usual Pathogens	Preferred IV Therapy	Alternate IV Therapy	PO Therapy or IV-to-PO Switch
Normal hosts* (Treat initially for MSSA; if later identified as MSRA, treat accordingly)	S. aureus (MSSA)	Nafcillin 2 gm (IV) q4h x 4-6 weeks **or** Meropenem 1 gm (IV) q8h x 4-6 weeks **or** Imipenem 1 gm (IV) q6h x 4-6 weeks	Linezolid 600 mg (IV) q12h x 4-6 weeks **or** Vancomycin 1 gm (IV) q12h x 4-6 weeks	Minocycline 100 mg (PO) q12h x 4-6 weeks **or** Cephalexin 1 gm (PO) q6h x 4-6 weeks **or** Linezolid 600 mg (PO) q12h x 4-6 weeks
	S. aureus (MRSA)	Vancomycin 1 gm (IV) q12h x 4-6 weeks **or** Linezolid 600 mg (IV) q12h x 4-6 weeks	Minocycline 100 mg (IV) q12h x 4-6 weeks	Linezolid 600 mg (PO) q12h x 4-6 weeks **or** Minocycline 100 mg (PO) q12h x 4-6 weeks

Acute Bacterial Endocarditis (ABE) (cont'd)

Subset	Usual Pathogens	Preferred IV Therapy	Alternate IV Therapy	PO Therapy or IV-to-PO Switch
IV drug abusers (Treat as MSSA before culture results; treat according to pathogen after culture results)	S. aureus (MSSA)	<u>Before culture results</u> Vancomycin 1 gm (IV) q12h **plus either** Gentamicin 120 mg (IV) q24h **or** Amikacin 500 mg (IV) q24h	<u>After culture results</u> Nafcillin 2 gm (IV) q4h x 4 weeks **or** Meropenem 1 gm (IV) q8h x 4 weeks **or** Imipenem 1 gm (IV) q6h x 4 weeks **or** Vancomycin 1 gm (IV) q12h x 4 weeks **or** Linezolid 600 mg (IV) q12h x 4 weeks	<u>After culture results</u> Linezolid 600 mg (PO) q12h x 4 weeks **or** Minocycline 100 mg (PO) q12h x 4 weeks **or** Cephalexin 1 gm (PO) q6h x 4 weeks
	S. aureus (MRSA)	<u>Before culture results</u> Treat the same as MSSA	<u>After culture results</u> Vancomycin 1 gm (IV) q12h x 4 weeks **or** Linezolid 600 mg (IV) q12h x 4 weeks **or** Minocycline 100 mg (IV) q12h x 4 weeks	<u>After culture results</u> Linezolid 600 mg (PO) q12h x 4 weeks **or** Minocycline 100 mg (PO) q12h x 4 weeks
	P. aeruginosa*	<u>Before culture results</u> Treat the same as MSSA	<u>After culture results</u> **One "A" drug + one "B" drug** **"A" Drugs** Piperacillin 4 gm (IV) q8h x 4-6 weeks **or** Cefepime 2 gm (IV) q8h x 4-6 weeks **or** Meropenem 1 gm (IV) q8h x 4-6 weeks **"B" Drugs** Amikacin 500 mg (IV) q24h x 4-6 weeks **or** Aztreonam 2 gm (IV) q8h x 4-6 weeks	<u>After culture results</u> Ciprofloxacin 750 mg (PO) q12h x 4-6 weeks

MSSA/MRSA = methicillin-sensitive/resistant S. aureus. Duration of therapy represents total time IV, PO, or IV + PO.
Most patients on IV therapy able to take PO meds should be switched to PO therapy after clinical improvement
* Treat only IV or IV-to-PO switch

Acute Bacterial Endocarditis

Diagnostic Considerations: Patients are critically ill and febrile (temperature ≥ 102°F). Vegetations are almost always present
Pitfalls: Obtain a baseline echocardiogram; watch for valve destruction, heart failure, ring/perivalvular abscess. Obtain cardiology consultation
Therapeutic Considerations: Treat for 4-6 weeks. Follow teichoic acid antibody levels weekly in S. aureus ABE, which fall (along with the ESR) with effective therapy
Prognosis: Related to extent of embolization/severity of heart failure

Acute Bacterial Endocarditis (IV Drug Abusers)

Diagnostic Considerations: IVDAs with S. aureus usually have mild ABE, permitting oral treatment
Pitfalls: IVDAs with new aortic or tricuspid regurgitation should be treated IV ± valve replacement
Therapeutic Considerations: After pathogen is isolated, may switch from IV to PO regimen to complete treatment course
Prognosis: Prognosis is better than for normal hosts (endocarditis usually milder) if not complicated by abscess, valve regurgitation, or heart failure

Prosthetic Valve Endocarditis (PVE)

Subset	Usual Pathogens	Before Culture Results	After Culture Results
Early PVE (< 60 days post-PVR)	S. aureus (MSSA/MRSA) Entero-bacteriaceae	Vancomycin 1 gm (IV) q12h **plus** Gentamicin 120 mg (IV) q24h	<u>MSSA/Enterobacteriaceae</u> Cefotaxime 3 gm (IV) q6h x 4-6 weeks **or** Ceftizoxime 4 gm (IV) q8h x 4-6 weeks **or** Cefepime 2 gm (IV) q8-12h x 4-6 weeks **or** Meropenem 1 gm (IV) q8h x 4-6 weeks <u>MRSA</u> Vancomycin 1 gm (IV) q12h x 4-6 weeks* **or** Linezolid 600 mg (IV or PO) q12h x 4-6 weeks **or** Minocycline 100 mg (IV or PO) q12h x 4-6 weeks
Late PVE (> 60 days post-PVR)	S. viridans S. epidermidis (MSSE/MRSE)	Linezolid 600 mg (IV or PO) q12h **or combination therapy with** Vancomycin 1 gm (IV) q12h **plus** Gentamicin 120 mg (IV) q24h	<u>S. viridans</u> Ceftriaxone 2 gm (IV) q24h x 4-6 weeks **or** Cefotaxime 3 gm (IV) q6h x 4-6 weeks **or** Ceftizoxime 4 gm (IV) q8h x 4-6 weeks <u>MSSE/MRSE</u> Linezolid 600 mg (IV or PO) q12h x 4-6 weeks **or** Vancomycin 1 gm (IV) q12h x 4-6 weeks*

MSSA/MRSA = methicillin-sensitive/resistant S. aureus; MSSE/MRSE = methicillin-sensitive/resistant S. epidermidis. Duration of therapy represents total time IV or IV + PO. Most patients on IV therapy able to take PO meds should be switched to PO therapy after clinical improvement
* ± Rifampin 300 mg (PO) q12h x 4-6 weeks

Clinical Presentation: Prolonged fevers and chills following prosthetic valve replacement (PVR)
Diagnosis: High-grade blood culture positivity (3/4 or 4/4) with endocarditis pathogen and no other source of infection

Early PVE (< 60 days post-PVR)

Diagnostic Considerations: Blood cultures persistently positive. Temperature usually ≤ 102°F
Pitfalls: Obtain baseline TTE/TEE. Premature closure of mitral leaflet is early sign of impending aortic valve regurgitation
Therapeutic Considerations: Patients improve clinically on treatment, but are not cured without valve replacement. Replace valve as soon as possible (no advantage in waiting)
Prognosis: Related to extent of embolization/severity of heart failure

Late PVE (> 60 days post-PVR)

Pitfalls: Culture of removed valve may be negative, but valve gram stain will be positive
Therapeutic Considerations: Late PVE resembles S. viridans SBE clinically. Valve removal for S. epidermidis PVE may be necessary for cure
Prognosis: Related to extent of embolization/severity of heart failure

Pericarditis/Myocarditis

Subset	Usual Pathogens	Preferred Therapy
Viral pericarditis/ myocarditis	Coxsackie virus	No treatment available
TB pericarditis	M. tuberculosis	Treat the same as pulmonary TB (p. 44)
Suppurative pericarditis	S. pneumoniae S. aureus	Treat the same as lung abscess/empyema (p. 49)

Clinical Presentation: Viral pericarditis presents with acute onset of fever/chest pain (made worse by sitting up) following a viral illness. Viral myocarditis presents with heart failure, arrhythmias ± emboli. TB pericarditis is indolent in presentation, with ↑ jugular venous distension (JVD), pericardial friction rub (40%), paradoxical pulse (25%), and chest x-ray with cardiomegaly ± left-sided pleural effusion. Suppurative pericarditis presents as acute pericarditis (patients are critically ill). Develops from contiguous (e.g., pneumonia) or hematogenous spread (e.g., S. aureus bacteremia)
Diagnostic Considerations: Pericarditis/effusion manifests cardiomegaly with decreased heart sounds ± tamponade. Diagnosis by culture/biopsy of pericardial fluid or pericardium for viruses, bacteria, or acid-fast bacilli (AFB). Diagnosis of myocarditis is clinical ± myocardial biopsy
Pitfalls: Consider other causes of pericardial effusion (malignancy, especially with bloody effusion, uremia, etc.). Rule out treatable non-viral causes of myocarditis (e.g., RMSF, Lyme disease, diphtheria)
Therapeutic Considerations: No specific treatment for viral myocarditis/pericarditis. TB pericarditis is treated the same as pulmonary TB ± pericardiectomy. Suppurative pericarditis is treated the same as lung abscess plus surgical drainage (pericardial window)
Prognosis: For viral pericarditis, the prognosis is good, but viral myocarditis may be fatal. For TB pericarditis, the prognosis is good if treated before constrictive pericarditis/adhesions develop. Suppurative pericarditis is often fatal without early pericardial window/antibiotic therapy

IV Line and Pacemaker Infections

Subset	Usual Pathogens	Preferred IV Therapy	Alternate IV Therapy	IV-to-PO Switch
Central IV line infection (temporary) (Treat initially for MSSA; if later identified as MRSA, treat accordingly)	S. aureus (MSSA) Entero-bacteriaceae	Cefepime 2 gm (IV) q12h x 2 weeks after line removal **or** Meropenem 1 gm (IV) q8h x 2 weeks after line removal **or** Imipenem 1 gm (IV) q6h x 2 weeks after line removal	Ceftizoxime 2 gm (IV) q8h x 2 weeks after line removal **or** Cefotaxime 2 gm (IV) q6h x 2 weeks after line removal	Clindamycin 300 mg (PO) q8h x 2 weeks after line removal **plus** Levofloxacin 500 mg (PO) q24h x 2 weeks after line removal
	S. aureus (MRSA)	Linezolid 600 mg (IV) q12h x 2 weeks after line removal **or** Vancomycin 1 gm (IV) q12h x 2 weeks after line removal	Minocycline 100 mg (IV) q12h x 2 weeks after line removal **or** Quinupristin/ dalfopristin 7.5 mg/kg (IV) q8h x 2 weeks after line removal	Linezolid 600 mg (PO) q12h x 2 weeks after line removal **or** Minocycline 100 mg (PO) q12h x 2 weeks after line removal
Central IV line infection (semi-permanent); Hickman/ Broviac (Treat initially for S. aureus; if later identified as S. epidermidis, treat accordingly)	S. aureus (MSSA/MRSA)	Linezolid 600 mg (IV) q12h x 2 weeks after line removal **or** Vancomycin 1 gm (IV) q12h x 2 weeks after line removal	Minocycline 100 mg (IV) q12h x 2 weeks after line removal **or** Quinupristin/ dalfopristin 7.5 mg/kg (IV) q8h x 2 weeks after line removal	Linezolid 600 mg (PO) q12h x 2 weeks after line removal **or** Minocycline 100 mg (PO) q12h x 2 weeks after line removal
	S. epidermidis (MSSE/MRSE)	Linezolid 600 mg (IV) q12h x 2 weeks after line removal **or** Vancomycin 1 gm (IV) q12h x 2 weeks after line removal	Cefepime 2 gm (IV) q12h x 2 weeks after line removal **or** Quinupristin/ dalfopristin 7.5 mg/kg (IV) q8h x 2 weeks after line removal	Linezolid 600 mg (PO) q12h x 2 weeks after line removal **or combination therapy with** Clindamycin 300 mg (PO) q8h x 2 weeks after line removal **plus** Levofloxacin 500 mg (PO) q24h x 2 weeks after line removal

IV Line and Pacemaker Infections (cont'd)

Subset	Usual Pathogens	Preferred IV Therapy	Alternate IV Therapy	IV-to-PO Switch
Pacemaker wire/generator infection (Treat initially for S. aureus; if later identified as S. epidermidis, treat accordingly)	S. aureus (MSSA/MRSA)	Linezolid 600 mg (IV) q12h x 2 weeks after wire/generator removal* **or** Vancomycin 1 gm (IV) q12h x 2 weeks after wire/generator removal*	Minocycline 100 mg (IV) q12h x 2 weeks after wire/generator removal* **or** Quinupristin/ dalfopristin 7.5 mg/kg (IV) q8h x 2 weeks after wire/generator removal*	Linezolid 600 mg (PO) q12h x 2 weeks after wire/generator removal* **or** Minocycline 100 mg (PO) q12h x 2 weeks after wire/generator removal*
	S. epidermidis (MSSE/MRSE)	Linezolid 600 mg (IV) q12h x 2 weeks after wire/generator removal **or** Vancomycin 1 gm (IV) q12h x 2 weeks after wire/generator removal	Cefepime 2 gm (IV) q12h x 2 weeks after wire/generator removal **or** Quinupristin/ dalfopristin 7.5 mg/kg (IV) q8h x 2 weeks after wire/generator removal	Linezolid 600 mg (PO) q12h x 2 weeks after wire/generator removal **or combination therapy with** Clindamycin 300 mg (PO) q8h x 2 weeks after wire/generator removal **plus** Levofloxacin 500 mg (PO) q24h x 2 weeks after wire/generator removal
Septic thrombo- phlebitis (Treat initially for MSSA; if later identified as MRSA, treat accordingly)	S. aureus (MSSA)	Nafcillin 2 gm (IV) q4h x 2 weeks* **or** Meropenem 1 gm (IV) q8h x 2 weeks* **or** Imipenem 1 gm (IV) q6h x 2 weeks* **or** Linezolid 600 mg (IV) q12h x 2 weeks*	Ceftizoxime 2 gm (IV) q8h x 2 weeks* **or** Cefotaxime 2 gm (IV) q6h x 2 weeks* **or** Quinupristin/ dalfopristin 7.5 mg/kg (IV) q8h x 2 weeks*	Linezolid 600 mg (PO) q12h x 2 weeks* **or combination therapy** Clindamycin 300 mg (PO) q8h x 2 weeks* **plus** Levofloxacin 500 mg (PO) q24h x 2 weeks*

IV Line and Pacemaker Infections (cont'd)

Subset	Usual Pathogens	Preferred IV Therapy	Alternate IV Therapy	IV-to-PO Switch
Septic thrombo-phlebitis (cont'd)	S. aureus (MRSA)	Linezolid 600 mg (IV) q12h x 2 weeks* **or** Vancomycin 1 gm (IV) q12h x 2 weeks*	Minocycline 100 mg (IV) q12h x 2 weeks* **or** Quinupristin/ dalfopristin 7.5 mg/kg (IV) q8h x 2 weeks*	Linezolid 600 mg (PO) q12h x 2 weeks* **or** Minocycline 100 mg (PO) q12h x 2 weeks*

MSSA/MRSA = methicillin-sensitive/resistant S. aureus; MSSE/MRSE = methicillin-sensitive/resistant S. epidermidis. Duration of therapy represents total time IV or IV + PO. Most patients on IV therapy able to take PO meds should be switched to PO therapy after clinical improvement
* *Obtain teichoic acid antibody titers after 2 weeks. If titers are 1:4 or less, 2 weeks of therapy is sufficient. If titers are > 1:4, rule out endocarditis and complete 4-6 weeks of therapy*

Central IV Line Infection (Temporary)
Clinical Presentation: Temperature ≥ 102°F ± IV site erythema
Diagnostic Considerations: Diagnosis by semi-quantitative catheter tip culture with ≥ 15 colonies plus blood cultures with same pathogen. If no other explanation for fever and line has been in place ≥ 7 days, remove line and obtain semi-quantitative catheter tip culture. Suppurative thrombophlebitis presents with hectic/septic fevers and pus at IV site ± palpable venous cord
Pitfalls: Temperature ≥ 102° F with IV line infection, in contrast to phlebitis
Therapeutic Considerations: Line removal is usually curative, but antibiotic treatment is usually given for 2 weeks after line removal
Prognosis: Good if line is removed before endocarditis/metastatic spread

Central IV Line Infection (Semi-Permanent) Hickman/Broviac
Clinical Presentation: Fever ± IV site erythema
Diagnostic Considerations: Positive blood cultures plus gallium scan pickup on catheter is diagnostic
Pitfalls: Antibiotics will lower temperature, but patient will usually not be afebrile without line removal
Therapeutic Considerations: Lines usually need to be removed for cure. Rifampin 600 mg (PO) q24h may be added to IV/PO regimen if pathogen is S. aureus
Prognosis: Good with organisms of low virulence

Pacemaker Wire/Generator Infection
Clinical Presentation: Persistently positive blood cultures without endocarditis in a pacemaker patient
Diagnostic Considerations: Positive blood cultures with gallium scan pickup on wire/pacemaker generator is diagnostic. Differentiate wire from pacemaker pocket infection by chest CT/MRI
Pitfalls: Positive blood cultures are more common in wire infections than pocket infections. Blood cultures may be negative in both, but more so with pocket infections
Therapeutic Considerations: Wire alone may be replaced if infection does not involve pacemaker generator. Replace pacemaker generator if involved; wire if uninvolved can usually be left in place
Prognosis: Good if pacemaker wire/generator replaced before septic complications develop

Septic Thrombophlebitis
Clinical Presentation: Temperature ≥ 102°F with local erythema and signs of sepsis
Diagnostic Considerations: Palpable venous cord and pus at IV site when IV line is removed
Pitfalls: Suspect diagnosis if persistent bacteremia and no other source of infection in a patient with

a peripheral IV
Therapeutic Considerations: Remove IV catheter. Surgical venotomy is usually needed for cure
Prognosis: Good if removed early before septic complications develop

Vascular Graft Infections

Subset	Usual Pathogens	Preferred IV Therapy	Alternate IV Therapy	IV-to-PO Switch
AV graft/shunt infection (Treat initially for MSSA, etc.; if later identified as MRSA, treat accordingly)	S. aureus (MSSA) Enterococci Entero-bacteriaceae	Vancomycin 1 gm (IV) x 1 dose*[†] **plus** Gentamicin 240 mg (IV) x 1 dose*[†]	Meropenem 1 gm (IV) x 1 dose*[†]	Levofloxacin 500 mg (IV or PO) x 1 dose*[†]
	S. aureus (MRSA)	Linezolid 600 mg (IV) x 1 dose*[†]	Vancomycin 1 gm (IV) x 1 dose*[†]	Linezolid 600 mg (PO) x 1 dose*[†]
Aortic graft infection	S. aureus (MSSA) Entero-bacteriaceae	Cefepime 2 gm (IV) q12h[†] **or** Meropenem 1 gm (IV) q8h[†] **or** Imipenem 1 gm (IV) q6h[†]	Ceftizoxime 2 gm (IV) q8h[†] **or** Cefotaxime 2 gm (IV) q6h[†]	Clindamycin 300 mg (PO) q8h[†] **plus** Levofloxacin 500 mg (PO) q24h[†]

MSSA/MRSA = methicillin-sensitive/resistant S. aureus. Duration of therapy represents total time IV or IV + PO. Most patients on IV therapy able to take PO meds should be switched to PO therapy after clinical improvement
*   Follow with maintenance dosing for renal failure (CrCl < 10 mL/min) and type of dialysis (see Chapter 7)
†   Treat until graft is removed/replaced

AV Graft Infection
Clinical Presentation: Persistent fever/bacteremia without endocarditis in a patient with an AV graft on hemodialysis
Diagnostic Considerations: Diagnosis by persistently positive blood cultures and gallium scan pickup over infected AV graft. Gallium scan will detect deep AV graft infection not apparent on exam
Pitfalls: Antibiotics will lower temperature, but patient will usually not become afebrile without AV graft replacement
Therapeutic Considerations: Graft usually must be removed for cure. MRSA is a rare cause of AV graft infection; if present, treat with linezolid 600 mg (IV or PO) q12h until graft is removed/replaced
Prognosis: Good if new graft does not become infected at same site

Aortic Graft Infection
Clinical Presentation: Persistently positive blood cultures without endocarditis in a patient with an aortic graft
Diagnostic Considerations: Diagnosis by positive blood cultures plus gallium scan pickup over infected aortic graft or abdominal CT/MRI scan
Pitfalls: Infection typically occurs at anastomotic sites
Therapeutic Considerations: Graft must be removed for cure. Operate as soon as diagnosis is

confirmed (no value in waiting for surgery). MRSA is a rare cause of AV graft infection; if present, treat with linezolid 600 mg (IV or PO) q12h until graft is replaced

Prognosis: Good if infected graft is removed before septic complications develop

Empiric Therapy of GI Tract Infections

Esophagitis

Subset	Usual Pathogens	Preferred IV Therapy	Alternate IV Therapy	PO Therapy or IV-to-PO Switch
Fungal	Candida albicans	Fluconazole 200 mg (IV) x 1 dose, then 100 mg (IV) q24h x 2-3 weeks **or** Itraconazole 200 mg (IV) q12h x 2 days, then 200 mg (IV) q24h for total of 2-3 weeks	Amphotericin B 1 mg/kg (IV) q24h x 2-3 weeks **or** Caspofungin 70 mg (IV) x 1 dose, then 50 mg (IV) q24h x 2-3 weeks **or** Voriconazole 400 mg (IV) x 1 dose, then 200 mg (IV) q12h x 2-3 weeks	Itraconazole 200 mg (IV) q12h x 2 days, then oral solution 200 mg (PO) q24h for total of 2-3 weeks* **or** Fluconazole 200 mg (PO) x 1 dose, then 100 mg (PO) q24h x 2-3 weeks* **or** Voriconazole 400 mg (PO) x 1 dose, then 200 mg (PO) q12h x 2-3 weeks*
Viral	HSV-1	Acyclovir 5 mg/kg (IV) q8h x 2-3 weeks	Not applicable	Valacyclovir 500 mg (PO) q12h x 2-3 weeks **or** Famciclovir 500 mg (PO) q12h x 2-3 weeks
	CMV	Ganciclovir 5 mg/kg (IV) q12h x 2-3 weeks	Not applicable	Foscarnet 90 mg (PO) q12h x 2-3 weeks **or** Valganciclovir 900 mg (PO) q24h x 2-3 weeks

Duration of therapy represents total time IV, PO, or IV + PO. Most patients on IV therapy able to take PO meds should be switched to PO therapy soon after clinical improvement (usually ≤ 72 hours)
* Loading dose is not needed PO if given IV with the same drug

Clinical Presentation: Pain on swallowing
Diagnosis: Stain/culture for fungi/HSV/CMV on biopsy specimen

Fungal (Candida) Esophagitis
Diagnostic Considerations: Rarely if ever in normal hosts. Usually associated with Candida in mouth. If patient is not an alcoholic or diabetic and is not receiving antibiotic therapy, test for HIV

Pitfalls: Candida esophagitis may extend into stomach and perforate. Treat early
Therapeutic Considerations: In normal hosts, treat for 1 week after clinical resolution. HIV patients respond more slowly than normal hosts and may need treatment for 2-3 weeks after clinical resolution
Prognosis: Related to degree of immunosuppression

Viral Esophagitis

Diagnostic Considerations: Rarely in normal hosts. May occur in non-HIV immunosuppressed patients
Pitfalls: Viral and non-viral esophageal ulcers look similar; need biopsy for viral diagnosis
Therapeutic Considerations: In normal hosts, treat for 1 week after clinical resolution. HIV patients respond more slowly than normal hosts and may need treatment for 2-3 weeks after clinical resolution
Prognosis: Related to degree of immunosuppression

Peptic Ulcer Disease

Subset	Usual Pathogens	Preferred Therapy
Peptic ulcer disease	Helicobacter pylori	Omeprazole 20 mg (PO) q12h x 2 weeks **plus** Clarithromycin 500 mg (PO) q12h x 2 weeks **plus** Amoxicillin 1 gm (PO) q8h x 2 weeks

Clinical Presentation: Periodic mid/upper abdominal pain relieved by meals. No fever
Diagnostic Considerations: Diagnosis by positive urea breath test
Pitfalls: Confirm diagnosis before starting therapy
Therapeutic Considerations: Regimens containing metronidazole or doxycycline are less effective
Prognosis: Excellent

Gastric Perforation

Subset	Usual Pathogens	Preferred IV Therapy	Alternate IV Therapy	IV-to-PO Switch
Gastric perforation	Oral anaerobes	Cefazolin 1 gm (IV) q8h x 2 weeks	Any β-lactam (IV) x 2 weeks	Amoxicillin 1 gm (PO) q8h x 2 weeks **or** Cephalexin 500 mg (PO) q6h x 2 weeks **or** Levofloxacin 500 mg (PO) q24h x 2 weeks

Duration of therapy represents total time IV or IV + PO. Most patients on IV therapy able to take PO meds should be switched to PO therapy after clinical improvement

Clinical Presentation: Presents acutely with fever and peritonitis
Diagnostic Considerations: Obtain CT/MRI of abdomen to determine site of perforation
Pitfalls: No need to cover B. fragilis with perforation of stomach/small intestine
Therapeutic Considerations: Obtain surgical consult for possible repair
Prognosis: Good if repaired

Infectious Diarrhea/Typhoid (Enteric) Fever

Subset	Usual Pathogens	Preferred Therapy	Alternate Therapy
Acute watery diarrhea	E. coli Campylobacter Yersinia Salmonella Vibrio sp.	Levofloxacin 500 mg (IV or PO) q24h x 5 days	Doxycycline 100 mg (IV or PO) q12h x 5 days **or** TMP-SMX 1 DS tablet (PO) q12h x 5 days
Antibiotic-associated diarrhea/colitis (AAD/AAC)	Clostridium difficile	<u>AAD:</u> Vancomycin 125 mg (PO) q6h x 7-10 days <u>AAC:</u> Metronidazole 1 gm (IV) q24h or 500 mg (IV) q12h until cured	<u>AAD:</u> Metronidazole 250 mg (PO) q6h x 7-10 days <u>AAC:</u> Metronidazole 500 mg (PO) q12h until cured
Typhoid (enteric) fever	Salmonella typhi/non-typhi	Any quinolone (IV or PO) x 10-14 days **or** TMP-SMX 5 mg/kg (IV or PO) q6h x 10-14 days	Chloramphenicol 500 mg (IV or PO) q6h x 10-14 days **or** Any 3rd generation cephalosporin (IV or PO) x 10-14 days
Chronic watery diarrhea	Giardia lamblia*	Metronidazole 250 mg (PO) q8h x 5 days	Albendazole 400 mg (PO) q24h x 5 days **or** Quinacrine 100 mg (PO) q8h x 5 days
	Cryptosporidia*	No good treatment	Paromomycin 500-750 mg (PO) q8h until response **or** Azithromycin 600 mg (PO) q24h x 4 weeks
	Cyclospora*	TMP-SMX 1 DS tablet (PO) q12h x 2-4 weeks	No good treatment
Acute dysentery	E. histolytica	Metronidazole 750 mg (PO) q8h x 10 days **followed by either** Iodoquinol 650 mg (PO) q8h x 20 days **or** Paromomycin 500 mg (PO) q8h x 7 days	Tinidazole 1 gm (PO) q12h x 3 days
	Shigella	Levofloxacin 500 mg (IV or PO) q24h x 3 days	TMP-SMX 1 DS tablet (PO) q12h x 3 days **or** Azithromycin 500 mg (IV or PO) q24h x 3 days

Duration of therapy represents total time IV, PO, or IV + PO. Most patients on IV therapy able to take PO meds should be switched to PO therapy soon after clinical improvement (usually < 72 hours)
* May also present as acute watery diarrhea

Acute Watery Diarrhea

Clinical Presentation: Acute onset of watery diarrhea without blood/mucus

Diagnostic Considerations: Diagnosis by culture of organism from stool specimens

Pitfalls: Recommended antibiotics are active against most susceptible bacterial pathogens causing diarrhea, but not viruses/parasites. Concomitant transient lactase deficiency may prolong diarrhea if dairy products are taken during an infectious diarrhea

Therapeutic Considerations: Avoid norfloxacin and ciprofloxacin due to resistance potential. V. cholerae may be treated with a single dose of any oral quinolone or doxycycline

Prognosis: Excellent. Most recover with supportive treatment

Antibiotic-Associated Diarrhea/Colitis (Clostridium difficile)

Clinical Presentation: Watery diarrhea following exposure to patients with C. difficile diarrhea or recent cancer/antibiotic therapy. Clinically indistinguishable from other toxigenic community-acquired watery diarrheas. Most often associated with clindamycin or beta-lactams. Rarely due to quinolones, aminoglycosides, linezolid, doxycycline, TMP-SMX, carbapenems, vancomycin, piperacillin/tazobactam, cefoperazone, or cefepime

Diagnostic Considerations: Watery diarrhea with positive C. difficile toxin in stool specimen. Temperature is usually < 102°F. In patients receiving enteral feeds and antibiotics, diarrhea is much more likely due to enteral feeds than C. difficile

Pitfalls: In a patient with C. difficile diarrhea, C. difficile colitis is suggested by the presence of abdominal pain and temperature > 102° F; confirm diagnosis with CT/MRI of abdomen

Therapeutic Considerations: Oral vancomycin is more often effective than oral metronidazole. C. difficile diarrhea begins to improve and usually resolves by 5-7 days, although some patients require 10 days of therapy. Do not continue treating C. difficile toxin-negative diarrhea with vancomycin or metronidazole. For relapses/recurrences, treat with vancomycin 250 mg (PO) q6h x 10-14 days. For C. difficile colitis, treat until colitis resolves with metronidazole 1 gm (IV) q24h or 500 mg (IV) q12h or 500 mg (PO) q6-12h. IV vancomycin is *not* useful for C. difficile diarrhea/colitis

Pitfalls: C. difficile toxin may remain positive in stools for weeks following treatment; do not treat positive stool toxin unless patient has persistent diarrhea

Prognosis: Good with early treatment. Worse if treated late or patient has colitis. Prognosis with C. difficile colitis is related to severity of the colitis

Typhoid (Enteric) Fever (Salmonella typhi/non-typhi)

Clinical Presentation: High fevers (> 102°F) increasing in a stepwise fashion accompanied by relative bradycardia in a patient with watery diarrhea/constipation, headache, abdominal pain, cough/sore throat ± Rose spots

Diagnostic Considerations: Most community-acquired watery diarrheas are not accompanied by temperatures > 102°F and relative bradycardia. Diagnosis is confirmed by demonstrating Salmonella in blood, bone marrow, Rose spots, or stool cultures. Culture of bone marrow is the quickest/most reliable method of diagnosis. WBC count is usually low/low normal. Leukocytosis should suggest another diagnosis or bowel perforation, which may occur during 2nd week of typhoid fever

Pitfalls: Rose spots are few/difficult to see and not present in all cases. Typhoid fever usually presents with constipation, not diarrhea. Suspect another diagnosis in the absence of headache

Therapeutic Considerations: 2nd generation cephalosporins, aztreonam, and aminoglycosides are ineffective. Since Salmonella strains causing enteric fever are intracellular pathogens, treat for a full 2 weeks to maximize cure rates/minimize relapses. Treat relapses with the suggested antibiotics x 2-3 weeks. Salmonella excretion into feces usually persists < 3 months. Persistent excretion > 3 months suggests a carrier state—rule out hepatobiliary/urinary calculi

Prognosis: Good if treated early. Poor with late treatment/bowel perforation

Chronic Watery Diarrhea

Clinical Presentation: Watery diarrhea without blood/mucus lasting > 1 month

Diagnostic Considerations: Diagnosis by demonstrating organisms/cysts in stool specimens. Multiple fresh daily stool samples often needed for diagnosis

Pitfalls: Concomitant transient lactase deficiency may prolong diarrhea if dairy products are taken during an infectious diarrhea

Therapeutic Considerations: Cryptosporidia and Cyclospora are being recognized increasingly in acute/chronic diarrhea in normal hosts

Prognosis: Excellent in well-nourished patients. Untreated patients may develop malabsorption

Giardia lamblia

Clinical Presentation: Acute/subacute onset of diarrhea, abdominal cramps, bloating, flatulence. Incubation period 1-2 weeks. Malabsorption may occur in chronic cases. No eosinophilia

Diagnostic Considerations: Diagnosis by demonstrating trophozoites or cysts in stool/antigen detection assay. If stool exam and antigen test are negative and Giardiasis is suspected, perform "string test"/duodenal aspirate and biopsy

Pitfalls: Eggs intermittently excreted into stool. Usually need multiple stool samples for diagnosis. Often accompanied by transient lactose intolerance

Therapeutic Considerations: Diarrhea may be prolonged if milk (lactose-containing) products are ingested after treatment/cure

Prognosis: Related to severity of malabsorption and health of host

Cryptosporidia

Clinical Presentation: Acute/subacute onset of diarrhea. Usually occurs in HIV/AIDS patients with CD_4 counts < 200. Biliary cryptosporidiosis is seen only in HIV; may present as acalculous cholecystitis or sclerosing cholangitis with RUQ pain, fever, ↑ alkaline phosphatase, but bilirubin is normal

Diagnostic Considerations: Diagnosis by demonstrating organism in stool/intestinal biopsy specimen. Cholera-like illness in normal hosts. Chronic watery diarrhea in compromised hosts

Pitfalls: Smaller than Cyclospora. Oocyst walls are smooth (not wrinkled) on acid fast staining

Prognosis: Related to adequacy of fluid replacement/underlying health of host

Cyclospora

Clinical Presentation: Acute/subacute onset of diarrhea. Incubation period 1-14 days

Diagnostic Considerations: Diagnosis by demonstrating organism in stool/intestinal biopsy specimen. Clinically indistinguishable from cryptosporidial diarrhea (intermittent watery diarrhea without blood or mucus). Fatigue/weight loss common

Pitfalls: Oocysts only form seen in stool and are best identified with modified Kinyoun acid fast staining. Acid fast fat globules stain pink with acid fast staining. "Wrinkled wall" oocysts are characteristic of Cyclospora, not Cryptosporidia. Oocysts are twice the size of similar appearing Cryptosporidia (~ 10 μm vs. 5 μm)

Prognosis: Related to adequacy of fluid replacement/underlying health of host

Acute Dysentery

Entamoeba histolytica

Clinical Presentation: Acute/subacute onset of bloody diarrhea/mucus. Fecal WBC/RBCs due to mucosal invasion. E. histolytica may also cause chronic diarrhea. Colonic ulcers secondary to E. histolytica are round and may form "collar stud" abscesses

Diagnostic Considerations: Diagnosis by demonstrating organism/trophozoites in stool/intestinal biopsy specimen. Serology is negative with amebic dysentery, but positive with extra-intestinal forms. Test to separate E. histolytica from non-pathogenic E. dispar cyst passers. On sigmoidoscopy, ulcers due to E. histolytica are round with normal mucosa in between, and may form "collar stud" abscesses. In contrast, ulcers due to Shigella are linear and serpiginous without normal intervening mucosa. Bloody dysentery is more subacute with E. histolytica compared to Shigella

Pitfalls: Intestinal perforation/abscess may complicate amebic colitis. Rule out infectious causes of

bloody diarrhea with mucus before diagnosing/treating inflammatory bowel disease (IBD). Obtain multiple stool cultures for bacterial pathogens/parasites. Do not confuse E. histolytica in stool specimens with E. hartmanni, a non-pathogen protozoa similar in appearance but smaller in size
Therapeutic Considerations: E. histolytica cyst passers should be treated, but metronidazole is ineffective against cysts. Use paromomycin 500 mg (PO) q8h x 7 days for asymptomatic cysts. Recommended antibiotics treat both luminal and hepatic E. histolytica
Prognosis: Good if treated early. Related to severity of dysentery/ulcers/extra-intestinal amebiasis

Shigella
Clinical Presentation: Acute onset of bloody diarrhea/mucus
Diagnostic Considerations: Diagnosis by demonstrating organism in stool specimens. Shigella ulcers in colon are linear, serpiginous, and rarely lead to perforation
Therapeutic Considerations: Shigella dysentery is more acute/fulminating than amebic dysentery. Shigella has no carrier state, unlike Entamoeba
Prognosis: Good if treated early. Severity of illness related to Shigella species: S. dysenteriae (most severe) > S. flexneri > S. boydii/S. sonnei (mildest)

Cholecystitis

Subset	Usual Pathogens	Preferred IV Therapy	Alternate IV Therapy	PO Therapy or IV-to-PO Switch
Normal host	E. coli Klebsiella Enterococci	Levofloxacin 500 mg (IV) q24h* **or** Piperacillin 4 gm (IV) q8h*	Cefazolin 1 gm (IV) q8h* **plus** Ampicillin 1 gm (IV) q4h*	Levofloxacin 500 mg (PO) q24h*
Emphy-sematous cholecystitis†	Clostridium perfringens	Meropenem 1 gm (IV) q8h x 1 week after cholecystectomy **or** Imipenem 1 gm (IV) q6h x 1 week after cholecystectomy **or** Ertapenem 1 gm (IV) q24h x 1 week after cholecystectomy	Piperacillin/ tazobactam 4.5 gm (IV) q8h x 1 week after cholecystectomy	Clindamycin 300 mg (PO) q8h x 1 week after cholecystectomy

Duration of therapy represents total time IV, PO, or IV + PO. Most patients on IV therapy able to take PO meds should be switched to PO therapy after clinical improvement
† *Treat only IV or IV-to-PO switch*
* *If no cholecystectomy, treat x 1-2 weeks. If cholecystectomy is peformed, treat x 1 week post-operatively*

Cholecystitis in Normal Hosts
Clinical Presentation: RUQ pain, fever usually ≤ 102°F, positive Murphy's sign, no percussion tenderness over right lower ribs
Diagnostic Considerations: Diagnosis by RUQ ultrasound/positive HIDA scan
Pitfalls: No need to cover B. fragilis
Therapeutic Considerations: Obtain surgical consult for possible cholecystectomy

Prognosis: Related to cardiopulmonary status

Emphysematous Cholecystitis
Clinical Presentation: Clinically presents as cholecystitis. Usually seen in diabetics
Diagnostic Considerations: RUQ/gallbladder gas on flat plate of abdomen
Pitfalls: Requires immediate cholecystectomy
Therapeutic Considerations: Usually a difficult/prolonged post-op course
Prognosis: Related to speed of gallbladder removal

Cholangitis

Subset	Usual Pathogens	Preferred IV Therapy	Alternate IV Therapy	IV-to-PO Switch
Normal host	E. coli Klebsiella Enterococci	Cefoperazone 2 gm (IV) q12h x 2 weeks **or** Meropenem 1 gm (IV) q8h x 2 weeks **or** Imipenem 1 gm (IV) q6h x 2 weeks	Levofloxacin 500 mg (IV) q24h x 2 weeks **or** Piperacillin 4 gm (IV) q8h x 2 weeks	Levofloxacin 500 mg (PO) q24h x 2 weeks

Duration of therapy represents total time IV or IV + PO. Most patients on IV therapy able to take PO meds should be switched to PO therapy after clinical improvement

Clinical Presentation: RUQ pain, fever > 102°F, positive Murphy's sign, percussion tenderness over right lower ribs
Diagnostic Considerations: Obstructed common bile duct on ultrasound/CT/MRI of abdomen
Pitfalls: Charcot's triad (fever, RUQ pain, jaundice) is present in only 50%
Therapeutic Considerations: Obtain surgical consult to relieve obstruction
Prognosis: Related to speed of surgical relief of obstruction

Gallbladder Wall Abscess/Perforation

Subset	Usual Pathogens	Preferred IV Therapy	Alternate IV Therapy	IV-to-PO Switch
Gallbladder wall abscess/ perforation	E. coli Klebsiella Enterococci	Cefoperazone 2 gm (IV) q12h x 2 weeks **or** Meropenem 1 gm (IV) q8h x 2 weeks **or** Imipenem 1 gm (IV) q6h x 2 weeks	Levofloxacin 500 mg (IV) q24h x 2 weeks **or** Piperacillin 4 gm (IV) q8h x 2 weeks	Levofloxacin 500 mg (PO) q24h x 2 weeks

Duration of therapy represents total time IV or IV + PO. Most patients on IV therapy able to take PO meds should be switched to PO therapy after clinical improvement

Clinical Presentation: RUQ pain, fever ≤ 102°F, positive Murphy's sign, no percussion tenderness over right lower ribs
Diagnostic Considerations: Diagnosis by CT/MRI of abdomen. Bile peritonitis is common
Pitfalls: Bacterial peritonitis may be present
Therapeutic Considerations: Obtain surgical consult for possible gallbladder removal. Usually a difficult and prolonged post-op course
Prognosis: Related to removal of gallbladder/repair of perforation

Acute Pancreatitis

Subset	Usual Pathogens	Preferred IV Therapy	Alternate IV Therapy	IV-to-PO Switch
Edematous pancreatitis	None	Not applicable	Not applicable	Not applicable
Hemorrhagic/ necrotizing pancreatitis	Entero- bacteriaceae B. fragilis	Meropenem 1 gm (IV) q8h x 2 weeks **or** Imipenem 1 gm (IV) q6h x 2 weeks **or** Ertapenem 1 gm (IV) q24h x 2 weeks	Piperacillin/ tazobactam 4.5 gm (IV) q8h x 2 weeks **or** Ampicillin/sulbactam 3 gm (IV) q6h x 2 weeks	Clindamycin 300 mg (PO) q8h x 2 weeks **plus** Levofloxacin 500 mg (PO) q24h x 2 weeks

Duration of therapy represents total time IV or IV + PO. Most patients on IV therapy able to take PO meds should be switched to PO therapy after clinical improvement

Edematous Pancreatitis
Clinical Presentation: Sharp abdominal pain with fever ≤ 102°F ± hypotension
Diagnostic Considerations: Diagnosis by elevated serum amylase and lipase levels with normal methemalbumin levels. May be drug-induced (e.g., steroids)
Pitfalls: Amylase elevation alone is not diagnostic of acute pancreatitis
Therapeutic Considerations: NG tube is not needed. Aggressively replace fluids
Prognosis: Good with adequate fluid replacement

Hemorrhagic/Necrotizing Pancreatitis
Clinical Presentation: Sharp abdominal pain with fever ≤ 102° F ± hypotension. Grey-Turner/Cullen's sign present in some
Diagnostic Considerations: Mildly elevated serum amylase and lipase levels with high methemalbumin levels
Pitfalls: With elevated lipase, amylase level is inversely related to severity of disease
Therapeutic Considerations: Obtain surgical consult for possible peritoneal lavage as adjunct to antibiotics. Serum albumin/dextran are preferred volume expanders
Prognosis: Poor with hypocalcemia or shock

Pancreatic Abscess

Subset	Usual Pathogens	Preferred IV Therapy	Alternate IV Therapy	IV-to-PO Switch
Pancreatic abscess	Entero-bacteriaceae B. fragilis	Meropenem 1 gm (IV) q8h x 2 weeks **or** Imipenem 1 gm (IV) q6h x 2 weeks **or** Ertapenem 1 gm (IV) q24h x 2 weeks	Piperacillin/ tazobactam 4.5 gm (IV) q8h x 2 weeks **or** Ampicillin/sulbactam 3 gm (IV) q6h x 2 weeks	Clindamycin 300 mg (PO) q8h x 2 weeks **plus** Levofloxacin 500 mg (PO) q24h x 2 weeks

Duration of therapy represents total time IV or IV + PO. Most patients on IV therapy able to take PO meds should be switched to PO therapy after clinical improvement

Clinical Presentation: Follows acute pancreatitis or develops in a pancreatic pseudocyst. Fevers usually ≥ 102°F
Diagnostic Considerations: CT/MRI of abdomen demonstrates pancreatic abscess
Pitfalls: Peritoneal signs are typically absent
Prognosis: Related to size/extent of abscess and adequacy of drainage

Liver Abscess

Subset	Usual Pathogens	Preferred IV Therapy	Alternate IV Therapy	PO Therapy or IV-to-PO Switch
Liver abscess	Entero-bacteriaceae Enterococci B. fragilis	Meropenem 1 gm (IV) q8h* **or** Imipenem 1 gm (IV) q6h* **or** Ertapenem 1 gm (IV) q24h* **or** Piperacillin/ tazobactam 4.5 gm (IV) q8h*	Levofloxacin 500 mg (IV) q24h* **plus either** Metronidazole 1 gm (IV) q24h* **or** Clindamycin 600 mg (IV) q8h*	Levofloxacin 500 mg (PO) q 24h* **plus either** Clindamycin 300 mg (PO) q8h* **or** Metronidazole 500 mg (PO) q12h*
	E. histolytica	See p. 173		

Duration of therapy represents total time IV, PO, or IV + PO. Most patients on IV therapy able to take PO meds should be switched to PO therapy after clinical improvement
* Treat until abscess(es) are no longer present or stop decreasing in size on CT scan

Clinical Presentation: Fever, RUQ tenderness, negative Murphy's sign, and negative right lower rib percussion tenderness
Diagnostic Considerations: Diagnosis by CT/MRI scan of liver and aspiration of abscess. CT shows multiple lesions in liver. Source is usually either the colon (diverticulitis or diverticular abscess with portal pyemia) or retrograde infection from the gallbladder (cholecystitis or gallbladder wall abscess)

Pitfalls: Bacterial abscesses are usually multiple and involve multiple lobes of liver; amebic abscesses are usually solitary and involve the right lobe of liver
Therapeutic Considerations: Liver laceration/trauma usually requires ~ 2 weeks of antibiotics
Prognosis: Good if treated early

Hepatosplenic Candidiasis

Subset	Usual Pathogens	Preferred IV Therapy	Alternate IV Therapy	IV-to-PO Switch
Hepato-splenic candidiasis	Candida albicans	Fluconazole 800 mg (IV) x 1 dose, then 400 mg (IV) q24h x 2-4 weeks **or** Caspofungin 70 mg (IV) x 1 dose, then 50 mg (IV) q24h x 2-4 weeks **or** Voriconazole 400 mg (IV) x 1 dose, then 200 mg (IV) q12h x 2-4 weeks	Amphotericin B 1 mg/kg (IV) q24h x 2-4 weeks **or** Itraconazole 200 mg (IV) q12h x 2 days, then 200 mg (IV) q24h x 2-4 weeks	Fluconazole 800 mg (PO) x 1 dose, then 400 mg (PO) q24h x 2-4 weeks* **or** Voriconazole 400 mg (PO) x 1 dose, then 200 mg (PO) q12h x 2-4 weeks* **or** Itraconazole 200 mg (PO) q12h x 2 days, then 200 mg (PO) q24h x 2-4 weeks*

Duration of therapy represents total time IV or IV + PO. Most patients on IV therapy able to take PO meds should be switched to PO therapy after clinical improvement
* Loading dose is not needed PO if given IV with the same drug

Clinical Presentation: New high spiking fevers with RUQ/LUQ pain after 2 weeks in a patient with afebrile leukopenia
Diagnostic Considerations: Diagnosis by abdominal CT/MRI showing mass lesions in liver/spleen
Pitfalls: Do not overlook RUQ tenderness and elevated alkaline phosphatase in leukopenic cancer patients as a clue to the diagnosis
Therapeutic Considerations: Treat until liver/spleen lesions resolve. Should be viewed as a form of disseminated disease
Prognosis: Related to degree/duration of leukopenia

Viral Hepatitis

Subset	Usual Pathogens	IV Therapy	PO/SQ Therapy
Acute	HAV, HBV, HCV, HDV, HEV, HFV	Not applicable	Not applicable
Chronic	HBV	Not applicable	Interferon alfa-2b 5 mu (SQ) q24h x 16 weeks **or** Lamivudine 100 mg (PO) q24h x 52 weeks **or** Famciclovir 500 mg (PO) q8h x 52 weeks
	HCV	Not applicable	Ribavirin 800-1400 mg (PO) q24h x 48 weeks *plus* pegylated interferon alfa-2b (Peg-Intron) 1.5 mcg/kg per week (SQ) x 48 weeks, using weight-based dosing:

	PEG Interferon alfa-2b		
Weight lb (kg)	Vial Size (mcg/mL)	Volume Used (mL)	Ribavirin Dose (mg)
<88 (<40)	100	0.5	800
88-111 (40-50) 112-141 (51-64)	160	0.4 0.5	800
142-166 (65-75) 167-187 (76-85)	240	0.4 0.5	1000
188-231 (86-105) >231 (>105)	300	0.5	1200 1400

or
Ribavirin 1000-1200 mg (PO) q24h x 48 weeks *plus* pegylated interferon alfa-2a (Pegasys) 180 mcg/week (SQ) x 48 weeks

Acute Viral Hepatitis
Clinical Presentation: Anorexia, malaise, RUQ tenderness, temperature ≤ 102°F ± jaundice
Diagnostic Considerations: Diagnosis by elevated IgM serology with markedly elevated serum transaminases (SGOT ≥ 1000). Serum alkaline phosphatase is normal/mildly elevated. Percussion tenderness over right lower ribs distinguishes liver from gallbladder problem
Pitfalls: In patients without jaundice (anicteric hepatitis), rule out other hepatitic viruses (EBV, CMV)
Therapeutic Considerations: Patients feel better after temperature falls/jaundice appears
Prognosis: Excellent for hepatitis A (does not progress to chronic active hepatitis). Hepatitis B and C may progress to chronic hepatitis/cirrhosis. Serum transaminases are not a good predictor/indicator of liver injury in hepatitis C

Chronic Viral Hepatitis
Clinical Presentation: Persistently elevated serum transaminases
Diagnostic Considerations: Liver biopsy is used to diagnose chronic viral hepatitis, and to differentiate chronic persistent hepatitis (CPH) from chronic active hepatitis (CAH). Hepatitis B is diagnosed by serum HBV DNA or PCR. Hepatitis C is diagnosed by serum HCV RNA levels
Pitfalls: Do not confuse viral hepatitis with lupoid/autoimmune hepatitis, which may present in similar fashion but with elevated ANAs. With HCV, rule out co-infection with HIV
Prognosis: CPH has a good prognosis. CAH has a worse prognosis and may progress to cirrhosis

Intraabdominal or Pelvic Peritonitis/Abscess

Subset	Usual Pathogens	Preferred IV Therapy	Alternate IV Therapy	PO Therapy or IV-to-PO Switch
Mild or moderate peritonitis (e.g, colitis, appendicitis, diverticulitis, septic pelvic thrombo-phlebitis[†])	Entero-bacteriaceae B. fragilis	Ceftizoxime 2 gm (IV) q8h x 2 weeks **or** Cefoxitin 2 gm (IV) q6h x 2 weeks	Moxifloxacin 400 mg (IV) q24h x 2 weeks **or** Ampicillin/sulbactam 1.5 gm (IV) q6h x 2 weeks	Moxifloxacin 400 mg (PO) q24h x 2 weeks **or combination therapy with** Levofloxacin 500 mg (PO) q24h x 2 weeks **plus** Clindamycin 300 mg (PO) q8h x 2 weeks
Severe peritonitis[‡] (e.g, colitis, appendicitis, diverticulitis, septic pelvic thrombo-phlebitis[†])	Entero-bacteriaceae B. fragilis	Meropenem 1 gm (IV) q8h x 2 weeks **or** Imipenem 1 gm (IV) q6h x 2 weeks **or** Ertapenem 1 gm (IV) q24h x 2 weeks **or** Piperacillin/ tazobactam 4.5 gm (IV) q8h x 2 weeks	Levofloxacin 500 mg (IV) q24h x 2 weeks **plus either** Clindamycin 600 mg (IV) q8h x 2 weeks **or** Metronidazole 1 gm (IV) q24h x 2 weeks	Levofloxacin 500 mg (PO) q24h x 2 weeks **plus either** Clindamycin 300 mg (PO) q8h x 2 weeks **or** Metronidazole 500 mg (PO) q12h x 2 weeks
Spontaneous bacterial peritonitis (SBP)[‡]	Entero-bacteriaceae	Levofloxacin 500 mg (IV) q24h x 2 weeks **or** Ceftriaxone 2 gm (IV) q24h x 2 weeks	Cefepime 2 gm (IV) q12h x 2 weeks	Levofloxacin 500 mg (PO) q24h x 2 weeks
Chronic non-bacterial (TB) peritonitis	M. tuberculosis	Not applicable		Treat the same as pulmonary TB (p. 44)
CAPD-associated peritonitis[‡]	S. epidermidis S. aureus Entero-bacteriaceae Non-fermentative gram (–) aerobic bacilli	<u>Before culture results</u> Vancomycin 1 gm (IV) loading dose* **plus** Gentamicin 5 mg/kg or 240 mg (IV) loading dose*	<u>After culture results</u> <u>*MSSA/Enterobacteriaceae*</u> Cefotaxime 2 gm (IV)* *or* ceftizoxime 2 gm (IV)* *or* cefepime 2 gm (IV)* *or* aztreonam 2 gm (IV)* <u>*MRSA*</u> Vancomycin (IV load given before culture results)* *or* linezolid 600 mg (IV or PO)*	

MSSA/MRSA = methicillin-sensitive/resistant S. aureus. Duration of therapy represents total time IV, PO, or IV + PO. Most patients on IV therapy able to take PO meds should be switched to PO therapy after clinical improvement

‡   Treat only IV or IV-to-PO switch

†   In addition to antibiotics, give heparin to maintain PTT ~ 2 times control x 7-14 days

*   Follow with maintenance dosing x 2 weeks after culture results are available. For maintenance dosing, use renal failure (CrCl < 10 mL/min) and post-peritoneal dialysis dosing (Chapter 7)

Intraabdominal or Pelvic Peritonitis/Abscess
(Colitis/Appendicitis/Diverticulitis/Septic Pelvic Thrombophlebitis)

Clinical Presentation: Spiking fevers with acute abdominal pain and peritoneal signs. In diverticulitis, the pain is localized over the involved segment of colon. Appendicitis ± perforation presents as RLQ pain/rebound tenderness or mass. Peri-diverticular abscess presents the same as intraabdominal/pelvic abscess, most commonly in the LLQ. Septic pelvic thrombophlebitis (SPT) presents as high spiking fevers unresponsive to antibiotic therapy following delivery/pelvic surgery

Diagnostic Considerations: Diagnosis by CT/MRI scan of abdomen/pelvis

Pitfalls: Tympany over liver suggests abdominal/visceral perforation. Pelvic peritonitis/abscess presents the same as intraabdominal abscess/peritonitis, but peritoneal signs are often absent

Therapeutic Considerations: Patients with ischemic/inflammatory colitis should be treated the same as peritonitis, depending on severity. Obtain surgical consult for repair/lavage or abscess drainage. In SPT, fever rapidly falls when heparin is added to antibiotics

Prognosis: Related to degree/duration of peritoneal spillage and rapidity/completeness of lavage. Prognosis for SPT is good if treated early and clots remain limited to pelvic veins

Spontaneous Bacterial Peritonitis (SBP)

Clinical Presentation: Acute or subacute onset of fever ± abdominal pain

Diagnostic Considerations: Diagnosis by positive blood cultures of SBP pathogens. For patients with abdominal pain, ascites, and a negative CT/MRI, paracentesis ascitic fluid with > 500 WBCs and > 100 PMNs predicts a positive ascitic fluid culture and is diagnostic of SBP. Some degree of splenic dysfunction usually exists, predisposing to infection with encapsulated organisms

Pitfalls: Do not overlook GI source of peritonitis (e.g, appendicitis, diverticulitis); obtain CT/MRI

Therapeutic Considerations: B. fragilis/anaerobes are not common pathogens in SBP, and B. fragilis coverage is unnecessary

Prognosis: Related to degree of hepatic/splenic dysfunction

Chronic Nonbacterial (TB) Peritonitis (Mycobacterium tuberculosis)

Clinical Presentation: Abdominal pain with fevers, weight loss, ascites over 1-3 months

Diagnostic Considerations: "Doughy consistency" on abdominal palpation. Diagnosis by AFB on peritoneal biopsy/culture

Pitfalls: Chest x-ray is normal in ~ 70%. Increased incidence in alcoholic cirrhosis

Therapeutic Considerations: Treated the same as pulmonary TB

Prognosis: Good if treated early

CAPD-Associated Peritonitis

Clinical Presentation: Abdominal pain + fever in a CAPD patient

Diagnostic Considerations: Diagnosis by gram stain/culture and ↑ WBC count in peritoneal fluid

Pitfalls: Fever is often absent

Therapeutic Considerations: Treat with systemic antibiotics, not with antibiotics into dialysate

Prognosis: Good with early therapy and removal of peritoneal catheter

Empiric Therapy of Genitourinary Tract Infections

Dysuria-Pyuria Syndrome (Acute Urethral Syndrome)

Subset	Usual Pathogens	IV Therapy	PO Therapy
Acute urethral syndrome	S. saprophyticus C. trachomatis E. coli (low concentration)	Not applicable	Doxycycline 100 mg (PO) q12h x 10 days **or** Levofloxacin 500 mg (PO) q24h x 7days

Clinical Presentation: Dysuria, frequency, urgency, lower abdominal discomfort, fevers < 102°F
Diagnostic Considerations: Diagnosis by symptoms of cystitis with pyuria and no growth or low concentration of E. coli ($\leq 10^3$ colonies/mL) by urine culture. Clue to S. saprophyticus is alkaline urinary pH and RBCs in urine
Pitfalls: Resembles "culture negative" cystitis
Therapeutic Considerations: S. saprophyticus is susceptible to most antibiotics used to treat UTIs
Prognosis: Excellent

Cystitis

Subset	Usual Pathogens	IV Therapy	PO Therapy
Bacterial	Enterobacteriaceae E. faecalis S. saprophyticus	Not applicable	Amoxicillin 1 gm (PO) x 1 dose **or** TMP-SMX 1 SS tablet (PO) x 1 dose
Fungal	Candida	Not applicable	Fluconazole 100 mg (PO) q24h x 7 days Alternate Itraconazole 100 mg (PO) q24h x 7 days **or** Voriconazole 200 mg (PO) q12h x 7 days

Bacterial Cystitis
Clinical Presentation: Dysuria, frequency, urgency, lower abdominal discomfort, fevers < 102°F
Diagnostic Considerations: Pyuria plus bacteriuria
Pitfalls: Single dose treatment is curative in acute uncomplicated cystitis in normal hosts. Compromised hosts (chronic steroids, diabetes, SLE, cirrhosis, multiple myeloma) become bacteremic/uroseptic easily; normal hosts do not develop urosepsis without instrumentation, stones, or anatomical abnormalities. For complicated hosts, treat with a quinolone or TMP-SMX x 1-2 weeks
Therapeutic Considerations: Pyridium 200 mg (PO) q8h after meals x 24-48h is useful to decrease dysuria (inform patients urine will turn orange)
Prognosis: Excellent in normal hosts

Candidal Cystitis
Diagnostic Considerations: Marked pyuria, urine nitrate negative ± RBCs. Speciate if not C. albicans
Pitfalls: Lack of response suggests non-C. albicans species or a "fungus ball" in renal collecting system
Therapeutic Considerations: If fluconazole fails, use itraconazole or voriconazole
Prognosis: Patients with impaired host defenses, abnormal collecting systems, cysts, renal disease or stones are prone to recurrent UTIs/urosepsis

Catheter-Associated Bacteriuria (CAB)

Subset	Usual Pathogens	IV Therapy	PO Therapy
Catheter-associated bacteriuria	E. coli E. faecalis	Not applicable	Nitrofurantoin 100 mg (PO) q12h x 5 days **or** Amoxicillin 500 mg (PO) q8h x 5 days
	E. faecium (VRE)	Not applicable	Nitrofurantoin 100 mg (PO) q12h x 5 days

Clinical Presentation: Indwelling urinary (Foley) catheter with bacteriuria and pyuria; no symptoms
Diagnostic Considerations: Pyuria plus bacteriuria. Usually afebrile or temperature < 101°F
Pitfalls: 95% of CAB represents colonization, not infection
Therapeutic Considerations: Compromised hosts (diabetes, SLE, chronic steroids, multiple myeloma, cirrhosis) require therapy for duration of catheterization
Prognosis: Excellent in normal hosts

Epididymitis

Subset	Usual Pathogens	Preferred IV Therapy	Alternate IV Therapy	PO Therapy or IV-to-PO Switch
Acute *Young males*	C. trachomatis	Doxycycline 200 mg (IV) q12h x 3 days, then 100 mg (IV) q12h x 4 days	Levofloxacin 500 mg (IV) q24h x 7 days	Doxycycline 200 mg (PO) q12h x 3 days, then 100 mg (PO) q12h x 4 days* **or** Azithromycin 1 gm (PO) x 1 dose **or** Levofloxacin 500 mg (PO) q24h x 7 days
Elderly males	P. aeruginosa	Cefepime 2 gm (IV) q8h x 10 days **or** Piperacillin 4 gm (IV) q8h x 10 days	Ciprofloxacin 400 mg (IV) q12h x 10 days	Ciprofloxacin 750 mg (PO) q12h x 10 days
Chronic	M. tuberculosis B. dermatiditis	Treat the same as pulmonary TB (p. 44) or pulmonary blastomycosis (p. 168)		

Duration of therapy represents total time IV, PO, or IV + PO. Most patients on IV therapy able to take PO meds should be switched to PO therapy soon after clinical improvement (usually < 72 hours)
* Loading dose is not needed PO if given IV with the same drug

Acute Epididymitis (Chlamydia trachomatis/Pseudomonas aeruginosa)
Clinical Presentation: Acute unilateral testicular pain ± fever
Diagnostic Considerations: Ultrasound to rule out torsion or tumor
Pitfalls: Rule out fever by absence of fever and ultrasound
Therapeutic Considerations: Young males respond to treatment slowly over 1 week. Elderly males respond to anti-Pseudomonal therapy within 72 hours
Prognosis: Excellent in young males. Related to health of host in elderly

Chronic Epididymitis (Mycobacterium tuberculosis/ Blastomyces dermatiditis)
Clinical Presentation: Chronic epididymoorchitis with epididymal nodules

Diagnostic Considerations: Diagnosis by AFB on biopsy/culture of epididymus. TB epididymitis is always associated with renal TB. Blastomyces epididymitis is a manifestation of systemic infection
Pitfalls: Vasculitis (e.g., polyarteritis nodosum) and lymphomas may present the same way
Therapeutic Considerations: Treated the same as pulmonary TB/blastomycosis
Prognosis: Good

Pyelonephritis/Renal TB

Subset	Usual Pathogens	Preferred IV Therapy	Alternate IV Therapy	PO Therapy or IV-to-PO Switch
Acute bacterial (Treat initially based on urine gram stain; see therapeutic considerations, p. 77)	Entero-bacteriaceae	Levofloxacin 500 mg (IV) q24h x 4 weeks **or** Ceftriaxone 1 gm (IV) q24h x 4 weeks	Aztreonam 2 gm (IV) q8h x 4 weeks **or** Gentamicin 240 mg (IV) q24h x 4 weeks	Levofloxacin 500 mg (PO) q24h x 4 weeks **or** Amoxicillin 1 gm (PO) q8h x 4 weeks
	Enterococcus faecalis	Ampicillin 1 gm (IV) q4h x 4 weeks **or** Linezolid 600 mg (IV) q12h x 4 weeks	Levofloxacin 500 mg (IV) q24h x 4 weeks	Amoxicillin 1 gm (PO) q8h x 4 weeks **or** Linezolid 600 mg (PO) q12h x 4 weeks **or** Levofloxacin 500 mg (PO) q24h x 4 weeks
	Enterococcus faecium (VRE)	Linezolid 600 mg (IV) q12h x 4 weeks **or** Doxycycline 200 mg (IV) q12h x 3 days, then 100 mg (IV) q12h x 4 weeks	Quinupristin/dalfopristin 7.5 mg/kg (IV) q8h x 4 weeks	Linezolid 600 mg (PO) q12h x 4 weeks **or** Doxycycline 200 mg (PO) q12h x 3 days, then 100 mg (PO) q12h x 4 weeks*
Chronic bacterial	Entero-bacteriaceae	<u>IV Therapy</u> Not applicable	<u>PO Therapy</u> Levofloxacin 500 mg (PO) q24h x 4-6 weeks **or** TMP-SMX 1 DS tab (PO) q12h x 4-6 weeks **or** Doxycycline 200 mg (PO) q12h x 3 days, then 100 mg (PO) q12h x 4-6 weeks total	
Renal TB	M. tuberculosis	<u>IV Therapy</u> Not applicable	Treated the same as pulmonary TB (p. 44)	

VRE = vancomycin-resistant enterococci. Duration of therapy represents total time IV, PO, or IV + PO. Most patients on IV therapy able to take PO meds should be switched to PO therapy after clinical improvement (usually < 72 hours)
* Loading dose is not needed PO if given IV with the same drug

Acute Bacterial Pyelonephritis (Enterobacteriaceae, E. faecalis/E. faecium)
Clinical Presentation: Unilateral CVA tenderness with fevers ≥ 102°F
Diagnostic Considerations: Bacteriuria plus pyuria with unilateral CVA tenderness and temperature ≥ 102°F. Bacteremia usually accompanies acute pyelonephritis; obtain blood and urine cultures
Pitfalls: Temperature decreases in 72 hours with or without antibiotic treatment. If temperature does not fall after 72 hours of antibiotic therapy, suspect renal/perinephric abscess

Therapeutic Considerations: Initial treatment is based on the urinary gram stain: If gram-negative bacilli, treat as Enterobacteriaceae. If gram-positive cocci in chains (enterococcus), treat as E. faecalis; if enterococcus is subsequently identified as E. faecium, treat accordingly. Acute pyelonephritis is usually treated initially for 1-3 days IV, then switched to PO to complete 4 weeks of antibiotics to minimize progression to chronic pyelonephritis. Obtain a CT/MRI in persistently febrile patients after 72 hours of antibiotics to rule out renal calculi, obstruction, abscess, or xanthomatous pyelonephritis

Prognosis: Excellent if first episode is adequately treated with antibiotics for 4 weeks

Chronic Bacterial Pyelonephritis (Enterobacteriaceae)

Clinical Presentation: Previous history of acute pyelonephritis with same symptoms as acute pyelonephritis but less CVA tenderness/fever

Diagnostic Considerations: Diagnosis by CT/MRI showing changes of chronic pyelonephritis plus bacteriuria/pyuria. Urine cultures may be intermittently negative before treatment. Chronic pyelonephritis is bilateral pathologically, but unilateral clinically

Pitfalls: Urine culture may be intermittently positive after treatment; repeat weekly x 4 to confirm urine remains culture-negative

Therapeutic Considerations: Treat x 4-6 weeks. Impaired medullary vascular blood supply/renal anatomical distortion makes eradication of pathogen difficult

Prognosis: Related to extent of renal damage

Renal TB (Mycobacterium tuberculosis)

Clinical Presentation: Renal mass lesion with ureteral abnormalities (pipestem, corkscrew, or spiral ureters) and sterile pyuria. Painless unless complicated by ureteral obstruction

Diagnostic Considerations: Combined upper/lower urinary tract abnormalities ± microscopic hematuria/urinary pH ≤ 5.5. Diagnosis by culture of TB from urine

Pitfalls: Chest x-ray is normal in 30%, but patients are PPD-positive. Rule out other infectious/inflammatory causes of sterile pyuria (e.g., Trichomonas, interstitial nephritis)

Therapeutic Considerations: Treat the same as pulmonary TB

Prognosis: Good if treated before renal parenchymal destruction/ureteral obstruction occur

Renal Abscess (Intrarenal/Perinephric)

Subset	Usual Pathogens	Preferred IV Therapy	Alternate IV Therapy	PO Therapy or IV-to-PO Switch
Cortical (Treat initially for MSSA; if later identified as MSRA, treat accordingly)	S. aureus	MSSA Nafcillin 2 gm (IV) q4h* or Ceftizoxime 2 gm (IV) q8h* or Clindamycin 600 mg (IV) q8h* MRSA Linezolid 600 mg (IV) q12h* or Minocycline 100 mg (IV) q12h*	MSSA Meropenem 1 gm (IV) q8h* or Imipenem 1 gm (IV) q6h* MRSA Vancomycin 1 gm (IV) q12h*	MSSA Clindamycin 300 mg (PO) q8h* MRSA Linezolid 600 mg (PO) q12h* or Minocycline 100 mg (PO) q12h*
Medullary	Entero-bacteriaceae	Levofloxacin 500 mg (IV) q24h*	TMP-SMX 2.5 mg/kg (IV) q6h*	Levofloxacin 500 mg (PO) q24h*

MSSA/MRSA = methicillin-sensitive/resistant S. aureus. Duration of therapy represents total time IV, PO, or IV + PO. Most patients on IV therapy able to take PO meds should be switched to PO therapy soon after clinical improvement
* Treat until renal abscess resolves completely or is no longer decreasing in size on CT/MRI

Clinical Presentation: Similar to pyelonephritis but fever remains elevated after 72 hours of antibiotics
Diagnostic Considerations: Obtain CT/MRI to diagnose perinephric/intra-renal abscess and rule out mass lesion. Cortical abscesses are usually secondary to hematogenous/contiguous spread. Medullary abscesses are usually due to extension of intrarenal infection
Pitfalls: Urine cultures may be negative with cortical abscesses
Therapeutic Considerations: Most large abscesses need to be drained. Multiple small abscesses are managed medically. Obtain urology consult
Prognosis: Related to degree of baseline renal dysfunction

Prostatitis/Prostatic Abscess

Subset	Usual Pathogens	Preferred IV Therapy	Alternate IV Therapy	PO Therapy or IV-to-PO Switch
Acute prostatitis/ acute prostatic abscess	Entero-bacteriaceae	Levofloxacin 500 mg (IV) q24h x 7 days **or** Ceftriaxone 1 gm (IV) q24h x 7 days	Aztreonam 2 gm (IV) q8h x 7 days **or** TMP-SMX 2.5 mg/kg (IV) q6h x 7 days	Levofloxacin 500 mg (PO) q24h x 2 weeks **or** Doxycycline 200 mg (PO) q12h x 3 days, then 100 mg (PO) q24h x 11 days **or** TMP-SMX 1 SS tablet (PO) q12h x 2 weeks
Chronic prostatitis	Entero-bacteriaceae	<u>IV Therapy</u> Not applicable	<u>PO Therapy</u> Levofloxacin 500 mg (PO) q24h x 1-3 months **or** Doxycycline 100 mg (PO) q24h x 1-3 months **or** TMP-SMX 1 DS tablet (PO) q12h x 1-3 months	

Duration of therapy represents total time IV, PO, or IV + PO. Most patients on IV therapy able to take PO meds should be switched to PO therapy soon after clinical improvement (usually < 72 hours)

Acute Prostatitis/Acute Prostatic Abscess (Enterobacteriaceae)
Clinical Presentation: Acute prostatitis presents as an acute febrile illness in males with dysuria and no CVA tenderness. Prostatic abscess presents with hectic/septic fevers without localizing signs
Diagnostic Considerations: Acute prostatitis is diagnosed by bacteriuria plus pyuria with exquisite prostate tenderness, and is seen primarily in young males. Positive urine culture is due to contamination of urine as it passes through infected prostate. Prostatic abscess is diagnosed by transrectal ultrasound or CT/MRI of prostate
Pitfalls: Do not overlook acute prostatitis in males with bacteriuria without localizing signs, or prostatic abscess in patients with a history of prostatitis
Therapeutic Considerations: Treat acute prostatitis for 2 full weeks to decrease progression to chronic prostatitis. Prostatic abscess is treated the same as acute prostatitis plus surgical drainage
Prognosis: Excellent if treated early with full course of antibiotics (plus drainage for prostatic abscess)

Chronic Prostatitis (Enterobacteriaceae)
Clinical Presentation: Vague urinary symptoms (mild dysuria ± low back pain), history of acute

prostatitis, and little or no fever

Diagnostic Considerations: Diagnosis by bacteriuria plus pyuria with "boggy prostate" ± mild tenderness. Urine/prostate expressate is culture positive. Chronic prostatitis with prostatic calcifications (rectal ultrasound) will not clear with antibiotics; treat with transurethral resection of prostate (TURP)

Pitfalls: Commonest cause of treatment failure is inadequate duration of therapy

Therapeutic Considerations: In sulfa-allergic patients, TMP alone may be used in place of TMP-SMX

Prognosis: Excellent if treated x 1-3 months. Prostatic abscess is a rare but serious complication (may cause urosepsis)

Urosepsis

Subset	Usual Pathogens	Preferred IV Therapy	Alternate IV Therapy	IV-to-PO Switch
Community-acquired (Treat initially based on urine gram stain)	Entero-bacteriaceae	Levofloxacin 500 mg (IV) q24h x 7 days **or** Ceftriaxone 1 gm (IV) q24h x 7 days	Gentamicin 240 mg (IV) q24h x 7 days **or** Aztreonam 2 gm (IV) q8h x 7 days	Levofloxacin 500 mg (PO) q24h x 7 days **or** TMP-SMX 1 SS tablet (PO) q12h x 7 days
	Enterococci (E. faecalis) Group B streptococci	Ampicillin 2 gm (IV) q4h x 7 days	Meropenem 1 gm (IV) q8h x 7 days **or** Imipenem 1 gm (IV) q6h x 7 days	Amoxicillin 1 gm (PO) q8h x 7 days **or** Levofloxacin 500 mg (PO) q24h x 7 days
Related to urological procedure (Treat initially for P. aeruginosa, etc; if later identified as non-aeruginosa Pseudomonas, treat accordingly)	P. aeruginosa Enterobacter Klebsiella Serratia	Cefepime 2 gm (IV) q8h x 7 days **or** Ciprofloxacin 400 mg (IV) q12h x 7 days	Piperacillin 4 gm (IV) q8h x 7 days **or** Aztreonam 2 gm (IV) q8h x 7 days **or** Gentamicin 240 mg (IV) q24h x 7 days	Ciprofloxacin 500 mg (PO) q12h x 7 days **or** Levofloxacin 500 mg (PO) q24h x 7 days
	Non-aeruginosa Pseudomonas (B. cepacia, S. maltophilia)	TMP-SMX 2.5 mg/kg (IV) q6h x 7 days	Meropenem 1 gm (IV) q8h x 7 days **or** Imipenem 1 gm (IV) q6h x 7 days	TMP-SMX 1 SS tablet (PO) q12h x 7 days **or** Levofloxacin 500 mg (PO) q24h x 7 days

Duration of therapy represents total time IV or IV + PO. Most patients on IV therapy able to take PO meds should be switched to PO therapy after clinical improvement.

Community-Acquired Urosepsis

Clinical Presentation: Sepsis from urinary tract source

Diagnostic Considerations: Blood and urine cultures positive for same uropathogen. If patient does not have diabetes, SLE, cirrhosis, myeloma, steroids, pre-existing renal disease or obstruction, obtain CT/MRI of GU tract to rule out abscess/obstruction. Prostatic abscess is rarely a cause of urosepsis

Pitfalls: Mixed gram-positive/negative urine cultures suggest specimen contamination or enterovesicular fistula

Therapeutic Considerations: Empiric treatment is based on urine gram stain. If gram-positive cocci, treat as Group B/D streptococci (not S. aureus/S. pneumoniae). If gram-negative bacilli, treat as

Enterobacteriaceae (not P. aeruginosa/B. fragilis)
Prognosis: Related to severity of underlying condition causing urosepsis and health of host

Urosepsis Following Urological Procedures
Clinical Presentation: Sepsis within 24 hours after GU procedure
Diagnostic Considerations: Blood and urine cultures positive for same uropathogen. Use pre-procedural urine culture to identify uropathogen and guide therapy
Pitfalls: If non-aeruginosa Pseudomonas in urine/blood, switch to TMP-SMX until susceptibility test results are available
Therapeutic Considerations: Empiric P. aeruginosa monotherapy will cover most other uropathogens
Prognosis: Related to severity of underlying condition causing urosepsis and health of host

Pelvic Inflammatory Disease (PID), Salpingitis, Tuboovarian Abscess, Endometritis/Endomyometritis, Septic Abortion

Subset	Usual Pathogens	Preferred IV Therapy	Alternate IV Therapy	PO Therapy or IV-to-PO Switch
Hospitalized patients[†]	B. fragilis Entero-bacteriaceae N. gonorrhoeae C. trachomatis	Doxycycline 200 mg (IV) q12h x 3 days, then 100 mg (IV) q12h x 11 days **plus either** Cefoxitin 2 gm (IV) q6h x 2 weeks **or** Clindamycin 600 mg (IV) q8h x 2 weeks	Doxycycline 200 mg (IV) q12h x 3 days, then 100 mg (IV) q12h x 11 days **plus** Ampicillin/sulbactam 3 gm (IV) q6h x 2 weeks 2nd Alternate Levofloxacin 500 mg (IV) q24h x 2 weeks **plus** Metronidazole 1 gm (IV) q24h x 2 weeks	Levofloxacin 500 mg (PO) q24h x 2 weeks **plus either** Doxycycline 200 mg (PO) q12h x 3 days, then 100 mg (PO) q12h x 11 days* **or** Metronidazole 500 mg (PO) q12h x 2 weeks
Outpatients (mild PID only)	N. gonorrhoeae C. trachomatis B. fragilis Entero-bacteriaceae	Levofloxacin 500 mg (PO) q24h x 14 days **plus either** Doxycycline 100 mg (PO) q12h x 14 days **or** Metronidazole 500 mg (PO) q12h x 14 days		

Duration of therapy represents total time IV, PO, or IV + PO. Most patients on IV therapy able to take PO meds should be switched to PO therapy after clinical improvement
† *Treat only IV or IV-to-PO switch for salpingitis, tuboovarian abscess, endometritis, endomyometritis, septic abortion, or severe PID*
* *Loading dose is not needed PO if given IV with the same drug*

Clinical Presentation: PID/salpingitis presents with cervical motion/adnexal tenderness, lower quadrant abdominal pain, and fever. Endometritis/endomyometritis presents with uterine tenderness ± cervical discharge/fever. Endomyometritis is the most common post-partum infection
Diagnostic Considerations: Unilateral lower abdominal pain in a female without a non-pelvic cause suggests PID/salpingitis

Pitfalls: Obtain CT/MRI of abdomen/pelvis to confirm diagnosis and rule out other pathology or tubo-ovarian abscess

Therapeutic Considerations: Tuboovarian abscess usually requires drainage/removal ± TAH/BSO, plus antibiotics (p. 80) x 1-2 weeks after drainage/removal. Septic abortion is treated the same as endometritis/endomyometritis plus uterine evacuation

Prognosis: Related to promptness of treatment/adequacy of drainage if tuboovarian abscess. Late complications of PID/salpingitis include tubal scarring/infertility

Empiric Therapy of Sexually Transmitted Diseases

Urethritis/Cervicitis

Subset	Usual Pathogens	IM Therapy	PO Therapy
Gonococcal	N. gonorrhoeae	Ceftriaxone 125 mg (IM) x 1 dose Alternate Any 3rd generation cephalosporin 250-500 mg (IM) x 1 dose	Azithromycin 2 gm (PO) x 1 dose **or** Levofloxacin 500 mg (PO) x 1 dose **or** Cefixime 400 mg (PO) x 1 dose
Non-gonococcal	C. trachomatis U. urealyticum M. genitalium	Not applicable	Doxycycline 100 mg (PO) q12h x 7 days **or** Azithromycin 1 gm (PO) x 1 dose **or** Levofloxacin 500 mg (PO) q24h x 7 days **or** Erythromycin 500 mg (PO) q6h x 7 days
	Trichomonas vaginalis	Not applicable	Metronidazole 2 gm (PO) x 1 dose **or** Metronidazole 500 mg (PO) q12h x 7 days

Gonococcal Urethritis/Cervicitis (Neisseria gonorrhoeae)

Clinical Presentation: Purulent penile/cervical discharge with burning/dysuria 3-5 days after contact

Diagnostic Considerations: Diagnosis in males by gram stain of urethral discharge showing gram-negative diplococci. In females, diagnosis requires culture of cervical discharge, not gram stain. Obtain throat/rectal culture for N. gonorrhoeae. Co-infections are common; obtain VDRL and HIV serologies

Pitfalls: Gram stain of cervical discharge showing gram-negative diplococci is not diagnostic of N. gonorrhoeae; must confirm by culture. N. gonorrhoeae infections are asymptomatic in 10%

Therapeutic Considerations: Failure to respond suggests re-infection or infection with another agent (e.g., Trichomonas, Ureaplasma). Treat pharyngeal/rectal GC the same as GC urethritis

Prognosis: Increased risk of disseminated infection with pharyngeal/rectal GC

Non-Gonococcal Urethritis/Cervicitis (Chlamydia/Ureaplasma/Mycoplasma)

Clinical Presentation: Non-purulent penile/cervical discharge + dysuria ~ 1 week after contact

Diagnostic Considerations: Diagnosis by positive chlamydial antigen test/Ureaplasma or Mycoplasma

culture of urethral/cervical discharge. Culture urethral/cervical discharge to rule out N. gonorrhoeae. Co-infections are common; obtain VDRL and HIV serologies
Pitfalls: C. trachomatis infections are asymptomatic in 25%
Therapeutic Considerations: Failure to respond to anti-Chlamydia therapy suggests re-infection or Trichomonas/Ureaplasma/Mycoplasma infection. Quinolones are also active against N. gonorrhoeae
Prognosis: Tubal scarring/infertility in chronic infection

Trichomonas Urethritis/Cervicitis (Trichomonas vaginalis)
Clinical Presentation: Frothy, pruritic, vaginal discharge; not foul smelling
Diagnostic Considerations: Trichomonas by wet mount/culture on special media
Pitfalls: Classic "strawberry cervix" is infrequently seen
Therapeutic Considerations: Use week-long regimen if single dose fails
Prognosis: Excellent if partner is also treated

Vaginitis/Balanitis

Subset	Usual Pathogens	IV Therapy	PO Therapy
Bacterial vaginosis/ vaginitis	Gardnerella vaginalis Mobiluncus Prevotella Mycoplasma hominis	Not applicable	Metronidazole 2 gm (PO) x 1 dose **or** Metronidazole 500 mg (PO) q12h x 7 days **or** Clindamycin 300 mg (PO) q12h x 7 days **or** Moxifloxacin 400 mg (PO) q24h x 7 days
Candida vaginitis/ balanitis	Candida	Not applicable	Fluconazole 100 mg (PO) q24h x 7 days **Alternate** Itraconazole 100 mg (PO) q24h x 7 days

Bacterial Vaginosis/Vaginitis
Clinical Presentation: Non-pruritic vaginal discharge with "fishy" odor
Diagnostic Considerations: Diagnosis by "clue cells" in vaginal fluid wet mount. Vaginal pH ≥ 4.5. "Fishy" odor emanates from smear of vaginal secretions when 10% KOH solution is added (positive "whiff test")
Pitfalls: Do not confuse "clue cells" with darkly staining bodies of H. ducreyi (chancroid)
Therapeutic Considerations: As an alternative to oral therapy, clindamycin cream 2% intravaginally qHS x 7 days or metronidazole gel 0.075% 1 application intravaginally q12h x 5 days can be used
Prognosis: Excellent

Candida Vaginitis/Balanitis
Clinical Presentation: Pruritic white plaques in vagina/glans penis
Diagnostic Considerations: Diagnosis by gram stain/culture of whitish plaques
Pitfalls: Rule out Trichomonas, which also presents with pruritus in females
Therapeutic Considerations: Treat both partners with oral anti-Candida therapy. Use itraconazole cream for non-albicans Candida
Prognosis: Good with systemic therapy. Diabetics/uncircumcised males may need prolonged therapy

Genital Vesicles

Subset	Usual Pathogens	IV Therapy	PO Therapy
Genital vesicles	HSV-2 (genital herpes)	Not applicable	Acyclovir 400 mg (PO) q8h x 7 days **or** Valacyclovir 1 gm (PO) q12h x 7 days **or** Famciclovir 250 mg (PO) q8h x 7 days

Clinical Presentation: Painful vesicles on genitals with painful bilateral regional adenopathy ± low-grade fever
Diagnostic Considerations: Diagnosis by clinical presentation/culture. "Satelliting" vesicles are characteristic of HSV-2
Pitfalls: Elevated IgG HSV-2 titer indicates past exposure, not acute infection
Therapeutic Considerations: If concomitant rectal herpes, increase acyclovir to 800 mg (PO) q8h x 7 days. For recurrent genital herpes, use acyclovir or valacyclovir (dose same as primary infection) for 7 days after each relapse. Recurrent episodes of HSV-2 are less painful than primary infection, and inguinal adenopathy is less prominent/painful
Prognosis: HSV-2 tends to recur, especially during the first year

Genital Ulcers

Subset	Usual Pathogens	IM Therapy	PO Therapy
Primary syphilis	Treponema pallidum	Benzathine penicillin 2.4 mu (IM) x 1 dose	Doxycycline 100 mg (PO) q12h x 2 weeks
Chancroid	Hemophilus ducreyi	Ceftriaxone 250 mg (IM) x 1 dose Alternate Any 3rd generation cephalosporin 250-500 mg (IM) x 1 dose	Azithromycin 1 gm (PO) x 1 dose **or** Levofloxacin 500 mg (PO) q24h x 3 days **or** Erythromycin base 500 mg (PO) q6h x 7 days

Primary Syphilis (Treponema pallidum)
Clinical Presentation: Painless, indurated ulcers (chancres) with bilateral painless inguinal adenopathy. Syphilitic chancres are elevated, clean and raised, but not undermined
Diagnostic Considerations: Diagnosis by spirochetes on darkfield examination of ulcer exudate. Elevated VDRL titers after 1 week
Pitfalls: VDRL titers fall slowly within 1 year; failure to decline suggests treatment failure/HIV
Therapeutic Considerations: Parenteral penicillin is the preferred antibiotic for all stages of syphilis. If treatment fails/VDRL does not decline, obtain HIV serology
Prognosis: Good with early treatment

Chancroid (Hemophilus ducreyi)
Clinical Presentation: Ragged, undermined, painful ulcer(s) + painful unilateral inguinal adenopathy
Diagnostic Considerations: Diagnosis by streptobacilli in "school of fish" configuration on gram-

stained smear of ulcer exudate/culture of H. ducreyi
Pitfalls: Co-infection is common; obtain VDRL and HIV serologies
Therapeutic Considerations: In HIV, multiple dose regimens or azithromycin is preferred. Resistance to erythromycin/ciprofloxacin has been reported
Prognosis: Good with early treatment

Suppurating Inguinal Adenopathy

Subset	Usual Pathogens	IV Therapy	PO Therapy
Lympho-granuloma venereum (LGV)	Chlamydia trachomatis (L_{1-3} serotypes)	Not applicable	Doxycycline 100 mg (PO) q12h x 3 weeks **or** Erythromycin 500 mg (PO) q6h x 3 weeks **or** Sulfisoxazole 500 mg (PO) q6h x 3 weeks
Granuloma inguinale (Donovanosis)	Calymmato-bacterium granulomatosis	Not applicable	Doxycycline 100 mg (PO) q12h x 3 weeks **or** Erythromycin 500 mg (PO) q6h x 3 weeks **or** TMP-SMX 1 DS tablet (PO) q12h x 3 weeks **or** Ciprofloxacin 500 mg (PO) q12h x 3 weeks

Lymphogranuloma Venereum (Chlamydia trachomatis) LGV
Clinical Presentation: Unilateral inguinal adenopathy ± discharge/sinus tract
Diagnostic Consideration: Diagnosis by very high Chlamydia trachomatis L_{1-3} titers. Do not biopsy site (often does not heal and may form a fistula). May present as FUO
Pitfalls: Initial papule not visible at clinical presentation
Therapeutic Considerations: Rectal LGV may require additional courses of treatment
Prognosis: Fibrotic perirectal/pelvic damage does not reverse with therapy

Granuloma Inguinale (Calymmatobacterium granulomatosis) Donovanosis
Clinical Presentation: Accentuated inguinal groove ± discharge. Pseudolymphadenopathy ("groove sign") due to prominent soft tissue swelling
Diagnostic Considerations: Donovan bodies ("puffed-wheat" appearance) in tissue biopsy
Pitfalls: No true inguinal adenopathy, as opposed to LGV infection
Therapeutic Considerations: Doxycycline or erythromycin preferred
Prognosis: Good if treated early

Genital/Perianal Warts (Condylomata Acuminata)

Subset	Pathogens	IV Therapy	Other Therapy
Genital/perianal warts	Human papilloma virus (HPV)	Not applicable	Podophyllin 10-25% in tincture of benzoin **or** Surgical/laser removal/cryotherapy with liquid nitrogen **or** Cidofovir gel (1%) daily at bedtime x 5 days every other week for 6 cycles

Clinical Presentation: Single/multiple verrucous genital lesions ± pigmentation usually without inguinal adenopathy

Diagnostic Considerations: Diagnosis by clinical appearance. Genital warts are usually caused by HPV types 11,16. Anogenital warts caused by HPV types 16,18,31,33,35 are associated with cervical neoplasia. Females with anogenital warts need serial cervical PAP smears to detect cervical dysplasia/neoplasia

Pitfalls: Most HPV infections are asymptomatic

Therapeutic Considerations: Cidofovir cures/halts HPV progression in 50% of cases

Prognosis: Related to HPV serotypes with malignant potential (HPV types 16,18,31,33,35)

Syphilis

Subset	Usual Pathogens	Preferred IV/IM Therapy	Alternate IV/IM Therapy	PO Therapy
Primary, secondary, or early latent (duration < 1 year) syphilis	Treponema pallidum	Benzathine penicillin 2.4 mu (IM) x 1 dose	Not applicable	Doxycycline 100 mg (PO) q12h x 2 weeks **or** Erythromycin 500 mg (PO) q6h x 2 weeks
Late latent (duration > 1 year) or tertiary syphilis	Treponema pallidum	Benzathine penicillin 2.4 mu (IM) weekly x 3 weeks	Not applicable	Doxycycline 100 mg (PO) q12h x 4 weeks
Neurosyphilis	Treponema pallidum	Penicillin G 4 mu (IV) q4h x 2 weeks	Procaine penicillin 2.4 mu (IM) q24h x 2 weeks **plus** Probenecid 500 mg (PO) q6h x 2 weeks **or monotherapy with** Ceftriaxone 1 gm (IV) q24h x 2 weeks	Doxycycline 100 mg (PO) q12h x 4 weeks **or** Minocycline 100 mg (PO) q12h x 4 weeks

Duration of therapy represents total time IV, IM, or PO. All stages of syphilis in HIV/AIDS patients usually respond to therapeutic regimens recommended for normal hosts. Syphilis in pregnancy should be treated according to the stage of syphilis; penicillin-allergic pregnant patients should be desensitized and treated with penicillin

Primary Syphilis (Treponema pallidum)

Clinical Presentation: Painless, indurated ulcer(s) (chancre) with bilateral painless inguinal adenopathy

Diagnostic Considerations: Diagnosis by spirochetes on darkfield examination of ulcer exudate. Elevated VDRL titers after 1 week

Pitfalls: VDRL titers fall slowly within 1 year; failure to decline suggests treatment failure

Therapeutic Considerations: Parenteral penicillin is the preferred antibiotic for all stages of syphilis; if treatment fails/VDRL does not decline, obtain HIV serology

Prognosis: Good with early treatment

Secondary Syphilis (Treponema pallidum)

Clinical Presentation: Facial/truncal macular, papular, papulosquamous, non-pruritic, tender, symmetrical rash which may involve the palms/soles. Usually accompanied by generalized adenopathy. Typically appears 4-10 weeks after primary chancre, although stages may overlap. Alopecia aereata, condyloma lata, mucous patches, iritis/uveitis may be present. Renal involvement ranges from mild proteinuria to nephrotic syndrome. Without treatment, spontaneous resolution occurs after 3-12 weeks

Diagnostic Considerations: Diagnosis by clinical findings and VDRL in high titers (≥ 1:256). After treatment, VDRL titers usually return to non-reactive within 2 years. Syphilitic hepatitis is characterized by elevated alkaline phosphatase > elevated SGOT

Pitfalls: Palmar/foot rashes are not due to 2° syphilis if VDRL is positive in low titer

Therapeutic Considerations: Parenteral penicillin is the preferred antibiotic for all stages of syphilis. VDRL titers that remain reactive after 2 years suggest reinfection and should be retreated

Prognosis: Excellent with early treatment

Latent Syphilis (Treponema pallidum)

Clinical Presentation: Patients are asymptomatic with elevated VDRL/FTA-ABS titers

Diagnostic Considerations: Diagnosis by positive serology ± prior history, but no signs/symptoms of syphilis. Asymptomatic syphilis < 1 year in duration is termed "early" latent syphilis; asymptomatic syphilis > 1 year/unknown duration is termed "late" latent syphilis. Secondary syphilis may relapse in up to 25% of patients with early latent syphilis, but relapse is rare in late latent syphilis. Evaluate patients for neurosyphilis

Pitfalls: FTA-ABS titers do not fall with treatment and may remain positive in low titer for life

Therapeutic Considerations: Parenteral penicillin is the preferred antibiotic for all stages of syphilis. Repeat VDRL titers at 6, 12, and 24 months; therapeutic response is defined as a 4-fold reduction in VDRL titers (2 tube dilutions).

Prognosis: Excellent even if treated late

Tertiary Syphilis (Treponema pallidum)

Clinical Presentation: May present with aortitis, neurosyphilis, iritis, or gummata 5-30 years after initial infection

Diagnostic Considerations: Diagnosis by history of syphilis plus positive VDRL/FTA-ABS with signs/symptoms of late syphilis

Pitfalls: Treat for signs of neurosyphilis on clinical exam or lumbar puncture, even if VDRL is non-reactive

Therapeutic Considerations: Parenteral penicillin is the preferred antibiotic for all stages of syphilis

Prognosis: Related to extent of end-organ damage

Neurosyphilis (Treponema pallidum)

Clinical Presentation: Patients are often asymptomatic, but may have ophthalmic/auditory symptoms, cranial nerve abnormalities, tabes dorsalis, paresis, psychosis, or signs of meningitis/dementia

Diagnostic Considerations: Diagnosis by elevated CSF VDRL titers; no need to obtain CSF FTA-ABS titers. CSF has pleocytosis, increased protein, and positive VDRL

Pitfalls: Persistent CSF abnormalities suggest treatment failure

Therapeutic Considerations: Parenteral penicillin is the preferred antibiotic for all stages of syphilis. CSF abnormalities should decrease in 6 months and return to normal after 2 years; repeat lumbar puncture 6 months after treatment. Failure rate with ceftriaxone is 20%

Prognosis: Related to extent of end-organ damage

Empiric Therapy of Bone and Joint Infections

Septic Arthritis/Bursitis

Subset	Usual Pathogens	Preferred IV Therapy	Alternate IV Therapy	PO Therapy or IV-to-PO Switch
Acute (Treat initially based on gram stain of synovial fluid. If gram positive cocci in clusters, treat initially for MSSA; if later identified as MSRA, treat accordingly)	S. aureus (MSSA)	Cefazolin 1 gm (IV) q8h x 3 weeks **or** Clindamycin 600 mg (IV) q8h x 3 weeks **or** Nafcillin 2 gm (IV) q4h x 3 weeks	Ceftizoxime 2 gm (IV) q8h x 3 weeks **or** Meropenem 1 gm (IV) q8h x 3 weeks **or** Imipenem 1 gm (IV) q6h x 3 weeks	Cephalexin 1 gm (PO) q6h x 3 weeks **or** Clindamycin 300 mg (PO) q8h x 3 weeks **or** Levofloxacin 500 mg (PO) q24h x 3 weeks
	S. aureus (MRSA)	Linezolid 600 mg (IV) q12h x 3 weeks **or** Quinupristin/ dalfopristin 7.5 mg/kg (IV) q8h x 3 weeks	Minocycline 100 mg (IV) q12h x 3 weeks **or** Vancomycin 1 gm (IV) q12h x 3 weeks	Linezolid 600 mg (PO) q12h x 3 weeks **or** Minocycline 100 mg (PO) q12h x 3 weeks
	Group A,B,C,G streptococci	Cefazolin 1 gm (IV) q8h x 2 weeks **or** Clindamycin 600 mg (IV) q8h x 2 weeks	Ceftizoxime 2 gm (IV) q8h x 2 weeks **or** Ceftriaxone 1 gm (IV) q24h x 2 weeks	Clindamycin 300 mg (PO) q8h x 2 weeks **plus** Cephalexin 500 mg (PO) q6h x 2 weeks
	Entero- bacteriaceae	Ceftriaxone 1 gm (IV) q24h x 2 weeks **or** Cefotaxime 2 gm (IV) q6h x 2 weeks **or** Cefepime 2 gm (IV) q12h x 2 weeks	Ceftizoxime 2 gm (IV) q8h x 2 weeks **or** Aztreonam 2 gm (IV) q8h x 2 weeks	Levofloxacin 500 mg (PO) q24h x 2 weeks **or** Ciprofloxacin 750 mg (PO) q12h x 2 weeks

Septic Arthritis/Bursitis (cont'd)

Subset	Usual Pathogens	Preferred IV Therapy	Alternate IV Therapy	PO Therapy or IV-to-PO Switch
Acute (cont'd)	P. aeruginosa	Piperacillin 4 gm (IV) q8h x 3 weeks **or** Cefepime 2 gm (IV) q8h x 3 weeks	Meropenem 1 gm (IV) q8h x 3 weeks **or** Imipenem 1 gm (IV) q6h x 3 weeks **or** Aztreonam 2 gm (IV) q8h x 3 weeks	Ciprofloxacin 750 mg (PO) q12h x 3 weeks
	N. gonorrhoeae	Ceftriaxone 1 gm (IV) q24h x 2 weeks **or** Ceftizoxime 2 gm (IV) q8h x 2 weeks	Levofloxacin 500 mg (IV) q24h x 2 weeks	Levofloxacin 500 mg (PO) q24h x 2 weeks **or** Cefixime 400 mg (PO) q12h x 2 weeks
	Brucella	Streptomycin 1 gm (IM) q24h x 3 weeks **plus** Doxycycline 200 mg (IV) q12h x 3 days, then 100 mg (IV) q12h for 3 week total course	Gentamicin 5 mg/kg (IV) q24h x 3 weeks **plus** Doxycycline 200 mg (IV) q12h x 3 days, then 100 mg (IV) q12h for 3-week total course	Doxycycline 200 mg (PO) q12h x 3 days, then 100 mg (PO) q12h for 3 weeks total* **plus** Rifampin 600 mg (PO) q24h x 3 weeks
	Salmonella	Levofloxacin 500 mg (IV) q24h x 2-3 weeks **or** Ceftriaxone 2 gm (IV) q24h x 2-3 weeks	Aztreonam 2 gm (IV) q8h x 2-3 weeks **or** TMP-SMX 2.5 mg/kg (IV) q6h x 2-3 weeks	Levofloxacin 500 mg (PO) q24h x 2-3 weeks **or** TMP-SMX 1 DS tablet (PO) q12h x 2-3 weeks

Septic Arthritis/Bursitis (cont'd)

Subset	Usual Pathogens	Preferred IV Therapy	Alternate IV Therapy	PO Therapy or IV-to-PO Switch
Secondary to animal bite wound	P. multocida S. moniliformis E. corrodens	Piperacillin/ tazobactam 4.5 gm (IV) q8h x 2 weeks **or** Ampicillin/ sulbactam 3 gm (IV) q6h x 2 weeks	Meropenem 1 gm (IV) q8h x 2 weeks **or** Imipenem 1 gm (IV) q6h x 2 weeks **or** Ertapenem 1 gm (IV) q24h x 2 weeks **or** Doxycycline 200 mg (IV) q12h x 3 days, then 100 mg (IV) q12h x 11 days	Amoxicillin/ clavulanic acid 875 mg (PO) q12h x 2 weeks **or** Doxycycline 200 mg (PO) q12h x 3 days, then 100 mg (PO) q12h x 11 days*
Fungal arthritis	Coccidioides immitis	Itraconazole 400 mg (IV) q24h x 6-12 months	Fluconazole 400-800 mg (IV) q24h x 6-12 months **or** Voriconazole 200 mg (IV) q12h x 6-12 months	Itraconazole 400 mg (PO) q24h x 6-12 months
	Sporothrix schenckii	Itraconazole 200 mg (IV) q24h x 3-6 months/until cured	Amphotericin B 0.5 mg/kg (IV) q24h until 2-2.5 gm given, **then** Itraconazole 200 mg (PO) q24h x 3-6 months/until cured	Itraconazole 200 mg (PO) q24h x 3-6 months/until cured
TB arthritis	M. tuberculosis	Not applicable	INH 300 mg (PO) q24h x 12 months **plus** Rifampin 600 mg (PO) q24h x 12 months <u>If multiresistant TB strain likely, also add</u> EMB 15 mg/kg (PO) q24h x 12 months **plus** PZA 25 mg/kg (PO) q24h x 12 months

MSSA/MRSA = methicillin-sensitive/resistant S. aureus. Duration of therapy represents total time IV, PO, or IV + PO.
Most patients on IV therapy able to take PO meds should be switched to PO therapy after clinical improvement
* Loading dose is not needed PO if given IV with the same drug

Acute Septic Arthritis/Bursitis
Clinical Presentation: Acute joint pain with fever. Septic joint unable to bear weight. Septic bursitis presents with pain on joint motion, but patient is able to bear weight

Diagnostic Considerations: Diagnosis by demonstrating organisms in synovial fluid by stain/culture. In septic bursitis (knee most common), there is pain on joint flexion (although the joint can bear weight), and synovial fluid findings are negative for septic arthritis. Except for N. gonorrhoeae, polyarthritis is not usually due to bacterial pathogens. Post-infectious polyarthritis is usually viral in origin, most commonly due to parvovirus B19, rubella, or HBV
Therapeutic Considerations: See specific pathogen, below. Treat septic bursitis as septic arthritis

Staphylococcus aureus

Diagnostic Considerations: Painful hot joint; unable to bear weight. Diagnosis by synovial fluid pleocytosis and positive culture for joint pathogen. Examine synovial fluid to rule out gout (doubly birefringent crystals) and pseudogout (calcium pyrophosphate crystals). May occur in setting of endocarditis with septic emboli to joints; other manifestations of endocarditis are usually evident
Pitfalls: Rule out causes of non-infectious arthritis (sarcoidosis, Whipple's disease, Ehlers-Danlos, etc.), which are less severe, but may mimic septic arthritis. In reactive arthritis following urethritis (C. trachomatis, Ureaplasma urealyticum, N. gonorrhoeae) or diarrhea (Shigella, Campylobacter, Yersinia, Salmonella), synovial fluid culture is negative, and synovial fluid WBCs counts are usually < 10,000/mm^3 with normal synovial fluid lactic acid and glucose. Do not overlook infective endocarditis in mono/polyarticular arthritis without apparent cause
Therapeutic Considerations: For MRSA septic arthritis, vancomycin penetration into synovial fluid is unreliable; use linezolid instead. Most believe immobilization of infected joint during therapy is helpful. Local installation of antibiotics into synovial fluid has no advantage over IV/PO antibiotics
Prognosis: Treat as early as possible to minimize joint damage. Repeated aspiration/open drainage may be needed to preserve joint function

Group A, B, C, G Streptococci

Diagnostic Considerations: Usually monoarticular. Not usually due to septic emboli from endocarditis
Prognosis: Related to extent of joint damage and rapidity of antibiotic treatment

Enterobacteriaceae

Diagnostic Considerations: Diagnosis by isolation of gram-negative bacilli from synovial fluid
Pitfalls: Septic arthritis involving an unusual joint (e.g., sternoclavicular, sacral) should suggest IV drug abuse until proven otherwise
Therapeutic Considerations: Joint aspiration is essential in suspected septic arthritis of the hip and may be needed for other joints; obtain orthopedic surgery consult. Local installation of antibiotics into joint fluid is of no proven value
Prognosis: Related to extent of joint damage and rapidity of antibiotic treatment

Pseudomonas aeruginosa

Diagnostic Considerations P. aeruginosa septic arthritis/osteomyelitis may occur after water contaminated puncture wound (e.g., nail puncture of heel through shoes). Sternoclavicular/sacroiliac joint involvement is common in IV drug abusers (IVDAs)
Pitfalls: Suspect IVDA in P. aeruginosa septic arthritis without a history of trauma
Therapeutic Considerations: If ciprofloxacin is used, treat with 750 mg (not 500 mg) dose for P. aeruginosa septic arthritis/osteomyelitis
Prognosis: Related to extent of joint damage and rapidity of antibiotic treatment

Neiserria gonorrhoeae

Diagnostic Considerations: Gonococcal arthritis may present as a monoarticular arthritis, or multiple joints may be affected as part of gonococcal arthritis-dermatitis syndrome (disseminated gonococcal infection). Bacteremia with positive blood cultures occurs early during rash stage while synovial fluid cultures are negative. Joint involvement follows with typical findings of septic arthritis and synovial fluid cultures positive for N. gonorrhoeae; blood cultures are negative at this stage. Acute tenosynovitis is

often a clue to gonococcal septic arthritis
Pitfalls: Spectinomycin is ineffective against pharyngeal gonorrhea
Therapeutic Considerations: Gonococcal arthritis-dermatitis syndrome is caused by very susceptible strains of N. gonorrhoeae. Cephalosporins also eliminate incubating syphilis
Prognosis: Excellent with arthritis-dermatitis syndrome; worse with only monoarticular arthritis

Brucella sp.
Diagnostic Considerations: Usually evidence of brucellosis elsewhere (meningitis, SBE, epididymoorchitis). Diagnosis by blood/joint cultures
Pitfalls: Brucella has predilection for bones/joints of spine
Therapeutic Considerations: Some patients may require 6 weeks of antibiotic therapy
Prognosis: Related to severity of infection and underlying health of host

Salmonella sp.
Diagnostic Considerations: Occurs in sickle cell disease and hemoglobinopathies. Diagnosis by blood/joint cultures
Pitfalls: S. aureus, not Salmonella, is the most common cause of septic arthritis in sickle cell disease
Prognosis: Related to severity of infection and underlying health of host

Septic Arthritis Secondary to Animal Bite Wound
Clinical Presentation: Penetrating bite wound into joint space
Diagnostic Considerations: Diagnosis by smear/culture of synovial fluid/blood cultures
Pitfalls: May develop metastatic infection from bacteremia
Therapeutic Considerations: Treat for at least 2 weeks of combined IV/PO therapy
Prognosis: Related to severity of infection and underlying health of host

Chronic Septic Arthritis
Clinical Presentation: Subacute/chronic joint pain with decreased range of motion and little or no fever. Able to bear weight on joint
Diagnostic Considerations: Diagnosis by smear/culture of synovial fluid/synovial biopsy

Coccidioides immitis
Diagnostic Considerations: Must grow organisms from synovium/synovial fluid for diagnosis
Pitfalls: Synovial fluid the same as in TB (lymphocytic pleocytosis, low glucose, increased protein)
Therapeutic Considerations: Oral therapy is preferred; same cure rates as amphotericin regimens. HIV/AIDS patients need life-long suppressive therapy
Prognosis: Related to severity of infection and underlying health of host

Sporothrix schenckii
Diagnostic Considerations: Usually a monoarticular infection secondary to direct inoculation/trauma
Pitfalls: Polyarticular arthritis suggests disseminated infection
Therapeutic Considerations: SSKI is useful for lymphocutaneous sporotrichosis, not bone/joint involvement
Prognosis: Excellent for localized disease (e.g., lymphocutaneous sporotrichosis). In disseminated disease, prognosis is related to host factors

Mycobacterium tuberculosis (TB)
Diagnostic Considerations: Clue is subacute/chronic tenosynovitis over involved joint. Unlike other forms of septic arthritis, which are usually due to hematogenous spread, TB arthritis is usually a complication of adjacent TB osteomyelitis. Synovial fluid findings include lymphocytic pleocytosis, low glucose, and increased protein

Pitfalls: Send synovial fluid for AFB smear/culture in unexplained chronic monoarticular arthritis
Therapeutic Considerations: TB arthritis is usually treated for 1 year
Prognosis: Related to severity of infection and underlying health of host

Lyme Disease/Lyme Arthritis

Subset	Usual Pathogens	Preferred IV Therapy	Alternate IV Therapy	PO Therapy or IV-to-PO Switch
Lyme disease/ arthritis	Borrelia burgdorferi	Ceftriaxone 1 gm (IV) q24h x 2 weeks	Ceftizoxime 2 gm (IV) q8h x 2 weeks	Amoxicillin 1 gm (PO) q8h x 2 weeks **or** Doxycycline 200 mg (PO) q12h x 3 days, then 100 mg (PO) q12h x 11 days

Duration of therapy represents total time IV, PO, or IV + PO. Most patients on IV therapy able to take PO meds should be switched to PO therapy after clinical improvement

Lyme Disease
Clinical Presentation: Can manifest acutely or chronically with local or disseminated disease following bite of tick infected with Borrelia spirochete. Erythema marginatum (expanding, erythematous, annular lesion with central clearing) occurs in ~ 75% within two weeks of tick bite, and may be associated with fever, headache, arthralgias/myalgias, meningismus. Other possible acute manifestations include meningitis, encephalitis, Bell's palsy, peripheral neuropathy, mild hepatitis, myocarditis with heart block, or arthritis. Chronic disease may present with arthritis, peripheral neuropathy, meningoencephalitis, or acrodermatitis chronica atrophicans (usually > 10 years after infection)
Diagnostic Considerations: Diagnosis by clinical presentation plus elevated IgM Lyme titers (IFA/ELISA). If Lyme titer is borderline or suspected to be a false-positive, obtain an IgM Western blot to confirm the diagnosis. IgM titers may take 4-6 weeks to increase after tick bite. Ixodes ticks are the principal vector; small rodents are the primary reservoir. In the United States, most cases occur in the coastal Northeast, upper Midwest, California, and western Nevada
Pitfalls: Rash is not always seen, and tick bite is often painless and goes unnoticed (tick often spontaneously falls off after 1-2 days of feeding). Do not overlook Lyme disease in patients with unexplained heart block in areas where Ixodes ticks are endemic
Therapeutic Considerations: B. burgdorferi is highly susceptible to all beta-lactams. For Bell's palsy or neuroborreliosis, minocycline (100 mg PO q12h x 2 weeks) may be preferred to doxycycline
Prognosis: Excellent in normal hosts

Lyme Arthritis
Clinical Presentation: Acute Lyme arthritis presents with joint pain, decreased range of motion, ability to bear weight on joint, and little or no fever. Chronic Lyme arthritis resembles rheumatoid arthritis
Diagnostic Considerations: Usually affects children and large weight-bearing joints (e.g., knee). Acute Lyme arthritis is diagnosed by clinical presentation plus elevated IgM Lyme titer. Chronic Lyme arthritis is suggested by rheumatoid arthritis-like presentation with negative ANA and rheumatoid factor, and positive IgG Lyme titer and synovial fluid PCR
Pitfalls: Acute Lyme arthritis joint is red but not hot, in contrast to septic arthritis. In chronic Lyme arthritis, a negative IgG Lyme titer essentially rules out chronic Lyme arthritis, but an elevated IgG Lyme titer indicates only past exposure to B. burgdorferi and is not diagnostic of Lyme arthritis. Joint fluid in chronic Lyme disease is usually negative by culture, but positive by PCR; synovial fluid PCR, however,

does not differentiate active from prior infection
Therapeutic Considerations: IgG Lyme titers remain elevated for life, and do not decrease with treatment. Joint symptoms often persist for months/years after effective antibiotic therapy due to autoimmune joint inflammation; treat with anti-inflammatory drugs, not repeat antibiotic courses
Prognosis: Good in normal hosts. Chronic/refractory arthritis may develop in genetically predisposed patients with DRW 2/4 HLA types

Infected Joint Prosthesis

Subset	Usual Pathogens	Preferred IV Therapy	Alternate IV Therapy	IV-to-PO Switch
Staphylococcal (Treat initially for MSSA; if later identified as MRSA or S. epidermidis, treat accordingly)	S. epidermidis (MSSE/MRSE)	Vancomycin 1 gm (IV) q12h* **or** Linezolid 600 mg (IV) q12h*	Cefotaxime 2 gm (IV) q6h* **or** Ceftizoxime 2 gm (IV) q8h*	Linezolid 600 mg (PO) q12h*
	S. aureus (MSSA)	Clindamycin 600 mg (IV) q8h* **or** Cefazolin 1 gm (IV) q8h* **or** Nafcillin 2 gm (IV) q4h*	Cefotaxime 2 gm (IV) q6h* **or** Ceftizoxime 2 gm (IV) q8h* **or** Meropenem 1 gm (IV) q8h* **or** Imipenem 1 gm (IV) q6h*	Clindamycin 300 mg (PO) q8h* **or** Cephalexin 1 gm (PO) q6h*
	S. aureus (MRSA)	Vancomycin 1 gm (IV) q12h* **or** Linezolid 600 mg (IV) q12h*	Minocycline 100 mg (IV) q12h* **or** Quinupristin/ dalfopristin 7.5 mg/kg (IV) q8h*	Minocycline 100 mg (PO) q12h* **or** Linezolid 600 mg (PO) q12h*

MSSA/MRSA – methicillin sensitive/resistant S. aureus; MSSE/MRSE – methicillin-sensitive/resistant S. epidermidis.
Duration of therapy represents total time IV or IV + PO. Most patients on IV therapy able to take PO meds should be switched to PO therapy after clinical improvement
* Treat for 1 week after joint prosthesis is replaced

Clinical Presentation: Pain in area of prosthesis with joint loosening/instability ± low-grade fevers
Diagnostic Considerations: Infected prosthesis is suggested by prosthetic loosening/lucent areas adjacent to prosthesis on plain films ± positive blood cultures. Diagnosis confirmed by bone scan. Use joint aspiration to identify organism
Pitfalls: An elevated ESR with prosthetic loosening suggests prosthetic joint infection. Mechanical loosening without infection is comon many years after joint replacement, but ESR is normal
Therapeutic Considerations: Infected prosthetic joints usually must be removed for cure. Replacement prosthesis may be inserted anytime after infected prosthesis is removed. To prevent infection of new joint prosthesis, extensive debridement of old infected material is important. If replacement of infected joint prosthesis is not possible, chronic suppressive therapy may be used with oral antibiotics; adding rifampin 600 mg (PO) q24h may be helpful
Prognosis: Related to adequate debridement of infected material when prosthetic joint is removed

Osteomyelitis

Subset	Usual Pathogens	Preferred IV Therapy	Alternate IV Therapy	PO Therapy or IV-to-PO Switch
Acute (Treat initially for MSSA; if later identified as MRSA or Enterobacteriaceae, treat accordingly)	S. aureus (MSSA)	Clindamycin 600 mg (IV) q8h x 4-6 weeks **or** Nafcillin 2 gm (IV) q4h x 4-6 weeks	Cefotaxime 2 gm (IV) q6h x 4-6 weeks **or** Ceftizoxime 2 gm (IV) q8h x 4-6 weeks	Clindamycin 300 mg (PO) q8h x 4-6 weeks **or** Cephalexin 1 gm (PO) q6h x 4-6 weeks
	S. aureus (MRSA)	Vancomycin 1 gm (IV) q12h x 4-6 weeks **or** Linezolid 600 mg (IV) q12h x 4-6 weeks	Minocycline 100 mg (IV) q12h x 4-6 weeks **or** Quinupristin/ dalfopristin 7.5 mg/kg (IV) q8h x 4-6 weeks	Linezolid 600 mg (PO) q12h x 4-6 weeks **or** Minocycline 100 mg (PO) q12h x 4-6 weeks
	Enterobacteriaceae	Ceftriaxone 1 gm (IV) q24h x 4-6 weeks **or** Levofloxacin 500 mg (IV) q24h x 4-6 weeks	Cefotaxime 2 gm (IV) q6h x 4-6 weeks **or** Ceftizoxime 2 gm (IV) q8h x 4-6 weeks	Levofloxacin 500 mg (PO) q24h x 4-6 weeks **or** Gatifloxacin 400 mg (PO) q24h x 4-6 weeks
Chronic *Diabetes mellitus*	Group A, B streptococci S. aureus (MSSA) E. coli P. mirabilis K. pneumoniae B. fragilis	Meropenem 1 gm (IV) q8h* **or** Imipenem 1 gm (IV) q6h* **or** Ertapenem 1 gm (IV) q24h* **or** Piperacillin/ tazobactam 4.5 mg (IV) q8h*	Ceftizoxime 2 gm (IV) q8h* **or** Ampicillin/ sulbactam 3 gm (IV) q6h* **or** Moxifloxacin 400 mg (IV) q24h* **or combination therapy with** Clindamycin 600 mg (IV) q8h* **plus** Levofloxacin 500 mg (IV) q24h*	Clindamycin 300 mg (PO) q8h* **plus** Levofloxacin 500 (PO) q24h* **or monotherapy with** Moxifloxacin 400 mg (PO) q24h*
		* Treat for 1 week after adequate debridement or amputation		

Osteomyelitis (cont'd)

Subset	Usual Pathogens	Preferred IV Therapy	Alternate IV Therapy	PO Therapy or IV-to-PO Switch
Chronic *Peripheral vascular disease (non-diabetics)*	S. aureus Group A, B streptococci Entero-bacteriaceae	Cefotaxime 2 gm (IV) q6h x 2-4 weeks **or** Ceftizoxime 2 gm (IV) q8h x 2-4 weeks	Clindamycin 600 mg (IV) q8h x 2-4 weeks **plus** Levofloxacin 500 mg (IV) q24h x 2-4 weeks	Clindamycin 300 mg (PO) q8h x 2-4 weeks **plus** Levofloxacin 500 mg (PO) q24h x 2-4 weeks
TB osteomyelitis	M. tuberculosis	Not applicable		Treat the same as pulmonary TB (p. 44)

MSSA/MRSA = methicillin-sensitive/resistant S. aureus. Duration of therapy represents total time IV, PO, or IV + PO. Most patients on IV therapy able to take PO meds should be switched to PO therapy soon after clinical improvement

Acute Osteomyelitis
Clinical Presentation: Tenderness over infected bone. Fever and positive blood cultures common
Diagnostic Considerations: Diagnosis by elevated ESR with positive bone scan. Bone biopsy is not needed for diagnosis. Bone scan is positive for acute osteomyelitis in first 24 hours
Pitfalls: Earliest sign on plain films is soft tissue swelling; bony changes evident after 2 weeks
Therapeutic Considerations: Treat 4-6 weeks with antibiotics. Debridement is not necessary for cure
Prognosis: Related to adequacy/promptness of treatment

Chronic Osteomyelitis
Diabetes Mellitus
Clinical Presentation: Afebrile or low-grade fever with normal WBC counts and deep penetrating ulcers ± draining sinus tracts
Diagnostic Considerations: Diagnosis by elevated ESR and bone changes on plain films. Bone scan is not needed for diagnosis. Bone biopsy is preferred method of demonstrating organisms, since blood cultures are usually negative and cultures from ulcers/sinus tracts are unreliable
Pitfalls: P. aeruginosa is a common colonizer and frequently cultured from deep ulcers/sinus tracts, but is not a pathogen in chronic osteomyelitis in diabetics
Therapeutic Considerations: Surgical debridement is needed for cure; antibiotics alone are ineffective. Revascularization procedures usually do not help, since diabetes is a microvascular disease. Do not culture penetrating foot ulcers/draining sinus tracts; culture results reflect superficial flora. Bone biopsy during debridement is the best way to identify pathogen; if biopsy not possible, treat empirically
Prognosis: Related to adequacy of blood supply/surgical debridement

Non-Diabetics with Peripheral Vascular Disease (PVD)
Clinical Presentation: Absent or low-grade fever with normal WBC counts ± wet/dry digital gangrene
Diagnostic Considerations: Diagnosis by clinical appearance of dusky/cold foot ± wet/dry gangrene. Chronic osteomyelitis secondary to PVD/open fracture is often polymicrobial
Pitfalls: Wet gangrene usually requires surgical debridement/antibiotic therapy; dry gangrene may not
Therapeutic Considerations: Surgical debridement needed for cure. Antibiotics alone are ineffective. Revascularization procedure may help treat infection by improving local blood supply
Prognosis: Related to degree of vascular compromise

TB Osteomyelitis (Mycobacterium tuberculosis)
Clinical Presentation: Presents similar to chronic bacterial osteomyelitis. Vertebral TB (Pott's disease) affects disk spaces early and presents with chronic back/neck pain ± inguinal/paraspinal mass

Diagnostic Considerations: Diagnosis by AFB on biopsy/culture of infected bone. PPD–positive
Pitfalls: Chest x-ray is normal in 50%. May be confused with cancer or chronic bacterial osteomyelitis
Therapeutic Considerations: Treated the same as TB arthritis
Prognosis: Good for non-vertebral TB/vertebral (if treated before paraparesis/paraplegia)

Empiric Therapy of Skin and Soft Tissue Infections

Cellulitis (Erysipelas/Impetigo)/Lymphangitis

Subset	Usual Pathogens	Preferred IV Therapy	Alternate IV Therapy	PO Therapy or IV-to-PO Switch
Above-the-waist (including mastitis) (Treat initially for Gp. A strep, MSSA; if later identified as MRSA, treat accordingly)	Group A streptococci S. aureus (MSSA)	Cefazolin 1 gm (IV) q8h x 2 weeks	Nafcillin 2 gm (IV) q4h x 2 weeks **or** Clindamycin 600 mg (IV) q8h x 2 weeks	Cephalexin 500 mg (PO) q6h x 2 weeks **or** Clindamycin 300 mg (PO) q6h x 2 weeks
	S. aureus (MRSA)	Vancomycin 1 gm (IV) q12h x 2 weeks **or** Linezolid 600 mg (IV) q12h x 2 weeks	Minocycline 100 mg (IV) q12h x 2 weeks **or** Quinupristin/ dalfopristin 7.5 mg/kg (IV) q8h x 2 weeks	Linezolid 600 mg (PO) q12h x 2 weeks **or** Minocycline 100 mg (PO) q12h x 2 weeks
Below-the-waist (Treat initially for Gp. A,B strep, etc.; if later identified as MRSA, treat accordingly)	Group A, B streptococci E. coli P. mirabilis K. pneumoniae S. aureus (MSSA)	Ceftizoxime 2 gm (IV) q8h x 2 weeks **or** Levofloxacin 750 mg (IV) q24h x 2 weeks	Cefotaxime 2 gm (IV) q6h x 2 weeks **or** Cefoxitin 2 gm (IV) q6h x 2 weeks	Cephalexin 500 mg (PO) q6h x 2 weeks **or combination therapy with** Clindamycin 300 mg (PO) q6h x 2 weeks **plus** Levofloxacin 750 mg (PO) q24h x 2 weeks
	S. aureus (MRSA)	Vancomycin 1 gm (IV) q12h x 2 weeks **or** Linezolid 600 mg (IV) q12h x 2 weeks	Minocycline 100 mg (IV) q12h x 2 weeks **or** Quinupristin/ dalfopristin 7.5 mg/kg (IV) q8h x 2 weeks	Linezolid 600 mg (PO) q12h x 2 weeks **or** Minocycline 100 mg (PO) q12h x 2 weeks

*MSSA/MRSA = methicillin-sensitive/resistant S. aureus. Duration of therapy represents total time IV, PO, or IV + PO.
Most patients on IV therapy able to take PO meds should be switched to PO therapy soon after clinical improvement*

Clinical Presentation: Cellulitis presents as warm, painful, non-pruritic skin erythema without discharge. Impetigo is characterized by vesiculopustular lesions, most commonly on the face/extremities. Erysipelas resembles cellulitis, but is raised and sharply demarcated. Mastitis presents as cellulitis/abscess of the breast, and is treated the same as cellulitis above-the-waist

Diagnostic Considerations: Diagnosis by clinical appearance ± culture of pathogen from aspirated skin lesion(s). Group B streptococci are important pathogens in diabetics. Lower extremity cellulitis tends to recur. Chronic edema of an extremity predisposes to recurrent/persistent cellulitis

Pitfalls: Streptococcal and staphylococcal cellulitis may be indistinguishable clinically, but regional adenopathy/lymphangitis favors Streptococci, and bullae favor S. aureus

Therapeutic Considerations: Lower extremity cellulitis requires ~ 1 week of antibiotics to improve. Patients with peripheral vascular disease, chronic venous stasis, alcoholic cirrhosis, and diabetes take 1-2 weeks longer to improve and often require 3-4 weeks of treatment. Treat mastitis as cellulitis above-the-waist, and drain surgically if an abscess is present

Prognosis: Related to degree of vascular insufficiency

Soft Tissue Infections

Subset	Usual Pathogens	Preferred IV Therapy	Alternate IV Therapy	IV-to-PO Switch
Mixed aerobic-anaerobic deep soft tissue infection	Entero-bacteriaceae Group A streptococci S. aureus Anaerobic streptococci Fusobacterium	Meropenem 1 gm (IV) q8h x 2 weeks **or** Imipenem 1 gm (IV) q6h x 2 weeks **or** Ertapenem 1 gm (IV) q24h x 2 weeks **or** Piperacillin/ tazobactam 4.5 gm (IV) q8h x 2 weeks	Clindamycin 600 mg (IV) q8h x 2 weeks **plus** Levofloxacin 750 mg (IV) q24h x 2 weeks **or monotherapy with** Cefoxitin 2 gm (IV) q6h x 2 weeks	Clindamycin 300 mg (PO) q8h x 2 weeks **plus** Levofloxacin 750 mg (PO) q24h x 2 weeks
Clostridial myonecrosis (gas gangrene)	Clostridia sp.	Penicillin G 10 mu (IV) q4h x 2 weeks **or** Clindamycin 600 mg (IV) q8h x 2 weeks **or** Piperacillin/ tazobactam 4.5 gm (IV) q8h x 2 weeks	Meropenem 1 gm (IV) q8h x 2 weeks **or** Imipenem 1 gm (IV) q6h x 2 weeks **or** Ertapenem 1 gm (IV) q24h x 2 weeks	Clindamycin 300 mg (PO) q8h x 2 weeks **plus** Levofloxacin 750 mg (PO) q24h x 2 weeks

Soft Tissue Infections (cont'd)

Subset	Usual Pathogens	Preferred IV Therapy	Alternate IV Therapy	IV-to-PO Switch
Necrotizing fasciitis/ synergistic gangrene	Group A streptococci Entero-bacteriaceae Anaerobic streptococci S. aureus (MSSA)	Meropenem 1 gm (IV) q8h x 2 weeks **or** Imipenem 1 gm (IV) q6h x 2 weeks **or** Ertapenem 1 gm (IV) q24h x 2 weeks **or** Piperacillin/ tazobactam 4.5 gm (IV) q8h x 2 weeks	Clindamycin 600 mg (IV) q8h x 2 weeks **plus** Levofloxacin 750 mg (IV) q24h x 2 weeks	Clindamycin 300 mg (PO) q8h x 2 weeks **plus** Levofloxacin 750 mg (PO) q24h x 2 weeks

Duration of therapy represents total time IV or IV + PO. Most patients on IV therapy able to take PO meds should be switched to PO therapy after clinical improvement

Mixed Aerobic/Anaerobic Deep Soft Tissue Infection
Clinical Presentation: Acutely ill patient with gross gas deep in soft tissues and usually high fevers
Diagnostic Considerations: Diagnosis by gram stain/culture of aspirated fluid. Patients usually have high fevers. Wound discharge is foul when present
Pitfalls: Gross crepitance/prominent gas in soft tissues on x-ray suggests a mixed aerobic/anaerobic necrotizing infection, not gas gangrene
Therapeutic Considerations: Prompt surgical debridement may be life-saving. Control/cure of infection requires surgical debridement and antibiotics
Prognosis: Related to severity of infection, adequacy of debridement, and underlying health of host

Gas Gangrene (Clostridial Myonecrosis)
Clinical Presentation: Fulminant infection of muscle with little or no fever. Infected area is extremely painful, indurated, and discolored with or without bullae
Diagnostic Considerations: Diagnosis is clinical. Aspiration of infected muscle shows few PMNs and gram-positive bacilli without spores. Gas gangrene is not accompanied by high fever. Patients are often apprehensive with relative bradycardia ± diarrhea. Wound discharge, if present, is sweetish and not foul. Rapidly progressive hemolytic anemia is characteristic
Pitfalls: Gas gangrene (clostridial myonecrosis) has little visible gas on plain film x-rays; abundant gas should suggest a mixed aerobic/anaerobic infection, not gas gangrene
Therapeutic Considerations: Surgical debridement is life-saving and the only way to control infection
Prognosis: Related to speed/extent of surgical debridement. Rapid progression/death may occur within hours

Necrotizing Fasciitis/Synergistic Gangrene
Clinical Presentation: Acutely ill patient with high fevers and extreme local pain without gas in tissues
Diagnostic Considerations: Diagnosis by CT/MRI of involved extremity showing infection confined to one or more muscle compartments/fascial planes. Patients are febrile and ill. Gas is not present on

exam or x-rays. May be polymicrobial or due to a single organism. Foul smelling exudate from infected soft tissues indicates anaerobes are present

Pitfalls: Extreme pain in patients with deep soft tissue infections should suggest a compartment syndrome/necrotizing fasciitis. No hemolytic anemia, diarrhea, or bullae as with gas gangrene

Therapeutic Considerations: Control/cure of infection requires surgical decompression of infected compartment, debridement of dead tissue in necrotizing fasciitis, and antimicrobial therapy

Prognosis: Related to rapidity/extent of surgical debridement

Skin Ulcers

Subset	Usual Pathogens	Preferred IV Therapy	Alternate IV Therapy	PO Therapy or IV-to-PO Switch
Decubitus ulcers *Above the waist*	Group A streptococci E. coli P. mirabilis K. pneumoniae S. aureus (MSSA)	Cefazolin 1 gm (IV) q8h*	Cefotaxime 2 gm (IV) q6h*	Cephalexin 500 mg (PO) q6h*
Below the waist	Group A streptococci E. coli P. mirabilis K. pneumoniae B. fragilis S. aureus (MSSA)	Ceftizoxime 2 gm (IV) q8h* **or** Cefoxitin 2 gm (IV) q6h*	Moxifloxacin 400 mg (IV) q24h* **or combination therapy with** Clindamycin 600 mg (IV) q6h* **plus** Levofloxacin 500 mg (IV) q24h*	Moxifloxacin 400 mg (PO) q24h* **or combination therapy with** Clindamycin 300 mg (PO) q8h* **plus** Levofloxacin 500 mg (PO) q24h*
Diabetic foot ulcers (chronic osteomyelitis)	Group A, B streptococci S. aureus (MSSA) E. coli P. mirabilis K. pneumoniae B. fragilis	Meropenem 1 gm (IV) q8h† **or** Imipenem 1 gm (IV) q6h† **or** Ertapenem 1 gm (IV) q24h† **or** Piperacillin/ tazobactam 4.5 gm (IV) q8h†	Ceftizoxime 2 gm (IV) q8h† **or** Ampicillin/sulbactam 3 gm (IV) q6h† **or** Moxifloxacin 400 mg (IV) q24h† **or combination therapy with** Clindamycin 600 mg (IV) q8h† **plus** Levofloxacin 500 mg (IV) q24h†	Clindamycin 300 mg (PO) q8h† **plus** Levofloxacin 500 mg (PO) q24h† **or monotherapy with** Moxifloxacin 400 mg (PO) q24h†

Skin Ulcers (cont'd)

Subset	Usual Pathogens	Preferred IV Therapy	Alternate IV Therapy	PO Therapy or IV-to-PO Switch
Ischemic foot ulcers	Group A streptococci E. coli S. aureus (MSSA)	Cefotaxime 2 gm (IV) q8h x 2 weeks **or** Ceftizoxime 2 gm (IV) q8h x 2 weeks **or** Cefoxitin 2 gm (IV) q6h x 2 weeks	Clindamycin 600 mg (IV) q8h x 2 weeks **plus** Levofloxacin 750 mg (IV) q24h x 2 weeks	Clindamycin 300 mg (PO) q8h x 2 weeks **plus** Levofloxacin 750 mg (PO) q24h x 2 weeks

MSSA = methicillin-sensitive S. aureus. Duration of therapy represents total time IV, PO, or IV + PO. Most patients on IV therapy able to take PO meds should be switched to PO therapy soon after clinical improvement (usually < 72 hrs)
* *Treat Stages I/II (superficial) decubitus ulcers with local care. Treat Stages III/IV (deep) decubitus ulcers with antibiotics for 1-2 weeks after adequate debridement*
† *Treat for 1 week after adequate debridement or amputation*

Decubitus Ulcers
Clinical Presentation: Painless ulcers with variable depth and infectious exudate ± fevers ≤ 102°F
Diagnostic Considerations: Diagnosis by clinical appearance. Obtain ESR/bone scan to rule out underlying osteomyelitis with deep (Stage III/IV) decubitus ulcers
Pitfalls: Superficial decubitus ulcers do not require systemic antibiotics
Therapeutic Considerations: Deep decubitus ulcers require antibiotics and debridement, superficial ulcers do not. Coverage for B. fragilis is needed for deep perianal decubitus ulcers. Good nursing care is important in preventing/limiting extension of decubitus ulcers
Prognosis: Related to fecal contamination of ulcer and bone involvement (e.g., osteomyelitis)

Diabetic Foot Ulcers/Chronic Osteomyelitis
Clinical Presentation: Ulcers/sinus tracts on bottom of foot/between toes; usually painless. Fevers ≤ 102°F and a foul smelling exudate are common
Diagnostic Considerations: In diabetics, deep, penetrating, chronic foot ulcers/draining sinus tracts are diagnostic of chronic osteomyelitis. ESR ≥ 100 mm/hr in a diabetic with a foot ulcer/sinus tract is diagnostic of chronic osteomyelitis. Foot films confirm chronic osteomyelitis. Bone scan is needed only in acute osteomyelitis
Pitfalls: Do not rely on culture results of deep ulcers/sinus tracts to choose antibiotic coverage, since cultures reflect skin colonization, not bone pathogens. Treat empirically
Therapeutic Considerations: B. fragilis coverage is required in deep penetrating diabetic foot ulcers/fetid foot infection. P. aeruginosa is often cultured from diabetic foot ulcers/sinus tracts, but represents colonization, not infection. P. aeruginosa is a "water" organism that colonizes feet from moist socks/dressings, irrigant solutions, or whirlpool baths. Surgical debridement is essential for cure of chronic osteomyelitis in diabetics. Treat superficial diabetic foot ulcers the same as cellulitis in non-diabetics (p. 96)
Prognosis: Related to adequacy of debridement of infected bone

Ischemic Foot Ulcers
Clinical Presentation: Ulcers often clean/dry ± digital gangrene. No fevers/exudate
Diagnostic Considerations: Diagnosis by clinical appearance/location in a patient with peripheral

vascular disease. Ischemic foot ulcers most commonly affect the toes, medial malleoli, dorsum of foot, or lower leg

Pitfalls: In contrast to ulcers in diabetics, ischemic ulcers due to peripheral vascular disease usually do not involve the plantar surface of the foot

Therapeutic Considerations: Dry gangrene should not be treated with antibiotics unless accompanied by signs of systemic infection. Wet gangrene should be treated as a mixed aerobic/anaerobic infection. Both dry/wet gangrene may require debridement for cure/control. Do not rely on ulcer cultures to guide treatment; treat empirically if necessary. Evaluate for revascularization

Prognosis: Related to degree of vascular insufficiency

Skin Abscesses/Infected Cysts
(Skin Pustules, Skin Boils, Furunculosis)

Subset	Usual Pathogens	Preferred IV Therapy	Alternate IV Therapy	PO Therapy or IV-to-PO Switch
Skin abscesses (Treat initially for MSSA; if later identified as MRSA, treat accordingly)	S. aureus (MSSA)	Clindamycin 600 mg (IV) q8h x 2 weeks	Cefazolin 1 gm (IV) q8h x 2 weeks **or** Nafcillin 2 gm (IV) q4h x 2 weeks	Cephalexin 500 mg (PO) q6h x 2 weeks **or** Clindamycin 300 mg (PO) q8h x 2 weeks
	S. aureus (MRSA)	Vancomycin 1 gm (IV) q12h x 2 weeks **or** Linezolid 600 mg (IV) q12h x 2 weeks	Minocycline 100 mg (IV) q12h x 2 weeks	Linezolid 600 mg (PO) q12h x 2 weeks **or** Minocycline 100 mg (PO) q12h x 2 weeks
Infected pilonidal cysts	Group A streptococci E. coli P. mirabilis K. pneumoniae S. aureus (MSSA)	Clindamycin 600 mg (IV) q8h x 2 weeks **plus** Levofloxacin 500 mg (IV) q24h x 2 weeks	Ceftizoxime 2 gm (IV) q8h x 2 weeks **or** Cefoxitin 2 gm (IV) q6h x 2 weeks	Clindamycin 300 mg (PO) q8h x 2 weeks **plus** Levofloxacin 500 mg (PO) q24h x 2 weeks
Hydradenitis suppurativa	S. aureus (MSSA)	Not applicable	TMP-SMX 1 SS tablet (PO) q12h x 2-4 weeks **or** Clindamycin 300 mg (PO) q8h x 2-4 weeks **or** Minocycline 100 mg (PO) q12h x 2-4 weeks	

MSSA/MRSA = methicillin-sensitive/resistant S. aureus. Duration of therapy represents total time IV, PO, or IV + PO. Most patients on IV therapy able to take PO meds should be switched to PO therapy soon after clinical improvement (usually < 72 hours)

Skin Abscesses

Clinical Presentation: Warm painful nodules ± bullae, low-grade fever ± systemic symptoms, no lymphangitis. Skin boils/furunculosis present as acute, chronic, or recurrent skin pustules, and remain localized without lymphangitis

Diagnostic Considerations: Specific pathogen diagnosed by gram stain of abscess. Recurring S.

aureus abscesses are not uncommon and should be drained. Blood cultures are rarely positive. Suspect Job's syndrome if recurring abscesses with peripheral eosinophilia. Skin boils/furunculosis are diagnosed by clinical appearance (skin pustules)
Pitfalls: Recurring S. aureus skin infections may occur on an immune basis, but immunologic studies are usually negative
Therapeutic Considerations: Repeated aspiration of abscesses may be necessary. Surgical drainage is required if antibiotics fail. Treat boils/furunculosis as in hydradenitis suppurativa
Prognosis: Excellent if treated early

Infected Pilonidal Cysts
Clinical Presentation: Chronic drainage from pilonidal cysts
Diagnostic Considerations: Diagnosis by clinical appearance. Deep/systemic infection is rare
Pitfalls: Culture of exudate is usually unhelpful
Therapeutic Considerations: Surgical debridement is often necessary
Prognosis: Good with adequate excision

Hydradenitis Suppurativa
Clinical Presentation: Chronic, indurated, painful, raised axillary/groin lesions ± drainage/sinus tracts
Diagnostic Considerations: Diagnosis by clinical appearance/location of lesions. Infections are often bilateral and tend to recur
Pitfalls: Surgical debridement is usually not necessary unless deep/extensive infection
Therapeutic Considerations: Most anti-S. aureus antibiotics have poor penetration and usually fail
Prognosis: Good with recommended antibiotics. Surgery, if necessary, is curative

Skin Vesicles (non-genital)

Subset	Usual Pathogens	IV Therapy	PO Therapy
Herpes simplex	Herpes simplex virus (HSV)	Not applicable	Acyclovir 400 mg (PO) q8h x 10 days **or** Valacyclovir 1 gm (PO) q12h x 10 days **or** Famciclovir 250 mg (PO) q8h x 10 days
Herpes zoster, dermatomal	Varicella zoster virus (VZV)	Not applicable	Acyclovir 800 mg (PO) 5x/day x 7 days **or** Famciclovir 500 mg (PO) q8h x 7 days **or** Valacyclovir 1 gm (PO) q8h x 7 days
Herpes whitlow	HSV-1	Not applicable	Acyclovir 400 mg (PO) q8h x 1-2 weeks **or** Valacyclovir 1 gm (PO) q12h x 1-2 weeks **or** Famciclovir 250 mg (PO) q8h x 1-2 weeks

Herpes Simplex (HSV)
Clinical Presentation: Painful, sometimes pruritic vesicles that form pustules or painful erythematous ulcers. Associated with fever, myalgias
Diagnostic Considerations: Diagnosis by clinical appearance and demonstration of HSV by culture of vesicle fluid/vesicle base. May be severe in HIV/AIDS

Pitfalls: Painful vesicular lesions surrounded by prominent induration distinguishes HSV from insect bites (pruritic) and cellulitis (no induration)

Therapeutic Considerations: Topical acyclovir ointment may be useful early when vesicles erupt, but is ineffective after vesicles stop erupting. For severe/refractory cases, use acyclovir 5 mg/kg (IV) q8h x 2-7 days, then if improvement, switch to acyclovir 400 mg (PO) q8h to complete 10-day course

Prognosis: Related to extent of tissue involvement/degree of cellular immunity dysfunction

Herpes Zoster (VZV)

Clinical Presentation: Painful, vesicular eruption in dermatomal distribution. Pain may be difficult to diagnose

Diagnostic Considerations: Diagnosis by appearance/positive Tzanck test of vesicle base scrapings

Pitfalls: Begin therapy within 2 days of vesicle eruption

Therapeutic Considerations: Higher doses of acyclovir are required for VZV than HSV. See p. 220 for disseminated VZV, ophthalmic nerve/visceral involvement, or acyclovir-resistant strains

Prognosis: Good if treated early. Some patients develop painful post-herpetic neuralgia of involved dermatomes

Herpes Whitlow

Clinical Presentation: Multiple vesicopustular lesions on fingers and hands. Lymphangitis, adenopathy, fever/chills are usually present, suggesting a bacterial infection

Diagnostic Considerations: Common in health care workers giving patients oral care/suctioning

Pitfalls: No need for antibiotics even though lesions appear infected with "pus"

Therapeutic Considerations: Never incise/drain herpes whitlow; surgical incision will flare/prolong the infection

Prognosis: Excellent, unless incision/drainage has been performed

Wound Infections (for rabies, see pp. 239, 246)

Subset	Usual Pathogens	Preferred IV Therapy	Alternate IV Therapy	PO Therapy or IV-to-PO Switch
Animal bite wounds	Group A streptococci P. multocida Capnocytophaga (DF2) S. aureus (MSSA)	Piperacillin/ tazobactam 4.5 gm (IV) q8h x 2 weeks **or** Ampicillin/ sulbactam 3 gm (IV) q6h x 2 weeks	Meropenem 1 gm (IV) q8h x 2 weeks **or** Imipenem 1 gm (IV) q6h x 2 weeks **or** Ertapenem 1 gm (IV) q24h x 2 weeks	Amoxicillin/ clavulanic acid 875 mg (PO) q12h x 2 weeks **or** Doxycycline 200 mg (PO) q12h x 3 days, then 100 mg (PO) q12h x 11 days
Human bite wounds	Oral anaerobes Group A streptococci E. corrodens S. aureus (MSSA)	Piperacillin/ tazobactam 4.5 gm (IV) q8h x 2 weeks **or** Ampicillin/ sulbactam 3 gm (IV) q6h x 2 weeks	Meropenem 1 gm (IV) q8h x 2 weeks **or** Imipenem 1 gm (IV) q6h x 2 weeks **or** Ertapenem 1 gm (IV) q24h x 2 weeks	Amoxicillin/ clavulanic acid 875 mg (PO) q12h x 2 weeks **or** Doxycycline 200 mg (PO) q12h x 3 days, then 100 mg (PO) q12h x 11 days

Wound Infections (cont'd) (for rabies, see pp. 239, 246)

Subset	Usual Pathogens	Preferred IV Therapy	Alternate IV Therapy	PO Therapy or IV-to-PO Switch
Cat scratch fever	Bartonella henselae	Doxycycline 200 mg (IV) q12h x 3 days, then 100 mg (IV) q12h x 4-8 weeks **or** Azithromycin 500 mg (IV) q24h x 4-8 weeks	Chloramphenicol 500 mg (IV) q6h x 4-8 weeks	Doxycycline 200 mg (PO) q12h x 3 days, then 100 mg (PO) q12h x 4-8 weeks* **or** Azithromycin 250 mg (PO) q24h x 4-8 weeks **or** Levofloxacin 500 mg (PO) q24h x 4-8 weeks
Burn wounds (severe)[†]	Group A streptococci Enterobacter P. aeruginosa	Cefepime 2 gm (IV) q8h x 2 weeks **or** Meropenem 1 gm (IV) q8h x 2 weeks	Piperacillin 4 gm (IV) q8h x 2 weeks **plus** Gentamicin 240 mg (IV) q24h x 2 weeks	Not applicable
Freshwater-exposed wounds	Aeromonas hydrophilia	Levofloxacin 500 mg (IV) q24h x 2 weeks **or** TMP-SMX 2.5 mg/kg (IV) q6h x 2 weeks	Aztreonam 2 gm (IV) q8h x 2 weeks **or** Gentamicin 240 mg (IV) q24h x 2 weeks **or** Ceftriaxone 1 gm (IV) q24h x 2 weeks	Levofloxacin 500 mg (PO) q24h x 2 weeks **or** TMP-SMX 1 SS tablet (PO) q12h x 2 weeks
Saltwater-exposed wounds	Vibrio vulnificus	Doxycycline 200 mg (IV) q12h x 3 days, then 100 mg (IV) q12h x 11 days **or** Levofloxacin 500 mg (IV) q24h x 2 weeks	Ceftriaxone 2 gm (IV) q12h x 2 weeks **or** Chloramphenicol 500 mg (IV) q6h x 2 weeks	Doxycycline 200 mg (PO) q12h x 3 days, then 100 mg (PO) q12h x 11 days* **or** Levofloxacin 500 mg (PO) q24h x 2 weeks

MSSA = methicillin-sensitive S. aureus. Duration of therapy represents total time IV, PO, or IV + PO. Most patients on IV therapy able to take PO meds should be switched to PO therapy soon after clinical improvement
† Treat only IV or IV-to-PO switch
* Loading dose is not needed PO if given IV with the same drug

Animal Bite Wounds (for rabies, see p. 239)
Clinical Presentation: Cellulitis surrounding bite wound
Diagnostic Considerations: Diagnosis by culture of bite wound exudate. Deep bites may also cause tendinitis/osteomyelitis, and severe bites may result in systemic infection with bacteremia
Pitfalls: Avoid erythromycin in penicillin-allergic patients (ineffective against P. multocida)
Therapeutic Considerations: For facial/hand bites, consult a plastic surgeon
Prognosis: Related to adequacy of debridement and early antibiotic therapy

Human Bite Wounds
Clinical Presentation: Cellulitis surrounding bite wound
Diagnostic Considerations: Diagnosis by culture of bite wound exudate. Infection often extends to involve tendon/bone
Pitfalls: Compared to animal bites, human bites are more likely to contain anaerobes, S. aureus, and Group A streptococci
Therapeutic Considerations: Avoid primary closure of human bite wounds
Prognosis: Related to adequacy of debridement and early antibiotic therapy

Cat Scratch Fever/Disease (Bartonella henselae)
Clinical Presentation: Subacute presentation of obscure febrile illness associated with cat bite/contact. Usually accompanied by adenopathy
Diagnostic Considerations: Diagnosis by wound culture/serology for Bartonella. Cat scratch fever/disease may follow a cat scratch, but a lick from a kitten contaminating an inapparent microlaceration is more common. May present as an FUO. Culture of exudate/node is unlikely to be positive, but silver stain of biopsy material shows organisms
Pitfalls: Rule out lymphoma, which may present in similar fashion
Therapeutic Considerations: Prolonged oral antibiotic therapy may be necessary. Treat until symptoms/signs resolve. Bartonella are sensitive in-vitro to cephalosporins and TMP-SMX, but these antibiotics are ineffective in-vivo
Prognosis: Related to health of host

Burn Wounds
Clinical Presentation: Severe (3rd/4th degree) burns ± drainage
Diagnostic Considerations: Semi-quantitative bacterial counts help differentiate colonization (low counts) from infection (high counts). Burn wounds quickly become colonized
Pitfalls: Treat only infected 3rd/4th degree burn wounds with systemic antibiotics
Therapeutic Considerations: Meticulous local care/eschar removal/surgical debridement is key in preventing and controlling infection
Prognosis: Related to severity of burns and adequacy of eschar debridement

Freshwater-Exposed Wounds (Aeromonas hydrophilia)
Clinical Presentation: Fulminant wound infection with fever and diarrhea
Diagnostic Considerations: Diagnosis by stool/wound/blood culture
Pitfalls: Suspect A. hydrophilia in wound infection with fresh water exposure followed by diarrhea
Therapeutic Considerations: Surgical debridement of devitalized tissue may be necessary
Prognosis: Related to severity of infection and health of host

Saltwater-Exposed Wounds (Vibrio vulnificus)
Clinical Presentation: Fulminant wound infection with fever, painful hemorrhagic bullae, diarrhea
Diagnostic Considerations: Diagnosis by stool/wound/blood culture. Vibrio vulnificus is a fulminant, life-threatening infection that may be accompanied by hypotension
Pitfalls: Suspect V. vulnificus in acutely ill patients with fever, diarrhea, and bullous lesions after salt

water exposure
Therapeutic Considerations: Surgical debridement of devitalized tissue may be necessary
Prognosis: Related to extent of infection and health of host

Superficial Fungal Infections of Skin and Nails

Subset	Usual Pathogens	Topical Therapy	PO Therapy
Cutaneous (local/non-disseminated) candidiasis	C. albicans	<u>Interdigital, other local</u> Clotrimazole 1% cream twice daily x 2-4 weeks	<u>Onychomycosis (nail infection)</u> Itraconazole 200 mg (PO) q12h x 1 week per month for 2 months <u>Cutaneous (local/non-disseminated) candidiasis</u> Fluconazole 400 mg (PO) x 1 dose, then 200 mg (PO) q24h x 2 weeks
Tinea corporis (body ringworm)	Trichophyton rubrum Epidermophyton floccosum Microsporum canis Trichophyton mentagrophytes	Clotrimazole 1% cream twice daily x 4-8 weeks **or** Miconazole 2% cream twice daily x 2 weeks **or** Econazole 1% cream twice daily x 2 weeks	Terbinafine 250 mg (PO) q24h x 4 weeks **or** Ketoconazole 200 mg (PO) q24h x 4 weeks **or** Fluconazole 200 mg (PO) weekly x 4 weeks
Tinea capitis (scalp ringworm)	Same as Tinea corporis, above	Selenium sulfide shampoo daily x 2-4 weeks	Same as Tinea corporis, above
Tinea cruris (jock itch)	T. cruris	Same as Tinea corporis, above	Same as Tinea corporis, above
Tinea pedis (athlete's foot)	Same as Tinea corporis, above	Same as Tinea corporis, above	Terbinafine 250 mg (PO) q24h x 2 weeks **or** Ketoconazole 200 mg (PO) q24h x 4 weeks **or** Itraconazole 200 mg (PO) q24h x 4 weeks
Tinea versicolor (pityriasis)	M. furfur (Pityrosporum orbiculare)	Clotrimazole cream (1%) or miconazole cream (2%) or ketoconazole cream (2%) daily x 7 days	Ketoconazole 200 mg (PO) q24h x 7 days **or** Itraconazole 200 mg (PO) q24h x 7 days **or** Fluconazole 400 mg (PO) x 1 dose

Superficial Fungal Infections of Skin and Nails (cont'd)

Subset	Usual Pathogens	Topical Therapy	PO Therapy
Tinea unguium (onycho-mycosis)	Epidermophyton floccosum Trichophyton mentagrophytes Trichophyton rubrum	Not applicable	Itraconazole 200 mg (PO) 1 week per month x 2 months (fingernail infection) or 3 months (toenail infection) **or** Terbinafine 250 mg (PO) q24h x 6 weeks (fingernail infection) or 12 weeks (toenail infection) **or** Fluconazole 200 mg (PO) 1 week per month x 3 months (fingernail infection) or 6 months (toenail infection)

Cutaneous (Local/Nondisseminated) Candidiasis
Clinical Presentation: Primary cutaneous findings include an erythematous rash with satellite lesions, which may be papular, pustular, or ulcerated. Lesions can be limited or widespread over parts of body. Chronic mucocutaneous candidiasis manifests as recurrent candidal infections of skin, nails, or mucous membranes
Diagnostic Considerations: Diagnosis by demonstrating organism by stain/culture in tissue specimen. In HIV/AIDS, Candida is very common on skin/mucous membranes
Pitfalls: Do not confuse with the isolated, multinodular lesions of disseminated disease, which may resemble ecthyma gangrenosa or purpura fulminans
Therapeutic Considerations: Diabetics and other compromised hosts may require prolonged therapy. In contrast to local disease, nodular cutaneous candidiasis represents disseminated disease (p. 187)
Prognosis: Related to extent of disease/host defense status

Tinea Corporis (Body Ringworm)
Clinical Presentation: Annular pruritic lesions on trunk/face with central clearing
Diagnostic Considerations: Diagnosis by clinical appearance/skin scraping
Pitfalls: Do not confuse with Erythema migrans, which is not pruritic
Therapeutic Considerations: If topical therapy fails, treat with oral antifungals
Prognosis: Excellent

Tinea Capitis (Scalp Ringworm)
Clinical Presentation: Itchy, annular scalp lesions
Diagnostic Considerations: Scalp lesions fluoresce with ultraviolet light. Culture hair shafts
Pitfalls: T. capitis is associated with localized areas of alopecia
Therapeutic Considerations: Selenium sulfide shampoo may be used first for 2-4 weeks. Treat shampoo failures with oral ketoconazole, terbinafine, or fluconazole
Prognosis: Excellent

Tinea Cruris (Jock Itch)
Clinical Presentation: Groin, inguinal, perineal, or buttock lesions that are pruritic and serpiginous with scaling borders/central clearing
Diagnostic Considerations: Diagnosis by clinical appearance/culture
Pitfalls: Usually spares penis/scrotum, unlike Candida

Therapeutic Considerations: In addition to therapy, it is important to keep area dry
Prognosis: Excellent

Tinea Pedis (Athlete's Foot)
Clinical Presentation: Painful cracks/fissures between toes
Diagnostic Considerations: Diagnosis by clinical appearance/skin scraping
Pitfalls: Must keep feet dry or infection will recur
Therapeutic Considerations: In addition to therapy, it is important to keep area dry
Prognosis: Excellent

Tinea Versicolor (Pityriasis)
Clinical Presentation: Oval hypo- or hyperpigmented scaly lesions that coalesce into large confluent areas typically on upper trunk; chronic/relapsing
Diagnostic Considerations: Diagnosis by clinical appearance and culture of affected skin lesions
Pitfalls: M. furfur also causes seborrheic dermatitis, but seborrheic lesions are typically on the face/scalp
Therapeutic Considerations: If topical therapy fails, treat with oral antifungals. Treat non-scalp seborrheic dermatitis with ketoconazole cream (2%) daily until cured
Prognosis: Excellent

Dermatophyte Nail Infections
Clinical Presentation: Chronically thickened, discolored nails
Diagnostic Considerations: Diagnosis by culture of nail clippings
Pitfalls: Nail clipping cultures often contaminated by bacterial/fungal colonizers. Green nail discoloration suggests P. aeruginosa, not a fungal nail infection; treat with ciprofloxacin 500 mg (PO) q12h x 2-3 weeks
Therapeutic Considerations: Prolonged therapy may be required until nail infection completely clears
Prognosis: Excellent if infection is totally eradicated from nail bed. New nail growth takes weeks

Skin Infestations

Subset	Usual Pathogens	IV/PO Therapy	Topical Therapy
Scabies	Sarcoptes scabiei	Not applicable	Treat whole body with Permethrin cream 5% (Elimite); leave on for 8-10 hours
Head lice	Pediculus humanus var. capitis	Not applicable	Shampoo with Permethrin 5% (Elimite) or 1% (NIX) cream x 10 minutes
Body lice	Pediculus humanus var. corporis	Not applicable	Body lice removed by shower. Removed clothes should be washed in hot water or sealed in bags for 1 month, or treated with DDT powder 10% or malathion powder 1%
Pubic lice (crabs)	Phthirus pubis	Not applicable	Permethrin 5% (Elimite) or 1% (NIX) cream x 10 minutes to affected areas

Scabies (Sarcoptes scabiei)
Clinical Presentation: Punctate, serpiginous, intensely pruritic black spots in webbed spaces of hands/feet and creases of elbows/knees
Diagnostic Considerations: Diagnosis by visualization of skin tracts/burrows. Incubation period up

to 6 weeks after contact. Spread by scratching from one part of body to another
Pitfalls: Mites are not visible, only their skin tracks
Therapeutic Considerations: Permethrin cream is usually effective. If itching persists after treatment, do not retreat (itching is secondary to hypersensitivity reaction of eggs in skin burrows). Treat close contacts. Vacuum bedding/furniture
Prognosis: Norwegian scabies is very difficult to eradicate

Head Lice (Pediculus humanus var. capitis)
Clinical Presentation: White spots may be seen on hair shafts of head/neck, but not eyebrows
Diagnostic Considerations: Nits on hair are unhatched lice eggs, seen as white dots attached to hair shaft. May survive away from body x 2 days
Pitfalls: May need to retreat in 7 days to kill any lice that hatched from surviving nits
Therapeutic Considerations: Shampoo with Permethrin 5% (Elimite) or 1% (NIX) cream kills lice/nits. Clothes and non-washables should be tied off in plastic bags x 2 weeks to kill lice. Alternately, wash and dry clothes/bed linens; heat from dryer/iron kills lice
Prognosis: Related to thoroughness of therapy

Body Lice (Pediculus humanus var. corporis)
Clinical Presentation: Intense generalized pruritus
Diagnostic Considerations: Smaller than head lice and more difficult to see. May survive away from body x 1 week
Pitfalls: Body lice live in clothes; leave only for a blood meal, then return to clothing
Therapeutic Considerations: Can survive in seams of clothing x 1 week
Prognosis: Good if clothes are also treated

Pubic Lice (Phthirus pubis) Crabs
Clinical Presentation: Genital pruritus
Diagnostic Considerations: Seen on groin, eyelashes, axilla. May survive away from body x 1 day
Pitfalls: Smaller than head lice, but easily seen
Therapeutic Considerations: Treat partners. Wash, dry, and iron clothes; heat from dryer/iron kills lice. Non-washables may be placed in a sealed bag x 7 days
Prognosis: Good if clothes are also treated

Ischiorectal/Perirectal Abscess

Subset	Pathogens	Preferred Therapy
Ischiorectal/ perirectal abscess	Enterobacteriaceae B. fragilis	Treat the same as mild/severe peritonitis (p. 72) ± surgical drainage depending on abscess size/severity

Clinical Presentation: Presents in normal hosts with perirectal pain, pain on defecation, leukocytosis, erythema/tenderness over abscess ± fever/chills. In febrile neutropenia, there is only tenderness
Diagnostic Considerations: Diagnosis by erythema/tenderness over abscess or by CT/MRI
Pitfalls: Do not confuse with perirectal regional enteritis (Crohn's disease) in normal hosts, or with ecthyma gangrenosum in febrile neutropenics
Therapeutic Considerations: Antibiotic therapy may be adequate for mild cases. Large abscesses require drainage plus antibiotics x 1-2 weeks post-drainage. With febrile neutropenia, use an antibiotic that is acitve against both P. aeruginosa and B. fragilis (e.g., meropenem, piperacillin/tazobactam)
Prognosis: Good with early drainage/therapy

Sepsis, Septic Shock, Febrile Neutropenia

Sepsis/Septic Shock

Subset	Usual Pathogens	Preferred IV Therapy	Alternate IV Therapy	IV-to-PO Switch
Unknown source (CNS source excluded)	Entero-bacteriaceae B. fragilis	Meropenem 1 gm (IV) q8h x 2 weeks **or** Imipenem 1 gm (IV) q6h x 2 weeks **or** Ertapenem 1 gm (IV) q24h x 2 weeks **or** Piperacillin/ tazobactam 4.5 gm (IV) q8h x 2 weeks	Levofloxacin 500 mg (IV) q24h x 2 weeks **plus either** Metronidazole 1 gm (IV) q24h x 2 weeks **or** Clindamycin 600 mg (IV) q8h x 2 weeks	Levofloxacin 500 mg (PO) q24h x 2 weeks **plus** Clindamycin 300 mg (PO) q8h x 2 weeks
SLE *Lungs or urinary tract focus*	S. pneumoniae H. influenzae Non-enterococcal streptococci Entero-bacteriaceae	Levofloxacin 500 mg (IV) q24h x 2 weeks **or** Ceftriaxone 2 gm (IV) q24h x 2 weeks	Cefepime 2 gm (IV) q12h x 2 weeks **or** Cefotaxime 2 gm (IV) q6h x 2 weeks	Levofloxacin 500 mg (PO) q24h x 2 weeks **or** Doxycycline 200 mg (PO) q12h x 3 days, then 100 mg (PO) q12h x 11 days
Skin or soft tissue focus (Treat initially for Gp. A strep, MSSA; if later identified as MRSA, treat accordingly)	Group A streptococci S. aureus (MSSA)	Cefotaxime 2 gm (IV) q6h x 2 weeks **or** Ceftizoxime 2 gm (IV) q8h x 2 weeks	Levofloxacin 750 mg (IV) q24h x 2 weeks **or** Nafcillin 2 gm (IV) q4h x 2 weeks	Levofloxacin 750 mg (PO) q24h x 2 weeks **or** Cephalexin 500 mg (PO) q6h x 2 weeks
	S. aureus (MRSA)	Vancomycin 1 gm (IV) q12h x 2 weeks **or** Linezolid 600 mg (IV) q12h x 2 weeks	Minocycline 100 mg (IV) q12h x 2 weeks **or** Quinupristin/ dalfopristin 7.5 mg/kg (IV) q8h x 2 weeks	Linezolid 600 mg (PO) q12h x 2 weeks **or** Minocycline 100 mg (PO) q12h x 2 weeks

Sepsis/Septic Shock (cont'd)

Subset	Usual Pathogens	Preferred IV Therapy	Alternate IV Therapy	IV-to-PO Switch
Multiple myeloma or CLL	S. pneumoniae H. influenzae N. meningitidis K. pneumoniae	Levofloxacin 500 mg (IV) q24h x 2 weeks **or** Ceftriaxone 2 gm (IV) q24h x 2 weeks	Cefepime 2 gm (IV) q12h x 2 weeks **or** Cefotaxime 2 gm (IV) q6h x 2 weeks **or** Ceftizoxime 2 gm (IV) q8h x 2 weeks	Levofloxacin 500 mg (PO) q24h x 2 weeks
Diabetes *Urinary tract focus*	Entero-bacteriaceae Group B streptococci	Levofloxacin 500 mg (IV) q24h x 2 weeks **or** Ceftriaxone 2 gm (IV) q24h x 2 weeks	Cefepime 2 gm (IV) q12h x 2 weeks	Levofloxacin 500 mg (PO) q24h x 2 weeks
Skin, soft tissue, abdominal focus	B. fragilis Anaerobes Gp A,B,C,D,G streptococci	Meropenem 1 gm (IV) q8h x 2 weeks **or** Imipenem 1 gm (IV) q6h x 2 weeks **or** Ertapenem 1 gm (IV) q24h x 2 weeks **or** Piperacillin/tazobactam 4.5 gm (IV) q8h x 2 weeks	Levofloxacin 500 mg (750 mg for complicated skin/soft tissue infections) (IV) q24h x 2 weeks **plus either** Clindamycin 600 mg (IV) q8h x 2 weeks **or** Metronidazole 1 gm (IV) q24h x 2 weeks	Levofloxacin 500 mg (750 mg for complicated skin/soft tissue infections) (PO) q24h x 2 weeks **plus either** Clindamycin 300 mg (PO) q6h x 2 weeks **or** Metronidazole 500 mg (PO) q6h x 2 weeks
Alcoholic cirrhosis	Entero-bacteriaceae Capnocyto-phaga (DF-2) P. multocida S. aureus Group A streptococci	Levofloxacin 500 mg (IV) q24h x 2 weeks **or** Ceftriaxone 2 gm (IV) q24h x 2 weeks	Cefepime 2 gm (IV) q12h x 2 weeks	Levofloxacin 500 mg (PO) q24h x 2 weeks

Sepsis/Septic Shock (cont'd)

Subset	Usual Pathogens	Preferred IV Therapy	Alternate IV Therapy	IV-to-PO Switch
HIV/AIDS *Lung focus (not PCP/TB)*	S. pneumoniae H. influenzae Salmonella Legionella	Levofloxacin 500 mg (IV) q24h x 2 weeks **or** Doxycycline 200 mg (IV) q12h x 3 days, then 100 mg (IV) q12h x 11 days	Ceftriaxone 2 gm (IV) q24h x 2 weeks **plus either** Doxycycline 200 mg (IV) q12h x 3 days, then 100 mg (IV) q12h x 11 days **or** Azithromycin 500 mg (IV) q24h x 1 week	Levofloxacin 500 mg (PO) q24h x 2 weeks **or** Doxycycline 200 mg (PO) q12h x 3 days, then 100 mg (PO) q12h x 11 days*
Steroids (chronic high dose)	Candida Aspergillus	Amphotericin B 1.5 mg/kg (IV) q24h until 1-2 grams given **or** Amphotericin B lipid formulation 5 mg/kg (IV) q24h x 3 weeks	Caspofungin 70 mg (IV) x 1 dose, then 50 mg (IV) q24h x 4 weeks **or** Voriconazole 400 mg (IV) x 1 dose, then 200 mg (IV) q12h x 4 weeks **or** Itraconazole 200 mg (IV) q12h x 2 days, then 200 mg (IV) q24h x 4 weeks	Voriconazole 400 mg (PO) x 1 dose, then 200 mg (PO) q12h x 4 weeks* **or** Itraconazole 200 mg (IV) q12h x 2 days, then 200 mg (PO) q24h x 4 weeks*
Hyposplenic function or asplenia	S. pneumoniae H. influenzae N. meningitidis	Levofloxacin 500 mg (IV) q24h x 2 weeks **or** Ceftriaxone 2 gm (IV) q24h x 2 weeks	Cefepime 2 gm (IV) q12h x 2 weeks **or** Cefotaxime 2 gm (IV) q6h x 2 weeks	Levofloxacin 500 mg (PO) q24h x 2 weeks **or** Amoxicillin 1 gm (PO) q8h x 2 weeks
Miliary (disseminated) TB	M. tuberculosis	Not applicable		Treat the same as pulmonary TB (p. 44)

MSSA/MRSA = methicillin-sensitive/resistant S. aureus. Duration of therapy represents total time IV or IV + PO. Most patients on IV therapy able to take PO meds should be switched to PO therapy after clinical improvement
* Loading dose is not needed PO if given IV with the same drug

Sepsis, Unknown Source (CNS Source Excluded)
Clinical Presentation: Abrupt onset of high spiking fevers, rigors ± hypotension

Diagnostic Considerations: Diagnosis suggested by high-grade bacteremia (2/4 - 4/4 positive blood cultures) with unexplained hypotension. Rule out pseudosepsis (GI bleed, myocardial infarction, pulmonary embolism, acute pancreatitis, adrenal insufficiency, etc.). Sepsis usually occurs from a GI, GU, or IV source, so coverage is directed against GI and GU pathogens if IV line infection is unlikely
Pitfalls: Most cases of fever/hypotension are *not* due to sepsis. Before the label of "sepsis" is applied to febrile/hypotensive patients, first consider treatable/reversible mimics (see above)
Therapeutic Considerations: Resuscitate shock patients initially with rapid volume replacement, followed by pressors, if needed. Do not give pressors before volume replacement or hypotension may continue/worsen. Use normal saline, plasma expanders, or blood for volume replacement, not D_5W. If patient is persistently hypotensive despite volume replacement, consider relative adrenal insufficiency: Obtain a serum cortisol level, then give cortisone 100 mg (IV) q6h x 24-72h; blood pressure will rise promptly if relative adrenal insufficiency is the cause of volume-unresponsive hypotension. Do not add/change antibiotics if patient is persistently hypotensive/febrile; look for GI bleed, myocardial infarction, pulmonary embolism, pancreatitis, undrained abscess, adrenal insufficiency, or IV line infection. Drain abscesses as soon as possible. Remove IV lines if the entry site is red or a central line has been in place for ≥ 7 days and there is no other explanation for fever/hypotension. In addition to antibiotic therapy, patients with severe sepsis and end-organ dysfunction may benefit from human activated protein C (Xigris), which reduced mortality by 6% (31% vs. 25%) at 28 days when given early at 24 mcg/kg/hr x 96 hours in randomized PROWESS trial (NEJM 2001;344:699-709), albeit at an increased risk of bleeding (3.5% vs 2.0% for placebo). Very expensive
Prognosis: Related to severity of septic process and underlying cardiopulmonary/immune status

Sepsis in SLE
Clinical Presentation: Usually presents with community-acquired pneumonia, urosepsis, or skin/soft tissue infections
Diagnostic Considerations: Differentiate SLE flare from infection by WBC count (↓ SLE; ↑ infection), SPEP (↑ alpha-2 globulin in SLE, not in infection), and by negative cultures in SLE flare. UTIs and skin/soft tissue infections are the most common sources of infection in SLE. Differentiate SLE cerebritis from meningitis by negative CSF gram stain and decreased CSF C_4 levels in SLE cerebritis. Differentiate SLE pneumonitis from community-acquired pneumonia by pleuritic chest pain with migratory infiltrates and pleural effusions in SLE pneumonitis
Pitfalls: CMV infection may induce a SLE flare
Therapeutic Considerations: Since SLE spares the liver, an elevated SGOT is a clue to acute CMV infection; obtain IgM CMV titers to confirm. Patients with SLE are not usually infected with B. fragilis/anaerobes, so anti-B. fragilis coverage is usually not needed
Prognosis: Related to severity of SLE and degree of immunosuppression

Sepsis in Multiple Myeloma/CLL
Clinical Presentation: Meningitis, community-acquired pneumonia, or bacteremia are most common
Diagnostic Considerations: Infections usually secondary to encapsulated respiratory tract organisms
Therapeutic Considerations: Anti-P. aeruginosa coverage is not needed unless patients are neutropenic
Prognosis: Good if treated early

Sepsis in Diabetes Mellitus
Clinical Presentation: Commonest acute infections are UTIs and skin/soft tissue infections. UTI presentation is similar to non-diabetics. Skin/soft tissue infections are much more severe in diabetics and often life-threatening
Diagnostic Considerations: UTIs/urinary tract focus is diagnosed by demonstrating same pathogen in urine/blood cultures. Skin/soft tissue infections are diagnosed clinically; for deep/severe infection, obtain a CT/MRI to assess for gas in tissue and compartment syndrome
Pitfalls: Mixed aerobic/anaerobic infections are common and life-threatening

Therapeutic Considerations: P. aeruginosa is frequently cultured from diabetic foot ulcers/sinus tracts as a skin colonizer, but is not a pathogen in bone biopsy cultures
Prognosis: Related to degree of renal dysfunction and severity of infection

Sepsis in Alcoholic Cirrhosis

Clinical Presentation: Acute or subacute onset of fever/hypotension ± abdominal pain
Diagnostic Considerations: Diagnosis by positive blood cultures of pathogens associated with cirrhosis. If abdominal pain with ascites and negative CT/MRI , paracentesis ascitic fluid > 500 WBCs with > 100 PMNs predicts positive ascitic fluid culture and is diagnostic of spontaneous bacterial peritonitis. Some degree of splenic dysfunction usually exists, predisposing to infection with encapsulated organisms. Patients with advanced cirrhosis may have overwhelming infection with Capnocytophaga or Pasteurella
Pitfalls: Do not overlook GI bleed as the source of fever/hypotension
Therapeutic Considerations: Source of sepsis is usually the abdomen (peritonitis); UTIs are an uncommon source of sepsis. Spontaneous bacterial peritonitis is usually due to Enterobacteriaceae; B. fragilis/anaerobes are not common pathogens in cirrhosis, and B. fragilis coverage is unnecessary
Prognosis: Related to degree of hepatic/splenic dysfunction

Sepsis in HIV/AIDS

Clinical Presentation: Severe sepsis is uncommon in HIV/AIDS
Diagnostic Considerations: Fever/hypotension suggests volume depletion after prolonged diarrhea or adrenal insufficiency secondary to CMV adrenalitis. HIV/AIDS patients with community-acquired pneumonia are not usually "septic," but may have severe pneumonia
Pitfalls: HIV/AIDS patients are often infected, but rarely septic
Therapeutic Considerations: B. fragilis/anaerobes are rarely a source of sepsis in HIV/AIDS. P. aeruginosa and S. aureus should be covered only in IV drug abusers with preterminal HIV/AIDS. P. aeruginosa is not a pathogen in HIV/AIDS patients with community-acquired pneumonia
Prognosis: Related to degree of immunosuppression (CD_4 count)

Sepsis in Patients on Chronic High-Dose Steroids (Candida, Aspergillus)

Clinical Presentation: Subacute onset of fever with disseminated infection in multiple organs
Diagnostic Considerations: Diagnosis by positive blood cultures for fungi or demonstration of invasive fungal infection from tissue biopsy specimens. Sepsis is most commonly due to fungemia
Pitfalls: Obtain blood cultures to diagnose fungemias and rule out bacteremias (uncommon)
Therapeutic Considerations: Use amphotericin B, caspofungin, itraconazole, or voriconazole for Candida or Aspergillus
Prognosis: Related to degree of immunosuppression

Sepsis in Hyposplenia/Asplenia

Clinical Presentation: Presents as overwhelming septicemia/shock with petechiae
Diagnostic Considerations: Diagnosis by gram stain of buffy coat of blood or by blood cultures. Organism may be stained/cultured from aspirated petechiae. Howell-Jolly bodies in the peripheral smear are a clue to decreased splenic function. Conditions associated with hyposplenism include sickle cell trait/disease, cirrhosis, rheumatoid arthritis, SLE, systemic necrotizing vasculitis, amyloidosis, celiac disease, chronic active hepatitis, Fanconi's syndrome, IgA deficiency, intestinal lymphangiectasia, intravenous gamma-globulin therapy, myeloproliferative disorders, non-Hodgkin's lymphoma, regional enteritis, ulcerative colitis, Sezary syndrome, splenic infarcts/malignancies, steroid therapy, systemic mastocytosis, thyroiditis, infiltrative diseases of spleen, mechanical compression of splenic artery/spleen, Waldenstrom's macroglobulinemia, hyposplenism of old age, congenital absence of spleen
Pitfalls: Suspect hyposplenia/asplenia in unexplained overwhelming infection
Therapeutic Considerations: In spite of early aggressive antibiotic therapy and supportive care, patients often die within hours from overwhelming infection, especially due to S. pneumoniae

Prognosis: Related to degree of splenic dysfunction

Miliary (Disseminated) TB (Mycobacterium tuberculosis)
Clinical Presentation: Unexplained, prolonged fevers without localizing signs
Diagnostic Considerations: Diagnosis by AFB on biopsy/culture of liver or bone marrow
Pitfalls: Chest x-ray is negative early in 1/3. Subtle miliary (2 mm) infiltrates on chest x-ray (1-4 weeks)
Therapeutic Considerations: Treated the same as pulmonary TB
Prognosis: Death within weeks without treatment

Febrile Neutropenia

Subset	Usual Pathogens	Preferred IV Therapy	Alternate IV Therapy	IV-to-PO Switch
Febrile leukopenia (without hypotension or septic shock)	P. aeruginosa Enterobacteriaceae	Cefepime 2 gm (IV) q8h until neutropenia resolves **or** Meropenem 1 gm (IV) q8h until neutropenia resolves **or** Imipenem 1 gm (IV) q6h until neutropenia resolves	Piperacillin 4 gm (IV) q8h until neutropenia resolves **plus either** Levofloxacin 500-750 mg (IV) q24h until neutropenia resolves **or** Aztreonam 2 gm (IV) q8h until neutropenia resolves **or** Amikacin 1 gm (IV) q24h until neutropenia resolves	Levofloxacin 750 mg (PO) q24h until neutropenia resolves

Duration of therapy represents total time IV or IV + PO. Most patients on IV therapy able to take PO meds should be switched to PO therapy after clinical improvement

Clinical Presentation: Incidence of infection rises as PMN counts fall below 1000/mm^3
Diagnostic Considerations: Febrile neutropenia ± positive blood cultures. After blood cultures are drawn, anti-P. aeruginosa coverage should be initiated. Do not overlook ischiorectal or perirectal abscess as sources of fever. Post-chemotherapy cancer patients with leukopenia are commonly febrile/infected, but not often septic. Sepsis in the setting of febrile neutropenia suggests IV line sepsis
Pitfalls: Suspect fungemia if abrupt rise in temperature occurs after 2 weeks of appropriate anti-P. aeruginosa antibiotic therapy. Fungemias usually do not occur in first 2 weeks of neutropenia
Therapeutic Considerations: If a patient is neutropenic for > 2 weeks and develops RUQ/LUQ pain/increased alkaline phosphatase, suspect hepatosplenic candidiasis; confirm diagnosis with abdominal CT/MRI showing mass lesions in liver/spleen and treat as systemic/invasive candidiasis (p. 70). S. aureus is not a common pathogen in neutropenic compromised hosts without central IV lines, and B. fragilis/anaerobes are not usual pathogens in febrile neutropenia. If IV line infection/perirectal abscess are ruled out, consider tumor fever or drug fever before changing antibiotic therapy. If febrile neutropenia persists after 1-2 weeks of antibiotic therapy, treat empirically for Aspergillus with amphotericin B, caspofungin, voriconazole, or itraconazole
Prognosis: Related to degree and duration of neutropenia

Toxin-Mediated Infectious Diseases

Toxin-Mediated Infectious Diseases

Subset	Usual Pathogens	IV Therapy	PO/IM Therapy or IV-to-PO Switch
Toxic shock syndrome (TSS)* (Treat initially for MSSA; if later identified as MRSA, treat accordingly)	S. aureus (MSSA)	<u>Preferred IV Therapy</u> Cefazolin 1 gm (IV) q8h x 2 weeks <u>Alternate IV Therapy</u> Nafcillin 2 gm (IV) q4h x 2 weeks **or** Clindamycin 600 mg (IV) q8h x 2 weeks	Cephalexin 500 mg (PO) q6h x 2 weeks **or** Clindamycin 300 mg (PO) q6h x 2 weeks
	S. aureus (MRSA)	<u>Preferred IV Therapy</u> Vancomycin 1 gm (IV) q12h x 2 weeks **or** Linezolid 600 mg (IV) q12h x 2 weeks <u>Alternate IV Therapy</u> Minocycline 100 mg (IV) q12h x 2 weeks **or** Quinupristin/dalfopristin 7.5 mg/kg (IV) q8h x 2 weeks	Linezolid 600 mg (PO) q12h x 2 weeks **or** Minocycline 100 mg (PO) q12h x 2 weeks
Botulism (food, infant, wound)	Clostridium botulinum	<u>Preferred Therapy</u> 2 vials of type-specific trivalent (types A,B,E) or polyvalent (types A,B,C,D,E) antitoxin (IV)	<u>Alternate Therapy</u> Amoxycillin 1 gm (PO) q8h x 7 days (wound botulism only)
Tetanus	Clostridium tetani	<u>Preferred Therapy</u> Tetanus immune globulin (TIG) antitoxin 3000-10,000 units (IM) (50% into deltoid, 50% into wound site) **plus either** Penicillin G 4 mu (IV) q4h x 10 days **or** Doxycycline 200 mg (IV or PO) q12h x 3 days, then 100 mg (IV or PO) x 7 days	<u>Alternate Therapy</u> Tetanus immune globulin (TIG) antitoxin 3000-10,000 units (IM) (50% into deltoid, 50% into wound site) **plus** Metronidazole 1 gm (IV) q12h x 10 days

Toxin-Mediated Infectious Diseases (cont'd)

Subset	Usual Pathogens	Preferred Therapy	Alternate Therapy
Diphtheria (pharyngeal, nasal, wound)	Coryne-bacterium diphtheriae	Diphtheria antitoxin (IV) over 1 hour (pharyngeal diphtheria = 40,000 units; nasopharyngeal diphtheria = 60,000 units; systemic diphtheria or diphtheria > 3 days duration = 100,000 units) **plus either** Penicillin G 1 mu (IV) q4h x 14 days **or** Erythromycin 500 mg (IV) q6h x 14 days	Diphtheria antitoxin (IV) over 1 hour (pharyngeal diphtheria = 40,000 units; nasopharyngeal diphtheria = 60,000 units; systemic diphtheria or diphtheria > 3 days duration = 100,000 units) **plus** Procaine penicillin 600,000 units (IM) q24h x 14 days

MSSA/MRSA = methicillin-sensitive/resistant S. aureus. Duration of therapy represents total time IV, PO, or IV + PO. Most patients on IV therapy able to take PO meds should be switched to PO therapy after clinical improvement
* Treat only IV or IV-to-PO switch

Toxic Shock Syndrome (S. aureus)

Clinical Presentation: Scarletiniform rash ± hypotension. Spectrum ranges from minimal infection to multiorgan system failure/shock. ↑ CPK common

Diagnostic Considerations: Diagnosis by clinical presentation with mucous membrane, renal, liver, and skin involvement/culture of TSS-1 toxin-producing strain of S. aureus from mouth, nares, vagina, or wound

Pitfalls: Toxic shock syndrome wound discharge is clear, not purulent

Therapeutic Considerations: Remove source of toxin production if possible (e.g., remove tampon, drain collections). Support organ dysfunction until recovery

Prognosis: Good in early/mild form. Poor in late/multisystem disease form

Botulism (Clostridium botulinum)

Clinical Presentation: Descending symmetrical paralysis beginning with cranial nerve involvement, induced by botulinum toxin. Onset begins with blurry vision, followed rapidly by ocular muscle paralysis, difficulty speaking, and inability to swallow. Respiratory paralysis may occur in severe cases. Mental status is unaffected. Usual incubation period is 10-12 hours. Incubation is shortest for Type E strain (hours), longest for Type A strain (up to 10 days), and is inversely proportional to the quantity of toxin consumed (food botulism). Wound botulism (Types A or B) may follow C. botulinum entry into IV drug abuser injection site, surgical or traumatic wounds. Infant (< 1 year) botulism (most commonly Type A or B) is acquired from C. botulinum containing honey. Patients with botulism are afebrile, and have profuse vomiting without diarrhea

Diagnostic Considerations: Detection of botulinum toxin from stool, serum, or food (especially home canned foods with neutral or near neutral pH [~ 7] or smoked fish [Type E]) is diagnostic of food botulism. Wound botulism is diagnosed by culturing C. botulinum from the wound or by detecting botulinum toxin in the serum

Pitfalls: Clinical diagnosis based on descending paralysis with cranial nerve involvement in an afebrile patient must be differentiated from Guillain-Barre (fever, ascending paralysis, sensory component) and polio (fever, pure ascending motor paralysis). Do not diagnose botulism in the absence of ocular/pharyngeal paralysis

Therapeutic Considerations: Antitoxin neutralizes only unbound toxin, and does not reverse toxin-induced paralysis. Botulism is a toxin-mediated infection and antibiotic therapy (wound botulism) is adjunctive. Guanidine has been used with variable effect. Ventilator support is needed for respiratory paralysis

Prognosis: Good if treated early, before respiratory paralysis

Tetanus (Clostridium tetani)

Clinical Presentation: Begins with jaw stiffness/difficulty chewing induced by C. tetani toxin (tetanospasmin). Trismus rapidly follows with masseter muscle spasm, followed by spasm of the abdominal/back muscles. Rigidity and convulsions may occur. Patients are afebrile unless there is hypothalamic involvement (central fever), in which case fevers may exceed 106^{0}F. Usual incubation period is 3-21 days

Diagnostic Considerations: Diagnosis suggested by muscle spasms/rigidity in a patient with trismus

Pitfalls: In rabies, muscle spasms are localized and usually involve the face/neck, rather than primary involvement of the extremities, as in tetanus

Therapeutic Considerations: Tetanus is self-limited with intensive supportive care. Sedation is important, and avoidance of all stimuli is mandatory to reduce the risk of convulsions. Avoid unnecessary handling/movement of patient. Antitoxin is effective only in neutralizing unbound toxin. Tracheostomy/respiratory support can be life-saving in severe cases

Prognosis: Good if not complicated by spinal fractures, aspiration pneumonia, or CNS involvement (hyperpyrexia, hyper/hypotension)

Diphtheria (Corynebacterium diphtheriae)

Clinical Presentation: Within 1 week following insidious onset of sore throat without fever, pharyngeal patches coalesce to form a gray diphtheric membrane (surrounded by a red border), which is adherent/bleeds easily when removed. Membrane begins unilaterally; may extend to the soft palate, uvula and contralateral posterior pharynx; are accompanied by prominent bilateral anterior adenopathy; become necrotic (green/black); and have a foul odor (fetor oris). Submandibular edema ("bull neck") and hoarseness (laryngeal stridor) precede respiratory obstruction/death. Cutaneous diphtheria may follow C. diphtheriae contaminated wounds (traumatic, surgical) or insect/human bites, and is characterized by a leathery eschar (cutaneous membrane) covering a deep punched out ulcer. Serosanguineous discharge is typical of nasal diphtheria (membrane in nares). Diphtheric myocarditis may complicate any form of diphtheria (most commonly follows pharyngeal form), and usually occurs in the second week, but may occur up to 8 weeks after infection begins. Diphtheric polyneuritis is a common complication. Cardiac/neurologic complications are due to elaboration of a potent toxin

Diagnostic Considerations: Diagnosis is suggested by unilateral membranous pharyngitis/palatal paralysis, absence of fever, and relative tachycardia. Diagnosis is confirmed by culture of C. diphtheriae from nares, membrane, or wound

Pitfalls: Differentiated from Arcanobacterium (Corynebacterium) haemolyticum (which also forms a pharyngeal membrane) by culture and absence of scarletiniform rash with C. diphtheriae

Therapeutic Considerations: Antibiotic therapy treats the infection and stops additional toxin production. Antitoxin is effective against unbound toxin, but will not reverse toxin-mediated myocarditis/neuropathy. Serum sickness is common 2 weeks after antitoxin. Respiratory/cardiac support may be life-saving

Prognosis: Poor with airway obstruction or myocarditis. Myocarditis may occur despite early treatment

Chapter 3

Initial Therapy of Isolates Pending Susceptibility Testing

Burke A. Cunha, M.D.

Introduction

When bacteria are isolated from a body site and reported, the clinical significance of the organism should be determined before deciding on potential antibiotic treatment.

The tables in this chapter serve as a guide to the clinical significance of bacterial and fungal isolates recovered from various body sites, including CSF, blood, sputum, urine, stool, and wound. In general, isolates listed as pathogens (P) should be treated with antibiotics, while those listed as non-pathogens (NP), colonizers (C), or skin contaminants (C*) ordinarily should not. The antibiotics recommended in this section should be effective initial therapy pending susceptibility testing.

Isolates by Gram Stain, Arrangement, Oxygen Requirements

AEROBIC ISOLATES

*   Enterobacteriaceae (oxidase negative, catalase positive)
**   Oxidase negative

CAPNOPHILIC ISOLATES[+]

GRAM-NEGATIVE BACILLI

+   Capnophilic organisms grow best under increased CO_2 tension

ANAEROBIC ISOLATES[++]

GRAM-POSITIVE COCCI (CHAINS)

GRAM-POSITIVE BACILLI

GRAM-NEGATIVE BACILLI

++ Microaerophilic organisms. Grow best under decreased O_2 concentration

YEASTS/FUNGI

Alphabetical Index of Isolates

Table 1. Clinical Significance of AEROBIC Isolates Pending Susceptibility Testing

	GRAM-POSITIVE COCCI (CLUSTERS)			
Isolate	Isolate Significance	Preferred Therapy	Alternate Therapy	Comments
Staphylococcus aureus (MSSA/MRSA)	• CSF = C*, P (CNS shunts) • Blood = C*, P (from soft tissue/bone infection, abscess, IV line infection, ABE, PVE) • Sputum = C, P (S. aureus pneumonia is rare; usually only after viral influenza) • Urine = C, P (S. aureus in urine is usually due to skin contamination or rarely overwhelming S. aureus bacteremia) • Stool = C, P (enterocolitis) • Wound = C, P (cellulitis, abscess)	**MSSA** Nafcillin (IV) Cefazolin (IV) Clindamycin (IV/PO) **MRSA** Vancomycin (IV) Linezolid (IV/PO)	**MSSA** Any 2nd, 3rd generation cephalosporin (IV) (except ceftazidime, ceftriaxone) Imipenem (IV) Meropenem (IV) Ertapenem (IV) Linezolid (IV/PO) **MRSA** Quinupristin/dalfopristin (IV) Minocycline (IV/PO)	For oral treatment, 1st generation cephalosporins are better tolerated and have more reliable blood levels than oral anti-staphylococcal penicillins (e.g., dicloxacillin). MRSA in-vitro susceptibility testing is unreliable; treat infection empirically. Do not treat MRSA colonization, which is responsible for most MRSA isolates. Cannot substitute doxycycline for minocycline. Ciprofloxacin, ceftazidime, imipenem use associated with increased prevalence of MRSA
Staphylococcus epidermidis (MSSE/MRSE) or coagulase-negative staphylococci	• CSF = C*, P (CNS shunts) • Blood = C*, P (from IV lines, infected implants, PVE, rarely native valve SBE) • Sputum = C • Urine = C (may be reported as S. saprophyticus; request novobiocin sensitivity to differentiate from other coagulase-negative staph) • Stool = NP • Wound = C, P (infected foreign body drainage)	**MSSE** Vancomycin (IV) Linezolid (IV/PO) Imipenem (IV) Meropenem (IV) Ertapenem (IV) **MRSE** Vancomycin (IV) ± rifampin (PO) Linezolid (IV/PO)	**MSSE** Clindamycin (IV/PO) Levofloxacin (IV/PO) **MRSE** Quinupristin/dalfopristin (IV)	Usually non-pathogenic in absence of prosthetic/implant materials. Common cause of PVE; rare cause of native valve SBE. Treat foreign body-related infection until foreign body is removed

C = colonizer; C* = skin contaminant; NP = non-pathogen; P = pathogen at site; (IV/PO) = IV or PO. See p. 1 for all other abbreviations

Table 1. Clinical Significance of AEROBIC Isolates Pending Susceptibility Testing (cont'd)

Isolate	Isolate Significance	Preferred Therapy	Alternate Therapy	Comments
GRAM-POSITIVE COCCI (CLUSTERS)				
Staphylococcus saprophyticus (coagulase-negative staphylococci)	• CSF = NP • Blood = NP • Sputum = NP • Urine = P (cystitis, pyelonephritis) • Stool = NP • Wound = NP	Amoxicillin (PO) TMP-SMX (PO) Nitrofurantoin (PO)	Any quinolone (PO) Any 1st generation cephalosporin (PO)	S. saprophyticus UTI is associated with a urinary "fishy odor," alkaline urine pH, and microscopic hematuria. Novobiocin sensitivity differentiates coagulase-negative staphylococci (sensitive) from S. saprophyticus (resistant)
GRAM-POSITIVE COCCI (CHAINS)				
Enterococcus faecalis	• CSF = NP (except from S. stercoralis hyperinfection or V-P shunt infection) • Blood = C*, P (from GI/GU source, SBE) • Sputum = NP • Urine = C, P (cystitis, pyelonephritis) • Stool = NP • Wound = C, P (cellulitis)	<u>Non-SBE</u> Amp/Sulb (IV) Amoxicillin (PO) Imipenem (IV) Meropenem (IV) Piperacillin (IV) Linezolid (IV/PO) <u>SBE</u> Gentamicin (IV) plus either ampicillin (IV) or vancomycin (IV) Imipenem (IV) Meropenem (IV) Piperacillin (IV) Linezolid (IV/PO)	<u>Non-SBE</u> Any quinolone (IV/PO) Cefoperazone (IV) Chloramphenicol (IV) Nitrofurantoin (PO) (UTIs only) <u>SBE</u> Any quinolone (IV/PO) Cefoperazone (IV)	Sensitive to ampicillin, not penicillin. Cause of intermediate (in-between ABE and SBE) endocarditis, hepatobiliary infections, and UTIs. Enterococci (E. faecalis, E. faecium) are the only cause of SBE from GI/GU sources. Permissive pathogen (i.e., usually does not cause infection alone) in the abdomen/pelvis. Cefoperazone is the only cephalosporin with anti-E. faecalis activity (MIC ~ 32 mcg/mL). Quinupristin/dalfopristin is not active against E. faecalis
Enterococcus faecium (VRE)	• CSF = NP (except from S. stercoralis hyperinfection or V-P shunt infection) • Blood = C*, P (from GI/GU source, SBE) • Sputum = C • Urine = C, P (cystitis, pyelo) • Stool = NP • Wound = C, P (cellulitis)	<u>Non-SBE</u> Doxycycline (IV/PO) Chloramphenicol (IV) <u>SBE</u> Linezolid (IV/PO)	<u>Non-SBE</u> Quinupristin/dalfopristin (IV) Nitrofurantoin (PO) (UTIs only) <u>SBE</u> Quinupristin/dalfopristin (IV)	Same spectrum of infection as E. faecalis. Colonization is more common than infection. Fecal carriage is intermittent but prolonged. In-vitro antibiotic sensitivity predicts in-vivo efficacy. Increased prevalence of E. faecium (VRE) infections related to IV vancomycin use, not PO vancomycin

C = colonizer; C* = skin contaminant; NP = non-pathogen at site; P = pathogen at site; (IV/PO) = IV or PO. See p. 1 for all other abbreviations

Table 1. Clinical Significance of AEROBIC Isolates Pending Susceptibility Testing (cont'd)

	GRAM-POSITIVE COCCI (CHAINS)		
Isolate	Isolate Significance	Preferred Therapy	Alternate Therapy	Comments

Isolate	Isolate Significance	Preferred Therapy	Alternate Therapy	Comments
Group A streptococci	• CSF = C*, P (rare cause of meningitis) • Blood = P (from skin/soft tissue infection) • Sputum = P (rare cause of CAP) • Urine = NP • Stool = NP • Wound = C, P (cellulitis) • Throat = C, P (pharynx is colonized with Group A streptococci in ~ 30% of patients with EBV mono)	Amoxicillin (PO) Clindamycin (IV/PO) Any β-lactam (IV/PO)	Penicillin (PO) Clarithromycin XL (PO) Azithromycin (PO)	For Group A streptococcal pharyngitis, amoxicillin is preferred over penicillin. Clindamycin is best for elimination of carrier states, and for penicillin-allergic patients with streptococcal pharyngitis. Any β-lactam is equally effective against Group A streptococcus. Nafcillin is the most active anti-staphylococcal penicillin against Group A streptococcus. Erythromycin is no longer reliable against Group A streptococcus due to increasing resistance. Doxycycline has little/no activity against Group A streptococcus
Group B streptococci (S. agalactiae)	• CSF = P (ABM) • Blood = P (from IV line/urine source, SBE) • Sputum = NP • Urine = P (CAB, UTIs, especially in diabetics, elderly) • Stool = NP • Wound = C, P (diabetic foot infections)	Non-SBE, non-CNS Clindamycin (IV/PO) Any 1st,2nd,3rd generation cephalosporin (IV/PO) SBE Penicillin (IV) Ceftriaxone (IV) Vancomycin (IV) CNS Penicillin (IV) Ceftriaxone (IV)	Non-SBE, non-CNS Vancomycin (IV) Amoxicillin (PO) SBE Imipenem (IV) Meropenem (IV) Ertapenem (IV) Linezolid (IV/PO) CNS Chloramphenicol (IV) Linezolid (IV/PO)	Cause of UTIs and IV line infections in diabetics and the elderly. Cause of neonatal meningitis. Infection is uncommon in the general population. Rarely a cause of SBE in non-pregnant adults. Aminoglycosides are ineffective

C = colonizer; C* = skin contaminant; NP = non-pathogen at site; P = pathogen at site; (IV/PO) = IV or PO. See p. 1 for all other abbreviations

Table 1. Clinical Significance of AEROBIC Isolates Pending Susceptibility Testing (cont'd)

GRAM-POSITIVE COCCI (CHAINS)

Isolate	Isolate Significance	Preferred Therapy	Alternate Therapy	Comments
Group C, F, G streptococci	• CSF = P (meningitis) • Blood = P (from skin/soft tissue infection, SBE) • Sputum = P (rare cause of CAP) • Throat = C (especially with viral pharyngitis, P (pharyngitis in medical personnel) • Urine = NP • Stool = NP • Wound = P (cellulitis)	Penicillin (IV) Ampicillin (IV) Any 1st,2nd,3rd generation cephalosporin (IV) Clindamycin (IV/PO)	Vancomycin (IV) Amoxicillin (PO) Imipenem (IV) Meropenem (IV) Ertapenem (IV)	Group G streptococci cause pharyngitis, wound infections, and rarely SBE. Common pharyngeal colonizers in medical personnel
Streptococcus bovis	• CSF = NP • Blood = P (SBE from GI source) • Sputum = NP • Urine = NP • Stool = NP • Wound = NP	Ampicillin (IV) Any 1st,2nd,3rd generation cephalosporin (IV) Clindamycin (IV/PO)	Vancomycin (IV) Amoxicillin (PO)	Associated with GI malignancies. Non-enterococcal Group D streptococci (e.g., S. bovis) are sensitive to penicillin
Streptococcus viridans group (S. mitior, mlleri, mitis, mutans, oralis, sanguis, parasanguis, salivarius)	• CSF = NP • Blood = C*, P (1° bacteremia, SBE) • Sputum = NP • Urine = NP • Stool = NP • Wound = NP	Penicillin (IV) Ceftriaxone (IV)	Amoxicillin (PO) Any 1st,2nd,3rd generation cephalosporin (IV/PO) Imipenem (IV) Meropenem (IV) Ertapenem (IV) Vancomycin (IV)	S. viridans is commonly isolated from blood cultures. Low-grade blood culture positivity (1/4) indicates contamination during venipuncture. High-grade blood culture positivity (3/4 or 4/4) indicates SBE until proven otherwise. S. milleri is associated with metastatic abscesses

C = colonizer; C* = skin contaminant; NP = non-pathogen at site; P = pathogen at site; (IV/PO) = IV or PO. See p. 1 for all other abbreviations

Table 1. Clinical Significance of AEROBIC Isolates Pending Susceptibility Testing (cont'd)

GRAM-POSITIVE COCCI (PAIRS)

Isolate	Isolate Significance	Preferred Therapy	Alternate Therapy	Comments
Leuconostoc	• CSF = NP • Blood = P (PVE) • Sputum = NP • Urine = P (UTIs) • Stool = NP • Wound = NP	Penicillin (IV) Ampicillin (IV) Clindamycin (IV/PO)	Amoxicillin (PO) Erythromycin (IV) Minocycline (IV/PO) Clarithromycin XL (PO)	Coccobacillary forms resemble streptococci/enterococci. Cause of infection in compromised hosts. Rare cause of IV line infection. Vancomycin resistant
Streptococcus pneumoniae *PCN-sensitive or relatively resistant (MIC ≤ 2 mcg/mL)* *PCN-resistant (MIC > 2 mcg/mL)*	• CSF = P (ABM) • Blood = P (from respiratory tract source) • Sputum = C, P • Urine = NP • Stool = NP • Wound = P (cellulitis only in SLE)	<u>Sensitive or relatively PCN-resistant (MIC ≤ 2 mcg/mL)</u> Any 1ˢᵗ, 2ⁿᵈ, 3ʳᵈ gen. cephalosporin (IV/PO) Doxycycline (IV/PO) Levofloxacin (IV/PO) Gatifloxacin (IV/PO) Moxifloxacin (IV,PO) <u>Highly PCN-resistant (MIC > 2 mcg/mL)</u> Levofloxacin (IV/PO)	<u>Sensitive or relatively PCN-resistant</u> Amoxicillin (PO) Clindamycin (IV/PO) <u>Highly PCN-resistant</u> Vancomycin (IV) Cefepime (IV) Imipenem (IV) Meropenem (IV) Ertapenem (IV) Linezolid (IV/PO)	Moderately penicillin-resistant S. pneumoniae are still sensitive to β-lactams. Highly penicillin-resistant strains (MIC ≥ 6 mcg/mL) are uncommon. Ciprofloxacin has limited anti-S. pneumoniae activity compared to "respiratory" quinolones. β-lactamase inhibitor combinations are ineffective against penicillin-resistant pneumococci, since resistance is due to changes in penicillin binding proteins (PBP's)

GRAM-NEGATIVE COCCI (PAIRS)

Isolate	Isolate Significance	Preferred Therapy	Alternate Therapy	Comments
Neisseria gonorrhoeae (GC)	• CSF = NP • Blood = P (from pharyngitis, proctitis, ABE) • Sputum = NP • Urine = P (urethritis) • Stool = NP • Wound = NP • Rectal discharge = P (GC proctitis)	<u>Penicillin-sensitive N. gonorrhoeae</u> Penicillin (IV/IM) Amoxicillin (PO) Any quinolone (IV/PO) <u>PPNG</u> Ceftriaxone (IV/IM) Any 1ˢᵗ, 2ⁿᵈ, 3ʳᵈ generation cephalosporin (IV/IM)	<u>Penicillin-sensitive N. gonorrhoeae</u> Doxycycline (IV/PO) <u>PPNG</u> Spectinomycin (IM) Levofloxacin (IV/PO) Ciprofloxacin (PO)	Cause of "culture negative" right-sided ABE. May be cultured from synovial fluid/blood in disseminated GC infection (arthritis-dermatitis syndrome). Treat possible Chlamydia trachomatis co-infection and sexual partners. Spectinomycin is ineffective against pharyngeal GC/incubating syphilis. PPNG are also tetracycline-resistant (TRNG)

C = colonizer; C* = skin contaminant; NP = non-pathogen at site; P = pathogen at site; (IV/PO) = IV or PO. See p. 1 for all other abbreviations

Table 1. Clinical Significance of AEROBIC Isolates Pending Susceptibility Testing (cont'd)

GRAM-NEGATIVE COCCI (PAIRS)

Isolate	Isolate Significance	Preferred Therapy	Alternate Therapy	Comments
Neisseria meningitidis	• CSF = P (ABM) • Blood = P (acute/chronic meningococcemia) • Sputum = C, P (only in closed populations, e.g., military recruits) • Urine C, P (urethritis rarely) • Stool = NP • Wound = NP	Penicillin (IV) Ampicillin (IV) Any 3rd generation cephalosporin (IV)	Chloramphenicol (IV) Cefepime (IV) Meropenem (IV)	In ABM, do not decrease meningeal dose of β-lactam antibiotics as patient improves, since CSF penetration/concentration decreases as meningeal inflammation decreases. Chloramphenicol is an excellent choice for penicillin-allergic patients. Preferred meningococcal prophylaxis is an oral quinolone (single dose)

GRAM-POSITIVE BACILLI

Isolate	Isolate Significance	Preferred Therapy	Alternate Therapy	Comments
Arcanobacterium (Corynebacterium) haemolyticum	• CSF = NP • Blood = NF • Sputum = P (oropharyngeal secretions) • Urine = NP • Stool = NP • Wound = NP	Doxycycline (PO)	Erythromycin (PO) Azithromycin (PO) Any 1st 2nd 3rd generation cephalosporin (PO) Clarithromycin XL (PO)	Causes membranous pharyngitis with scarlet fever-like rash. Differentiate from C. diphtheriae by culture. Penicillin and ampicillin are less effective than erythromycin or doxycycline
Bacillus anthracis	• CSF = P (A3M) • Blood = P (septicemia; isolation required; dangerous) • Sputum = ? (mediastinitis; anthrax pneumonia rare) • Urine = NP • Stool = NP • Wound = P (ulcer; isolation required; dangerous)	Penicillin (IV) Ampicillin (IV) Doxycycline (IV/PO)	Any quinolone (IV/PO) Amoxicillin (PO)	Doxycycline may be used for outbreak prophylaxis. Streptobacillary configuration in blood. Causes hemorrhagic meningitis, wound infections, and bacteremia. Quinolones have in-vitro activity, but in-vivo experience is limited. Alert microbiology laboratory of potentially biohazardous specimens. Do not culture

C = colonizer; C* = skin contaminant; NP = non-pathogen at site; P = pathogen at site; (IV/PO) = IV or PO. See p. 1 for all other abbreviations

Table 1. Clinical Significance of AEROBIC Isolates Pending Susceptibility Testing (cont'd)

GRAM-POSITIVE BACILLI

Isolate	Isolate Significance	Preferred Therapy	Alternate Therapy	Comments
Bacillus cereus, subtilis, megaterium	• CSF = NP • Blood = C* P (leukopenic compromised hosts) • Sputum = NP • Urine = NP • Stool = NP • Wound = NP	Vancomycin (IV) Clindamycin (IV/PO)	Imipenem (IV) Meropenem (IV) Any quinolone (IV/PO)	Soil organisms not commonly pathogenic for humans. Suspect pseudoinfection if isolated from clinical specimens. Look for soil/dust contamination of blood culture tube top/apparatus. Rare pathogen in leukopenic compromised hosts
Corynebacterium diphtheriae	• CSF = NP • Blood = NP • Sputum = P (oropharyngeal secretions) • Urine = NP • Stool = NP • Wound = P (wound diphtheria)	Penicillin (IV) Erythromycin (IV) Clindamycin (IV/PO)	Doxycycline (IV/PO) Clarithromycin XL (PO) Rifampin (PO)	Administer diphtheria antitoxin as soon as possible (p. 117). Antibiotic therapy is adjunctive, since diphtheria is a toxin-mediated disease. Patients may die unexpectedly from toxin-induced myocarditis during recovery
Corynebacterium jeikeium (CDC group JK)	• CSF = C* P (CSF shunts) • Blood = C* P (from IV lines) • Sputum = NP • Urine = NP • Stool = NP • Wound = C	Vancomycin (IV) Linezolid (IV/PO)	Quinupristin/ dalfopristin (IV)	Cause of IV line/foreign body infections. In-vitro testing is not always reliable. Highly resistant to most anti-gram positive antibiotics
Erysipelothrix rhusiopathiae	• CSF = NP • Blood = P (from SBE) • Sputum = NP • Urine = NP • Stool = NP • Wound = P (chronic erysipelas-like skin lesions)	Penicillin (IV) Ampicillin (IV)	Any 3rd generation cephalosporin (IV) Any quinolone (IV/PO)	Cause of "culture-negative" SBE. One of the HACEK organisms. Resistant to clindamycin and metronidazole

C = colonizer; C* = skin contaminant; NP = non-pathogen at site; P = pathogen at site; (IV/PO) = IV or PO. See p. 1 for all other abbreviations

Table 1. Clinical Significance of AEROBIC Isolates Pending Susceptibility Testing (cont'd)

GRAM-POSITIVE BACILLI

Isolate	Isolate Significance	Preferred Therapy	Alternate Therapy	Comments
Listeria monocytogenes	• CSF = P (ABM) • Blood = P (1° bacteremia, SBE) • Sputum = NP • Urine = NP • Stool = NP • Wound = NP	Ampicillin (IV) Amoxicillin (PO) Chlo-amphenicol (IV) <u>CNS</u> Ampicillin (IV) TMP-SMX (IV/PO) Chlo-amphenicol (IV) <u>SBE</u> Ampicillin (IV)	Doxycycline (IV/PO) Levofloxacin (IV/PO) Erythromycin (IV) Linezolid (IV/PO)	Listeria ABM is common in T-cell deficiencies (e.g., lymphoma). Causes SBE in normal hosts, and is the commonest cause of bacteremia in non-neutropenic cancer patients. 3rd generation cephalosporins are ineffective against Listeria
Nocardia asteroides, brasiliensis	• CSF = P (brain abscess) • Blood = P (from lung/soft tissue source) • Sputum = P (pneumonia, lung abscess) • Urine = NP • Stool = NP • Wound = P (skin lesions from direct inoculation or dissemination)	TMP-SMX (IV/PO) Minocycline (IV/PO)	Imipenem (IV) plus either amikacin (IV) or any 3rd generation cephalosporin (IV)	Branched, filamentous, beady hyphae are typical, but coccobacillary and bacillary forms are also common. Nocardia are gram-positive, aerobic, and acid fast. Quinolones and macrolides are usually ineffective
Rhodococcus equi	• CSF = NP • Blood = P (from pneumonia, lung abscess) • Sputum = P (pneumonia with abscess/cavitation) • Urine = NP • Stool = NP • Wound = NP	Any quinolone (IV/PO) Vancomycin (IV)	Erythromycin (IV) Imipenem (IV) Meropenem (IV) Doxycycline (IV/PO) TMP-SMX (IV/PO)	Causes TB-like community-acquired pneumonia in AIDS patients. Filamentous bacteria break into bacilli/cocci. Aminoglycosides and β-lactams are relatively ineffective

C = colonizer; C* = skin contaminant; NP = non-pathogen at site; P = pathogen at site; (IV/PO) = IV or PO. See p. 1 for all other abbreviations

Table 1. Clinical Significance of AEROBIC Isolates Pending Susceptibility Testing (cont'd)

GRAM-NEGATIVE BACILLI

Isolate	Isolate Significance	Preferred Therapy	Alternate Therapy	Comments
Acinetobacter baumannii, Iwoffi, calcoaceticus, haemolyticus	• CSF = C* , P (ABM) • Blood = P (from IV line, lung, or urine source) • Sputum = C, P (VAP) • Urine = C, P (CAB) • Stool = NP • Wound = C (common), P (rare)	Imipenem (IV) Meropenem (IV) Cefepime (IV)	Ampicillin/sulbactam (IV) Piperacillin/tazobactam (IV) Any 3rd generation cephalosporin (IV) (except ceftazidime)	Usually associated with respiratory support equipment. Occurs in outbreaks of ventilator-associated pneumonia. Ertapenem is inactive
Actinobacillus actinomycetem-comitans	• CSF = NP • Blood = P (from abscess, SBE) • Sputum = NP • Urine = NP • Stool = NP • Wound = P (from abscess, draining fistulous tract)	Any quinolone (IV/PO) Any 3rd generation cephalosporin (IV/PO)	Penicillin (IV) + gentamicin (IV) TMP-SMX (IV/PO)	Cause of "culture-negative" SBE. One of the HACEK organisms. Found with Actinomyces in abscesses. Resistant to erythromycin and clindamycin
Aeromonas hydrophila	• CSF = NP • Blood = P (from wound, urine, or GI source) • Sputum = NP • Urine = C, P (CAB) • Stool = P (diarrhea) • Wound = P (cellulitis)	Gentamicin (IV) TMP-SMX (IV/PO) Any quinolone (IV/PO)	Doxycycline (IV/PO) Any 3rd generation cephalosporin (IV/PO) Imipenem (IV) Meropenem (IV) Aztreonam (IV)	Cause of wound infection, septic arthritis, diarrhea, and necrotizing soft tissue infection resembling gas gangrene
Alcaligenes (Achromobacter) xylosoxidans	• CSF = P (rarely ABM) • Blood = P (from urine) • Sputum = NP • Urine = P (CAB) • Stool = NP • Wound = P (cellulitis rare)	Imipenem (IV) Meropenem (IV) Any 3rd generation cephalosporin (IV/PO) Piperacillin (IV)	Any quinolone (IV/PO) Cefepime (IV) Aztreonam (IV) Ticarcillin/clavulanic acid (IV/PO)	Water-borne pathogen resembling Acinetobacter microbiologically. Resistant to aminoglycosides and 1st, 2nd generation cephalosporins

C = colonizer; C* = skin contaminant; NP = non-pathogen at site; P = pathogen at site; (IV/PO) = IV or PO. See p. 1 for all other abbreviations

Table 1. Clinical Significance of AEROBIC Isolates Pending Susceptibility Testing (cont'd)

GRAM-NEGATIVE BACILLI

Isolate	Isolate Significance	Preferred Therapy	Alternate Therapy	Comments
Bartonella henselae, quintana, bacilliformis	• CSF = NP • Blood = P (from skin source, SBE) • Sputum = NP • Urine = NP • Stool = NP • Wound = P (skin lesions)	Doxycycline (IV/PO), Azithromycin (PO)	Clarithromycin XL (PO) Levofloxacin (IV/PO)	Causes bacillary angiomatosis or verruga peruana in AIDS patients. Also the cause of Cat Scratch disease and Aroya fever. May present as FUO. TMP-SMX and cephalosporins are ineffective
Bordetella pertussis	• CSF = NP • Blood = P (from respiratory tract source) • Sputum = C, P (pertussis) • Urine = NP • Stool = NP • Wound = NP	Erythromycin (IV) Clarithromycin XL (PO) Azithromycin (IV/PO)	Levofloxacin (IV/PO) TMP-SMX (IV/PO)	Causes pertussis in children and incompletely/non-immunized adults. Macrolides remain the preferred therapy. Resistant to penicillins, cephalosporins, and aminoglycosides
Brucella abortus, canis, suis, melitensis	• CSF = P (meningitis) • Blood = P (from abscess, SBE) • Sputum = NP • Urine = P (pyelonephritis) • Stool = NP • Wound = NP	Doxycycline (IV/PO) + gentamicin (IV) Doxycycline + streptomycin (IM)	TMP-SMX (IV/PO) + gentamicin (IV) Doxycycline (IV/PO) + rifampin (PO) Levofloxacin (IV/PO) + rifampin (PO)	Causes prolonged relapsing infection. Zoonotic cause of brucellosis/Malta fever. Resistant to penicillins
Burkholderia (Pseudomonas) cepacia	• CSF = NP • Blood = P (usually from IV line/urinary tract infection) • Sputum = C (not a cause of VAP) • Urine = C • Stool = NP • Wound = NP	TMP-SMX (IV/PO)	Chloramphenicol (IV) Minocycline (IV/PO) Any quinolone (IV/PO) Cefepime (IV) Piperacillin (IV) Meropenem (IV)	Rare cause of urosepsis following urologic instrumentation. Common water-borne colonizer in intensive care units. Opportunistic pathogen in cystic fibrosis/bronchiectasis. Resistant to aminoglycosides

C = colonizer; C* = skin contaminant; NP = non-pathogen at site; P = pathogen at site; (IV/PO) = IV or PO. See p. 1 for all other abbreviations

Table 1. Clinical Significance of AEROBIC Isolates Pending Susceptibility Testing (cont'd)

GRAM-NEGATIVE BACILLI

Isolate	Isolate Significance	Preferred Therapy	Alternate Therapy	Comments
Burkholderia (Pseudomonas) pseudomallei	• CSF = NP • Blood = P (from septicemic melioidosis) • Sputum = P (chronic cavitary pneumonia) • Urine = NP • Stool = NP • Wound = NP	TMP-SMX (IV/PO) Ceftazidime (IV)	Imipenem (IV) Meropenem (IV) Chloramphenicol (IV)	Causes melioidosis, which resembles chronic fibrocaseating TB, but in lower lobe distribution. Resistant to aminoglycosides
Campylobacter fetus	• CSF = P (ABM) • Blood = P (from vascular source) • Sputum = NP • Urine = NP • Stool = NP • Wound = NP	Gentamicin (IV) Imipenem (IV) Meropenem (IV)	Chloramphenicol (IV) Ampicillin (IV) Any 3rd generation cephalosporin (IV)	Causes invasive infection with spread to CNS. CNS infection may be treated with meningeal doses of chloramphenicol, ampicillin, or a 3rd generation cephalosporin. Resistant to erythromycin
Campylobacter jejuni	• CSF = NP • Blood = P (from GI source) • Sputum = NP • Urine = NP • Stool = P (diarrhea) • Wound = NP	Any quinolone (IV/PO) Erythromycin (PO) Doxycycline (IV/PO)	Azithromycin (PO) Clarithromycin XL (PO)	Commonest cause of acute bacterial diarrhea. Resistant to TMP-SMX
Cardiobacterium hominis	• CSF = NP • Blood = P (from SBE) • Sputum = NP • Urine = NP • Stool = NP • Wound = NP	Penicillin (IV) + gentamicin (IV) Ampicillin (IV) + gentamicin (IV)	Any 3rd generation cephalosporin (IV) + gentamicin (IV)	Pleomorphic bacillus with bulbous ends. Often appears in clusters resembling rosettes. Cause of "culture-negative" SBE (one of the HACEK organisms). Rare cause of abdominal abscess. Grows best with CO_2 enhancement. Resistant to macrolides and clindamycin

C = colonizer; C* = skin contaminant; NP = non-pathogen at site; P = pathogen at site; (IV/PO) = IV or PO. See p. 1 for all other abbreviations

Table 1. Clinical Significance of AEROBIC Isolates Pending Susceptibility Testing (cont'd)

GRAM-NEGATIVE BACILLI

Isolate	Isolate Significance	Preferred Therapy	Alternate Therapy	Comments
Chromobacterium violaceum	• CSF = NP • Blood = P (from wound infection) • Sputum = NP • Urine = NP • Stool = NP • Wound = P (drainage from deep soft tissue infection)	Gentamicin (IV) Doxycycline (IV/PO)	Chloramphenicol (IV)	Cause of cutaneous lesions primarily in tropical/subtropical climates. Often mistaken for Vibrio or Alcaligenes. Resistant to β-lactams
Chryseobacterium (Flavobacterium) meningosepticum	• CSF = P (ABM) • Blood = P (from IV line infection, PVE) • Sputum = NP • Urine = C, P (from urologic instrumentation) • Stool = NP • Wound = C, P (cellulitis)	CNS TMP-SMX (IV/PO) Non-CNS Vancomycin (IV) + rifampin (PO) Levofloxacin (IV/PO)	CNS Chloramphenicol (IV) Non-CNS Clarithromycin XL (PO) + rifampin (PO) Clindamycin (IV/PO)	Rare cause of ABM in newborns and PVE in adults. Only unencapsulated Flavobacterium species. Clindamycin, clarithromycin, and vancomycin are useful only in non-CNS infections. Resistant to aztreonam and carbapenems
Citrobacter diversus, freundii, koseri	• CSF = C*, P (from NS procedure) • Blood = C* (from IV line/ urinary tract infection) • Sputum = C (not pneumonia) • Urine = C, P (from urologic instrumentation) • Stool = NP • Wound = C, P (rarely in comprom sed hosts)	Any quinolone (IV/PO) Imipenem (IV) Meropenem (IV) Ertapenem (IV) Cefepime (IV)	Aztreonam (IV) Piperacillin/tazobactam (IV) Any 3rd generation cephalosporin (IV)	Common wound/urine colonizer. Rare pathogen in normal hosts. Often aminoglycoside resistant (C. freundii is usually more resistant than C. koseri)

C = colonizer; C* = skin contaminant; NP = non-pathogen at site; P = pathogen at site; (IV/PO) = IV or PO. See p. 1 for all other abbreviations

Table 1. Clinical Significance of AEROBIC Isolates Pending Susceptibility Testing (cont'd)

GRAM-NEGATIVE BACILLI

Isolate	Isolate Significance	Preferred Therapy	Alternate Therapy	Comments
Edwardsiella tarda	• CSF = NP • Blood = P (from liver abscess) • Sputum = NP • Urine = NP • Stool = NP • Wound C, P (wound infection)	Ampicillin (IV) Amoxicillin (PO) Levofloxacin (IV/PO)	Doxycycline (IV/PO) Any 3rd generation cephalosporin (IV/PO)	Cause of bacteremia, usually from liver abscess or wound source
Enterobacter agglomerans, aerogenes, cloacae	• CSF = C*, P (from NS procedure) • Blood = C*, P (from IV line/ urinary tract infection) • Sputum = C (not a cause of pneumonia) • Urine = C, P (post-urologic instrumentation) • Stool = NP • Wound = C, P (rarely in compromised hosts)	Cefepime (IV) Levofloxacin (IV/PO) Aztreonam (IV)	Piperacillin/tazobactam (IV) Imipenem (IV) Meropenem (IV) Ertapenem (IV)	Not a cause of community-acquired or nosocomial pneumonia. Common colonizer of respiratory secretions and wound/urine specimens. Treatment of Enterobacter colonizers with ceftazidime or ciprofloxacin may cause multi-drug resistance
Escherichia coli	• CSF = P (ABM) • Blood = P (from GI/GU source) • Sputum = P (rarely CAP from urinary source, VAP) • Urine = C, P (CAB, cystitis, pyelonephritis) • Stool = C, P (diarrhea) • Wound = P (cellulitis)	Amoxicillin (PO) TMP-SMX (IV/PO) Any 1st,2nd,3rd generation cephalosporin (IV/PO) Any quinolone (IV/PO)	Aztreonam (IV) Gentamicin (IV) Nitrofurantoin (PO) (UTIs only)	Common pathogen, usually from GI/ GU source. Most strains are resistant to ampicillin and 1st generation cephalosporins. ESBL-producing E. coli are best treated with cefepime, imipenem, or meropenem

C = colonizer; C* = skin contaminant; NP = non-pathogen at site; P = pathogen at site; (IV/PO) = IV or PO. See p. 1 for all other abbreviations

Table 1. Clinical Significance of AEROBIC Isolates Pending Susceptibility Testing (cont'd)

GRAM-NEGATIVE BACILLI

Isolate	Isolate Significance	Preferred Therapy	Alternate Therapy	Comments
Francisella tularensis	• CSF = NP • Blood = P (isolation required; dangerous) • Sputum = P (tularemic pneumonia; isolation required; dangerous) • Urine = NP • Stool = NP • Wound = P (isolation required; dangerous)	Doxycycline (IV/PO) Gentamicin (IV/IM) Streptomycin (IM)	Chloramphenicol (IV/PO) Any quinolone (IV/PO)	Six clinical tularemia syndromes. Alert microbiology laboratory of potentially biohazardous specimens. Do not culture. Resistant to penicillins and cephalosporins
Hafnia alvei	• CSF = C, P (from NS procedure) • Blood = C*, P (from IV line/ urinary tract infection) • Sputum = C (not pneumonia) • Urine = C, P (post-urologic instrumentation) • Stool = NP • Wound = C, P (rarely in compromised hosts)	Cefepime (IV) Any quinolone (IV/PO) Aztreonam (IV)	Piperacillin/tazobactam (IV) Imipenem (IV) Meropenem (IV)	Formerly Enterobacter hafnia. Uncommon nosocomial pathogen. Rarely pathogenic in normal hosts. Cause of UTIs in compromised hosts
Helicobacter (Campylobacter) pylori	• CSF = NP • Blood = NP • Sputum = NP • Urine = NP • Stool = P (from upper GI tract biopsy specimens, not stool) • Wound = NP	Omeprazole (PO) + clarithromycin XL (PO) Omeprazole (PO) + amoxicillin (PO) Metronidazole (PO) + amoxicillin (PO) + bismuth subsalicylate (PO)	Doxycycline (PO) + metronidazole (PO) + bismuth subsalicylate (PO)	Do not treat H. pylori gastritis, only peptic ulcer disease and MALT lymphomas. Optimal therapy awaits definition. Treat until cured. Some strains of clarithromycin-resistant H. pylori may respond to re-treatment with higher clarithromycin doses. TMP-SMX is ineffective

C = colonizer; C* = skin contaminant; NP = non-pathogen; P = pathogen at site; (IV/PO) = IV or PO. See p. 1 for all other abbreviations

Table 1. Clinical Significance of AEROBIC Isolates Pending Susceptibility Testing (cont'd)

GRAM-NEGATIVE BACILLI

Isolate	Isolate Significance	Preferred Therapy	Alternate Therapy	Comments
Hemophilus influenzae, parainfluenzae, aphrophilus, paraphrophilus	• CSF = P (ABM) • Blood = P (from respiratory tract or cardiac source) • Sputum = C, P (CAP) • Urine = NP • Stool = NP • Wound = NP	**Ampicillin-sensitive H. influenzae** Any 2nd,3rd generation cephalosporin (IV/PO) Doxycycline (IV/PO) Any quinolone (IV/PO) **Ampicillin-resistant H. influenzae** Any 2nd,3rd generation cephalosporin (IV/PO) Doxycycline (IV/PO) Any quinolone (IV/PO)	**For all Hemophilus species** Chloramphenicol (IV) TMP-SMX (IV/PO) Azithromycin (PO) Aztreonam (IV) **Ampicillin-resistant H. influenzae** Imipenem (IV) Meropenem (IV) Ertapenem (IV) Aztreonam (IV) Cefepime (IV)	1st generation cephalosporins, erythromycin, and clarithromycin have limited anti-H. influenzae activity; doxycycline and azithromycin are better. Hemophilus species are common colonizers of the respiratory tract. Rarely a cause of "culture-negative" SBE (H. parainfluenzae/aphrophilus are HACEK organisms). Growth enhanced with CO_2. Penicillin has little anti-H. influenzae activity
Kingella (Moraxella) kingae	• CSF = NP • Blood = P (from skeletal or cardiac source) • Sputum = C • Urine = NP • Stool = NP • Wound = NP	Ampicillin (IV) + any aminoglycoside (IV)	Any 3rd generation cephalosporin (IV) + any aminoglycoside (IV) Imipenem (IV) Meropenem (IV) Levofloxacin (IV/PO)	Common colonizer of respiratory tract, but rarely a respiratory pathogen. Causes septic arthritis/osteomyelitis in children and endocarditis in adults (one of HACEK organisms). Oxidase positive. Growth enhanced with CO_2
Klebsiella pneumoniae, oxytoca	• CSF = P (ABM) • Blood = P (from respiratory, GI, GU source) • Sputum = C, P (CAP/VAP) • Urine = C (CAB), P • Stool = NP • Wound = C, P (cellulitis)	Any 3rd generation cephalosporin (IV,PO) Cefepime (IV) Imipenem (IV) Meropenem (IV) Ertapenem (IV) Any quinolone (IV/PO)	Piperacillin/tazobactam (IV) Aztreonam (IV)	TMP-SMX may be ineffective in systemic infection, but is acceptable for UTIs. Anti-pseudomonal penicillins have limited anti-Klebsiella activity. ESBL-producing Klebsiella are best treated with cefepime, imipenem, ertapenem, or meropenem

C = colonizer; C* = skin contaminant; NP = non-pathogen at site; P = pathogen at site; (IV/PO) = IV or PO. See p. 1 for all other abbreviations

Table 1. Clinical Significance of AEROBIC Isolates Pending Susceptibility Testing (cont'd)

GRAM-NEGATIVE BACILLI

Isolate	Isolate Significance	Preferred Therapy	Alternate Therapy	Comments
Klebsiella ozaenae, rhinoscleromatis	• CSF = NP • Blood = NP • Sputum = NP • Urine = NP • Stool = NP • Wound = P (rhinoscleromatis lesions)	Any quinolone (PO)	TMP-SMX (PO) + rifampin (PO)	Skin infection usually requires prolonged treatment for cure (weeks-to-months)
Legionella sp.	• CSF = NP • Blood = NP • Sputum = P (CAP or VAP) • Urine = NP • Stool = NP • Wound = NP	Any quinolone (IV/PO) Doxycycline (IV/PO)	Erythromycin (IV) Azithromycin (IV/PO) Clarithromycin XL (PO)	Anti-Legionella activity: Levofloxacin > ciprofloxacin > doxycycline > erythromycin. Erythromycin failures are not uncommon. In compromised hosts (e.g., organ transplants), optimal treatment is levofloxacin + azithromycin. Rarely a cause of culture-negative SBE/ PVE
Leptospira interrogans	• CSF = P (ABM) • Blood = P (1° bacteremia) • Sputum = NP • Urine = P (excreted in urine) • Stool = NP • Wound = NP	Doxycycline (IV/PO) Penicillin G (IV)	Amoxicillin (PO)	Blood/urine cultures may be positive during initial/bacteremic phase, but are negative during immune phase. Relapse is common. Resistant to chloramphenicol
Moraxella (Branhamella) catarrhalis	• CSF = NP • Blood = P (rarely from CAP) • Sputum = C, P (CAP) • Urine = NP • Stool = NP • Wound = NP	Doxycycline (IV/PO) Any 2nd, 3rd generation cephalosporin (IV/PO) Any quinolone (IV/PO)	TMP-SMX (IV/PO) Clarithromycin XL (PO) Azithromycin (PO)	Almost all strains are β-lactamase positive and resistant to penicillin/ampicillin. β-lactamase-resistant β-lactams are effective

C = colonizer; C* = skin contaminant; NP = non-pathogen at site; P = pathogen at site; (IV/PO) = IV or PO. See p. 1 for all other abbreviations

Table 1. Clinical Significance of AEROBIC Isolates Pending Susceptibility Testing (cont'd)

GRAM-NEGATIVE BACILLI

Isolate	Isolate Significance	Preferred Therapy	Alternate Therapy	Comments
Morganella morgani	• CSF = NP • Blood = P (from GU source) • Sputum = NP • Urine = P (CAB, cystitis, pyelonephritis) • Stool = NP • Wound = P (cellulitis rare)	Levofloxacin (IV/PO) Any 3rd generation cephalosporin (IV) Cefepime (IV) Imipenem (IV) Meropenem (IV) Ertapenem (IV)	Any aminoglycoside (IV) Aztreonam (IV)	Common uropathogen. Causes bacteremia with urosepsis. Rare cause of wound infections
Ochrobactrum anthropi (CDC group Vd)	• CSF = NP • Blood = P (from IV line infections) • Sputum = C • Urine = C • Stool = C • Wound = C	Any quinolone (IV/PO) TMP-SMX (IV/PO)	Any aminoglycoside (IV) Imipenem (IV) Meropenem (IV)	Pathogen in compromised hosts. Oxidase and catalase positive. Resistant to β-lactams
Pasteurella multocida	• CSF = P (ABM) • Blood = P (from respiratory source, bite wound/abscess) • Sputum = C, P (CAP) • Urine = C, P (pyelonephritis) • Stool = NP • Wound = P (human/animal bites)	Amoxicillin (PO) Doxycycline (IV/PO) Penicillin G (IV)	Ampicillin/sulbactam (IV) Piperacillin/tazobactam (IV) Any quinolone (IV/PO)	Common cause of infection following dog/cat bites. Many antibiotics are effective, but erythromycin is ineffective
Plesiomonas shigelloides	• CSF = NP • Blood = P (from GU source) • Sputum = NP • Urine = NP • Stool = P (diarrhea) • Wound = NP	Any quinolone (PO) TMP-SMX (PO)	Doxycycline (PO) Aztreonam (PO)	Infrequent cause of diarrhea, less commonly dysentery. Oxidase positive. β-lactamase strains are increasing. Resistant to penicillins

C = colonizer; C* = skin contaminant; NP = non-pathogen at site; P = pathogen at site; (IV/PO) = IV or PO. See p. 1 for all other abbreviations

Table 1. Clinical Significance of AEROBIC Isolates Pending Susceptibility Testing (cont'd)

GRAM-NEGATIVE BACILLI

Isolate	Isolate Significance	Preferred Therapy	Alternate Therapy	Comments
Proteus mirabilis, vulgaris	• CSF = NP • Blood = P (from urinary source) • Sputum = C • Urine = C, P (from urologic instrumentation) • Stool = NP • Wound = C, P (wound infection)	P. mirabilis, indole (–) Ampicillin (IV) Any 1st, 2nd, 3rd gen. cephalosporin (IV/PO) P. vulgaris, indole (+) Any 3rd generation cephalosporin (IV/PO) Cefepime (IV) Any quinolone (IV/PO)	P. mirabilis, indole (–) TMP-SMX (IV/PO) Amoxicillin (PO) P. vulgaris, indole (+): Aztreonam (IV) Imipenem (IV) Meropenem (IV) Ertapenem (IV) Any aminoglycoside (IV)	Usually a uropathogen. Most antibiotics are effective against P. mirabilis (indole-negative), but indole-positive Proteus require potent antibiotics to treat non-UTIs
Providencia rettgeri, stuartii	• CSF = NP • Blood = C*, P (from GU source) • Sputum = NP • Urine = C, P • Stool = NP • Wound = C, P (rare)	Any quinolone (IV/PO) Any 3rd generation cephalosporin (IV/PO) Cefepime (IV) Imipenem (IV) Meropenem (IV) Ertapenem (IV)	Any aminoglycoside (IV) Aztreonam (IV) Piperacillin/tazobactam (IV)	Almost always a uropathogen. Formerly classified as indole-positive Proteus
Pseudomonas aeruginosa	• CSF = NP • Blood = P (from respiratory, GU source) • Sputum = C (usually), P (rarely indicates VAP) • Urine = C, P (from urologic instrumentation) • Stool = NP • Wound = C (almost always)	Monotherapy Cefepime (IV) Meropenem (IV) Piperacillin (IV) Amikacin (IV) Combination therapy Levofloxacin (IV) plus either cefepime (IV) or piperacillin (IV) or meropenem (IV) Meropenem (IV) + cefepime (IV)	Monotherapy Any aminoglycoside (IV) Aztreonam (IV) Polymyxin B (IV) Combination therapy Piperacillin (IV) plus either amikacin (IV) or cefepime (IV)	For serious P. aeruginosa infection, double-drug therapy is preferred. All double anti-P. aeruginosa regimens are equally effective. Individual differences in activity (MICs) are unimportant if combination therapy is used

C = colonizer; C* = skin contaminant; NP = non-pathogen; P = pathogen at site; (IV/PO) = IV or PO. See p. 1 for all other abbreviations

Table 1. Clinical Significance of AEROBIC Isolates Pending Susceptibility Testing (cont'd)

GRAM-NEGATIVE BACILLI

Isolate	Isolate Significance	Preferred Therapy	Alternate Therapy	Comments
Pseudomonas (Chryseomonas) luteola (CDC group Ve-1)	• CSF = NP • Blood = P (from IV line infection) • Sputum = NP • Urine = NP • Stool = NP • Wound = NP	Imipenem (IV) Meropenem (IV) Cefepime (IV)	Piperacillin/tazobactam (IV) Aztreonam (IV)	Opportunistic pathogen primarily in compromised hosts
Pseudomonas (Flavimonas) oryzihabitans (CDC group Ve-2)	• CSF = P (NS procedures) • Blood = P (from IV line infection) • Sputum = NP • Urine = NP • Stool = NP • Wound = P (rare)	Imipenem (IV) Meropenem (IV) Cefepime (IV)	Any 3rd generation cephalosporin (IV) Piperacillin/tazobactam (IV) Aztreonam (IV)	Rare cause of central IV line infections in compromised hosts (usually in febrile neutropenics). Rare cause of peritonitis in CAPD patients. Oxidase negative, unlike other Pseudomonas species
Salmonella typhi, non-typhi	• CSF = NP • Blood = P (from GI source) • Sputum = NP • Urine = P (only with enteric fever) • Stool = C (carrier), P (gastroenteritis, enteric fever) • Wound = NP	Any quinolone (IV/PO) Any 3rd generation cephalosporin (IV)	Chloramphenicol (IV) TMP-SMX (IV/PO) Doxycycline (IV/PO)	Carrier state is best eliminated by a quinolone or TMP-SMX. If drug therapy fails to eliminate carrier state, look for hepatic/bladder calculi for persistent focus. Many strains are resistant to ampicillin/amoxicillin

C = colonizer; C* = skin contaminant; NP = non-pathogen at site; P = pathogen at site; (IV/PO) = IV or PO. See p. 1 for all other abbreviations

Table 1. Clinical Significance of AEROBIC Isolates Pending Susceptibility Testing (cont'd)

		GRAM-NEGATIVE BACILLI		
Isolate	Isolate Significance	Preferred Therapy	Alternate Therapy	Comments
Serratia marcescens	• CSF = P (from NS procedures) • Blood = P (from IV line or urinary source) • Sputum = C, P (rarely in VAP) • Urine = C, P (post-urologic instrumentation) • Stool = NP • Wound = C, P (rare)	Any 3rd generation cephalosporin (IV/PO) (except ceftazidime) Any quinolone (IV/PO) Cefepime (IV)	Imipenem (IV) Meropenem (IV) Ertapenem (IV) Gentamicin (IV) Aztreonam (IV) Piperacillin/tazobactam (IV)	Enterobacteriaceae. Associated with water sources. Common colonizer of respiratory secretions/urine in ICU. Serratia nosocomial pneumonia and PVE are rare. Cause of septic arthritis, osteomyelitis, and SBE (IV drug abusers). Among aminoglycosides, gentamicin has the greatest anti-Serratia activity
Shigella boydii, sonnei, flexneri, dysenteriae	• CSF = NP • Blood = P (from GI source) • Sputum = NP • Urine = NP • Stool = P (Shigella dysentery) • Wound = NP	Any quinolone (IV/PO)	TMP-SMX (IV/PO) Azithromycin (IV/PO)	No carrier state. Severity of dysentery varies with the species: S. dysenteriae (most severe) > S. flexneri > S. sonnei/boydii (least severe)
Stenotrophomonas (Xanthomonas, Pseudomonas) maltophilia	• CSF = C, P (from NS procedures) • Blood = C*, P (from IV line infection, GU source) • Sputum = C (not VAP) • Urine = C, P (from urologic instrumentation) • Stool = NP • Wound = C, P (rarely in compromised hosts)	TMP-SMX (IV/PO) Chloramphenicol (IV)	Imipenem (IV) Minocycline (IV/PO) Aztreonam (IV) Any quinolone (IV/PO)	Not a cause of community-acquired or nosocomial pneumonia. Potential pulmonary pathogen only in bronchiectasis/cystic fibrosis. Resistant to aminoglycosides

C = colonizer; C* = skin contaminant; NP = non-pathogen at site; P = pathogen at site; (IV/PO) = IV or PO. See p. 1 for all other abbreviations

Table 1. Clinical Significance of AEROBIC Isolates Pending Susceptibility Testing (cont'd)

GRAM-NEGATIVE BACILLI

Isolate	Isolate Significance	Preferred Therapy	Alternate Therapy	Comments
Streptobacillus moniliformis	• CSF = P (brain abscess) • Blood = P (from wound) • Sputum = P (lung abscess) • Urine = NP • Stool = NP • Wound = P (from rat bite)	Penicillin (IV) Ampicillin (IV) Amoxicillin (PO)	Doxycycline (IV/PO) Erythromycin (IV) Clindamycin (IV/PO)	Cause of Haverhill fever and rat-bite fever, with abrupt onset of severe headache/arthralgias after bite wound has healed. No regional adenopathy. Arthritis in 50%. May cause SBE
Vibrio cholerae	• CSF = NP • Blood = P (from GI source) • Sputum = NP • Urine = NP • Stool = P (cholera) • Wound = NP	Doxycycline (IV/PO) Any quinolone (IV/PO)	TMP-SMX (IV/PO)	No carrier state. Treat for 3 days. Single-dose therapy is often effective. Resistant to ampicillin
Vibrio parahaemolyticus	• CSF = NP • Blood = P (from GI source) • Sputum = NP • Urine = NP • Stool = P (diarrhea) • Wound = P	Doxycycline (IV/PO)	Any quinolone (IV/PO)	Most cases of gastroenteritis caused by V. parahaemolyticus are self-limited and require no treatment
Vibrio vulnificus, alginolyticus	• CSF = NP • Blood = P (from GI/wound source) • Sputum = NP • Urine = NP • Stool = P (diarrhea) • Wound = P (water-contaminated wound)	Doxycycline (IV/PO) Any quinolone (IV/PO)	Piperacillin/tazobactam (IV) Ampicillin/sulbactam (IV)	Causes necrotizing soft tissue infection resembling gas gangrene. Patients are critically ill with fever, bullous lesions, diarrhea, and hypotension. Treat wound infection, bacteremia. Aminoglycoside susceptibilities are unpredictable

C = colonizer; C* = skin contaminant; NP = non-pathogen at site; P = pathogen at site; (IV/PO) = IV or PO. See p. 1 for all other abbreviations

Table 1. Clinical Significance of AEROBIC Isolates Pending Susceptibility Testing (cont'd)

		GRAM-NEGATIVE BACILLI		
Isolate	Isolate Significance	Preferred Therapy	Alternate Therapy	Comments
Yersinia enterocolitica	• CSF = NP • Blood = P (from GI source) • Sputum = NP • Urine = NP • Stool = P (diarrhea) • Wound = NP	Any quinolone (IV/PO) Gentamicin (IV) Doxycycline (IV/PO)	TMP-SMX (IV/PO) Any 3rd generation cephalosporin (IV/PO)	Cause of diarrhea with abdominal pain. If pain in is right lower quadrant, may be mistaken for acute appendicitis
Yersinia pestis	• CSF = NP • Blood = P (septicemic plague; isolation required; dangerous) • Sputum = P (pneumonic plague; isolation required; dangerous) • Urine = NP • Stool = NP • Wound = P (lymph nodes, lymph node drainage; bubonic plague; isolation required; dangerous)	Doxycycline (IV/PO) Streptomycin (IM)	Chloramphenicol (IV/PO) Gentamicin (IV)	Cause of bubonic, septicemic, and pneumonic plagues. Doxycycline may be used for prophylaxis. Alert microbiology laboratory of potentially biohazardous specimens. Do not culture

C = colonizer; C* = skin contaminant; NP = non-pathogen at site; P = pathogen at site; (IV/PO) = IV or PO. See p. 1 for all other abbreviations

Table 1. Clinical Significance of AEROBIC Isolates Pending Susceptibility Testing (cont'd)

SPIROCHETES

Isolate	Isolate Significance	Preferred Therapy	Alternate Therapy	Comments
Borrelia burgdorferi	• CSF = P (neuroborreliosis) • Blood = P (rarely isolated; requires special media) • Sputum = NP • Urine = NP • Stool = NP • Wound = P (rarely isolated from erythema migrans lesions)	Doxycycline (PO) Amoxicillin (PO)	Any cephalosporin (PO) Azithromycin (PO) Erythromycin (PO)	Cause of Lyme disease. β-lactams and doxycycline are effective. Azithromycin is less likely to fail than erythromycin. Minocycline may be better than doxycycline for CNS Lyme disease. Amoxicillin/doxycycline are effective for erythema migrans
Borrelia recurrentis	• CSF = P (ABM) • Blood = P (1° bacteremia) • Sputum = NP • Urine = NP • Stool = NP • Wound = NP	Doxycycline (IV/PO) Azithromycin (IV/PO)	Erythromycin (IV) Penicillin (IV) Ampicillin (IV) Any 1st, 2nd, 3rd generation cephalosporin (IV/PO)	Cause of relapsing fever. May be recovered from septic metastatic foci. Septic emboli may cause sacroiliitis, SBE, myositis, orchitis, or osteomyelitis
Spirillum minus	• CSF = NP • Blood = P (from wound source, SBE) • Sputum = NP • Urine = NP • Stool = NP • Wound = P (from rat bite)	Penicillin (IV) Amoxicillin (PO)	Doxycycline (IV/PO) Any quinolone (IV/PO)	Cause of rat-bite fever. Bite wound heals promptly, but 1-4 weeks later becomes painful, purple and swollen, and progresses to ulceration and eschar formation. Painful regional adenopathy. Central maculopapular rash is common (rarely urticarial). Arthralgias/arthritis is rare compared to rat-bite fever from Streptobacillus moniliformis. Rarely causes SBE

C = colonizer; C* = skin contaminant; NP = non-pathogen at site; P = pathogen at site; (IV/PO) = IV or PO. See p. 1 for all other abbreviations

Table 2. Clinical Significance of CAPNOPHILIC Isolates Pending Susceptibility Testing

GRAM-NEGATIVE BACILLI

Isolate	Isolate Significance	Preferred Therapy	Alternate Therapy	Comments
Capnocytophaga carimorsus (CDC group DF-2)	• CSF = NP • Blood = P (from GI source, bite wound) • Sputum = NP • Urine = NP • Stool = NP • Wound = P (from dog/cat bite)	Ampicillin/sulbactam (IV) Piperacillin/tazobactam (IV) Imipenem (IV) Meropenem (IV) Ertapenem (IV)	Clindamycin (IV/PO) Any quinolone (IV/PO) Doxycycline (IV/PO)	Associated with animal bites or cancer. May cause fatal septicemia in cirrhotics/asplenics. Resistant to aminoglycosides, metronidazole, TMP-SMX, and aztreonam
Capnocytophaga ochraceus (CDC group DF-1)	• CSF = NP • Blood = P (from GI, wound, abscess source) • Sputum = NP • Urine = NP • Stool = NP • Wound = P	Ampicillin/sulbactam (IV) Piperacillin/tazobactam (IV) Imipenem (IV) Meropenem (IV) Ertapenem (IV)	Clindamycin (IV/PO) Any quinolone (IV/PO) Doxycycline (IV/PO)	Thin, spindle-shaped bacilli resemble Fusobacteria morphologically. "Gliding motility" seen in hanging drop preparations. Cause of septicemia, abscesses, and wound infections. Resistant to aminoglycosides, metronidazole, TMP-SMX, and aztreonam
Eikenella corrodens	• CSF = NP • Blood = P (SBE in IV drug abusers) • Sputum = NP • Urine = NP • Stool = NP • Wound = P (IV drug abusers)	Penicillin (IV) Ampicillin (IV) Imipenem (IV) Meropenem (IV) Ertapenem (IV)	Doxycycline (IV/PO) Amoxicillin (PO) Ampicillin/sulbactam (IV) Piperacillin/tazobactam (IV)	Cause of "culture-negative" SBE (one of the HACEK organisms). Resistant to clindamycin and metronidazole

C = colonizer; C* = skin contaminant; NP = non-pathogen at site; P = pathogen at site; (IV/PO) = IV or PO. See p. 1 for all other abbreviations

Table 3. Clinical Significance of ANAEROBIC Isolates Pending Susceptibility Testing

Isolate	Isolate Significance	Preferred Therapy	Alternate Therapy	Comments
GRAM-POSITIVE COCCI (CHAINS)				
Peptococcus	• CSF = P (brain abscess) • Blood = P (from GI/pelvic source) • Sputum = C, P (aspiration pneumonia, lung abscess) • Urine = NP • Stool = NP • Wound = P (rarely a sole pathogen)	Penicillin (IV) Ampicillin (IV) Amoxicillin (PO) Clindamycin (IV/PO)	Chloramphenicol (IV) Erythromycin (IV) Imipenem (IV) Meropenem (IV) Ertapenem (IV) Moxifloxacin (IV/PO)	Normal flora of mouth, GI tract, and pelvis. Associated with mixed aerobic/anaerobic dental, abdominal, and pelvic infections, especially abscesses
Pepto-streptococcus	• CSF = P (brain abscess) • Blood = P (GI/pelvic source) • Sputum = C, P (aspiration pneumonia, lung abscess) • Urine = NP • Stool = NP • Wound = P (rarely a sole pathogen)	Penicillin (IV) Ampicillin (IV) Amoxicillin (PO) Clindamycin (IV/PO)	Chloramphenicol (IV) Erythromycin (IV) Imipenem (IV) Meropenem (IV) Ertapenem (IV) Moxifloxacin (IV/PO)	Normal flora of mouth, GI tract, and pelvis. Associated with mixed aerobic/anaerobic dental, abdominal, and pelvic infections, especially abscesses
GRAM-POSITIVE BACILLI				
Actinomyces israelii, odontolyticus	• CSF = P (brain abscess) • Blood = NP • Sputum = C, P (lung abscess) • Urine = NP • Stool = NP • Wound = P (fistulas/underlying abscess)	Amoxicillin (PO) Doxycycline (PO)	Erythromycin (PO) Clindamycin (PO)	Anaerobic and non-acid fast. Usually presents as cervical, facial, thoracic, or abdominal masses/fistulas. Prolonged (6-12 month) treatment is needed for cure. Unlike Nocardia, Actinomyces rarely causes CNS infections. May be cultured from polymicrobial brain abscess of pulmonary origin. Quinolones, aminoglycosides, metronidazole, and TMP-SMX have little activity

C = colonizer; C* = skin contaminant; NP = non-pathogen at site; P = pathogen at site; (IV/PO) = IV or PO. See p. 1 for all other abbreviations

Table 3. Clinical Significance of ANAEROBIC Isolates Pending Susceptibility Testing (cont'd)

GRAM-POSITIVE BACILLI

Isolate	Isolate Significance	Preferred Therapy	Alternate Therapy	Comments
Arachnia propionica	• CSF = P (brain abscess) • Blood = P (from dental, GI, lung source) • Sputum = C, P (lung abscess) • Urine = NP • Stool = NP • Wound = NP	Clindamycin (IV/PO) Ampicillin (IV) + gentamicin (IV)	Erythromycin (IV)	Polymicrobial pathogen in dental, lung, and brain abscesses
Bifidobacterium sp.	• CSF = P (brain abscess) • Blood = NP • Sputum = C, P (lung abscess) • Urine = NP • Stool = NP • Wound = NP	Clindamycin (IV/PO) Ampicillin (IV) + gentamicin (IV)	Erythromycin (IV)	Usually part of polymicrobial infection
Clostridium botulinum	• CSF = NP • Blood = NP • Sputum = NP • Urine = NP • Stool = NP • Wound = P (wound botulism)	Penicillin (IV)	Clindamycin (IV/PO) Imipenem (IV) Meropenem (IV)	Give trivalent equine antitoxin (p. 116) as soon as possible. Antibiotic therapy is adjunctive
Clostridium difficile	• CSF = NP • Blood = P (rarely from GI source) • Sputum = NP • Urine = NP • Stool = C (normal fecal flora), P (antibiotic-associated diarrhea/colitis) • Wound = NP	Antibiotic-associated diarrhea (AAD) Vancomycin (PO) Antibiotic-associated colitis (AAC) Metronidazole (IV)	Antibiotic-associated diarrhea (AAD) Metronidazole (PO) Antibiotic-associated colitis (AAC) Metronidazole (PO)	For C. difficile diarrhea, PO vancomycin is more consistently effective than PO metronidazole. For C. difficile colitis, use IV or PO metronidazole (IV/PO vancomycin is ineffective). Diagnose AAD by stool C. difficile toxin assay, not stool culture

C = colonizer; C* = skin contaminant; NP = non-pathogen; P = pathogen at site; (IV/PO) = IV or PO. See p. 1 for all other abbreviations

Table 3. Clinical Significance of ANAEROBIC Isolates Pending Susceptibility Testing (cont'd)

	GRAM-POSITIVE BACILLI		
Isolate	Isolate Significance	Preferred Therapy	Alternate Therapy	Comments
Clostridium perfringens, septicum, novyi	• CSF = NP • Blood = P (from GI source/ malignancy) • Sputum = NP • Urine = NP • Stool = NP • Wound = P (gas gangrene)	Penicillin (IV) Imipenem (IV) Meropenem (IV) Ertapenem (IV) Piperacillin/tazobactam (IV)	Clindamycin (IV) Chloramphenicol (IV)	Usual cause of myonecrosis (gas gangrene). Surgical debridement is crucial; antibiotic therapy is adjunctive. Also causes emphysematous cholecystitis/ cystitis
Clostridium tetani	• CSF = NP • Blood = NP • Sputum = NP • Urine = NP • Stool = NP • Wound = P (wound tetanus)	Penicillin (IV) Clindamycin (IV)	Imipenem (IV) Meropenem (IV)	Prompt administration of tetanus immune globulin is crucial (p. 116). Antibiotic therapy is adjunctive
Eubacterium sp.	• CSF = P (brain abscess) • Blood = P (from dental, GI, GU, lung source) • Sputum = P (lung abscess) • Urine = NP • Stool = NP • Wound = NP	Clindamycin (IV/PO) Ampicillin (IV) + gentamicin (IV)	Erythromycin (IV)	Pathogen in lung/pelvic/brain abscesses, and chronic periodontal disease. Eubacterium bacteremias are associated with malignancies
Lactobacillus sp.	• CSF = P (ABM) • Blood = P (1° bacteremia, SBE, or from endometritis) • Sputum = NP • Urine = P (rare) • Stool = NP • Wound = NP	Clindamycin (IV/PO) Ampicillin (IV) + gentamicin (IV)	Erythromycin (IV)	Uncommon pathogen in normal/compromised hosts. Rare cause of SBE. Variably resistant to cephalosporins and quinolones. Resistant to metronidazole and vancomycin

C = colonizer; C* = skin contaminant; NP = non-pathogen at site; P = pathogen at site; (IV/PO) = IV or PO. See p. 1 for all other abbreviations

Table 3. Clinical Significance of ANAEROBIC Isolates Pending Susceptibility Testing (cont'd)

Isolate	Isolate Significance	Preferred Therapy	Alternate Therapy	Comments
GRAM-POSITIVE BACILLI				
Propionibacterium acnes	• CSF = C* = P (meningitis from NS shunts) • Blood = C* = P (from IV line infection, SBE) • Sputum = NP • Urine = NP • Stool = NP • Wound = C (acne)	Penicillin (IV) Clindamycin (IV/PO)	Doxycycline (IV/PO)	Common skin colonizer/blood culture contaminant. Rarely causes prosthetic joint infection, endocarditis, or CNS shunt infection
GRAM-NEGATIVE BACILLI				
Bacteroides fragilis group (B. distasonis, ovatus, thetaiotaomicron, vulgatus)	• CSF = P (meningitis from Strongyloides hyperinfection) • Blood = P (from GI/pelvic source) • Sputum = NP • Urine = NP, = P (only from colonic fistula) • Stool = NP • Wound = NP	Imipenem (IV) Meropenem (IV) Ertapenem (IV) Piperacillin/tazobactam (IV)	Ampicillin/sulbactam (IV) Clindamycin (IV/PO) + levofloxacin (IV/PO) Metronidazole (IV/PO) + levofloxacin (IV/PO) Moxifloxacin (IV/PO)	Major anaerobe below the diaphragm. Usually part of polymicrobial lower intra-abdominal and pelvic infections. Cefotetan is less effective against B. fragilis DOT strains (B. distasonis, B. ovatus, B. thetaiotaomicron). Resistant to penicillin
Fusobacterium nucleatum	• CSF = P (brain abscess) • Blood = P (from lung, GI source) • Sputum = P (aspiration pneumonia, lung abscess) • Urine = NP • Stool = NP • Wound = P (rarely)	Clindamycin (IV/PO) Piperacillin/tazobactam (IV) Ampicillin/sulbactam (IV)	Chloramphenicol (IV) Metronidazole (IV/PO)	Mouth flora associated with dental infections and anaerobic lung infections. F. nucleatum is associated with jugular vein septic phlebitis and GI cancer

C = colonizer; C* = skin contaminant; NP = non-pathogen at site; P = pathogen at site; (IV/PO) = IV or PO. See p. 1 for all other abbreviations

Table 3. Clinical Significance of ANAEROBIC Isolates Pending Susceptibility Testing (cont'd)

GRAM-NEGATIVE BACILLI

Isolate	Isolate Significance	Preferred Therapy	Alternate Therapy	Comments
Prevotella (Bacteroides) bivia	• CSF = NP • Blood = P (from dental, lung, pelvic source) • Sputum = P (lung abscess) • Urine = NP • Stool = NP • Wound = NP	Penicillin (IV/PO) Any β-lactam (IV/PO)	Any quinolone (IV/PO) Doxycycline (IV/PO) Clindamycin (IV/PO)	Cause of dental, oropharyngeal, and female genital tract infections
Prevotella (Bacteroides) melaninogenicus, intermedius	• CSF = P (brain abscess) • Blood = P (from oral/pulmonary source) • Sputum = P (from aspiration pneumonia, lung abscess) • Urine = NP • Stool = NP • Wound = NP	<u>Aspiration pneumonia/lung abscess</u> Any β-lactam (IV/PO) Any quinolone (IV/PO) <u>Brain abscess</u> Penicillin (IV)	<u>Aspiration pneumonia/lung abscess</u> Doxycycline (IV/PO) <u>Brain abscess</u> Chloramphenicol (IV)	Predominant anaerobic flora of mouth. Known as "oral pigmented" Bacteroides (e.g., B. melanogenicus). Antibiotics used to treat community-acquired pneumonia are effective against oral anaerobes (e.g., Prevotella) in aspiration pneumonia; does not require anti-B. fragilis coverage with clindamycin, metronidazole, or moxifloxacin

C = colonizer; C* = skin contaminant; NP = non-pathogen at site; P = pathogen at site; (IV/PO) = IV or PO. See p. 1 for all other abbreviations

Table 4. Clinical Significance of YEAST/FUNGI Pending Susceptibility Testing

YEAST/FUNGI

Isolate	Isolate Significance	Preferred Therapy	Alternate Therapy	Comments
Aspergillus fumigatus, flavus, niger	• CSF = P (only from disseminated infection) • Blood = P (1° fungemia or from pulmonary source) • Sputum = C, P (pneumonia) • Urine = NP • Stool = NP • Wound = NP	Amphotericin B (IV) Itraconazole (IV/PO) Caspofungin (IV) Voriconazole (IV/PO)	Amphotericin B lipid formulation (IV)	A. fumigatus is the usual cause of invasive aspergillosis. A. flavus/niger are usually airborne specimen contaminants. Aspergillus pneumonia and disseminated aspergillosis are common in patients receiving chronic steroids or immunosuppressive therapy (especially organ transplants). Recovery of Aspergillus from respiratory tract is not diagnostic of Aspergillus pneumonia; tissue biopsy is required for diagnosis
Candida non-albicans group (C. krusei, Lusitaniae, tropicalis, pseudotropicalis, glabrata, gilliermondii, lipolytica)	• CSF = P (only from disseminated infection) • Blood = P (1° candidemia or from IV line infection) • Sputum = NP • Urine = C (indwelling catheters), P (from cystitis, pyelonephritis) • Stool = C (source of candiduria) • Wound = NP	Itraconazole (IV/PO) Caspofungin (IV) Voriconazole (IV/PO)	Amphotericin B (IV/PO) Amphotericin B lipid formulation (IV/PO) Fluconazole (IV/PO)	Most non-C. albicans are fluconazole-resistant, especially C. lusitaniae and C. krusei. Non-C. albicans infections cause the same spectrum of disease as C. albicans

C = colonizer; C* = skin contaminant; NP = non-pathogen at site; P = pathogen at site; (IV/PO) = IV or PO. See p. 1 for all other abbreviations

Table 4. Clinical Significance of YEAST/FUNGI Pending Susceptibility Testing (cont'd)

		YEAST/FUNGI		
Isolate	Isolate Significance	Preferred Therapy	Alternate Therapy	Comments
Candida albicans	• CSF = P (only from disseminated infection) • Blood = P (1° candidemia or from IV line infection) • Sputum = C, P (only from disseminated infection) • Urine = C, P (from cystitis, pyelonephritis) • Stool = C (source of candiduria) • Wound = NP	Fluconazole (IV/PO) Itraconazole (IV/PO) Caspofungin (IV) Voriconazole (IV/PO)	Amphotericin B (IV/PO) Amphotericin B lipid formulation (IV)	Common colonizer of GI/GU tracts. Colonization is common in diabetics, alcoholics, and patients receiving steroids/antibiotics. Commonest cause of fungemia in hospitalized patients. Candidemia secondary to central IV lines does not indicate disseminated candidiasis. Primary Candida pneumonia does not occur; secondary Candida pneumonia rarely may complicate disseminated candidiasis
Cryptococcus neoformans	• CSF = P (meningitis, brain abscess) • Blood = P (from pulmonary source) • Sputum = P (pneumonia) • Urine = NP • Stool = NP • Wound = NP	**CNS** Amphotericin B (IV) ± flucytosine (PO) **Non-CNS** Amphotericin B (IV) Amphotericin B lipid formulation (IV)	**CNS** Fluconazole (IV/PO) Voriconazole (IV/PO) **Non-CNS** Itraconazole (IV/PO)	C. neoformans meningitis may occur with or without dissemination. Cryptococcal pneumonia frequently disseminates to CNS. C. neoformans in blood cultures occurs in compromised hosts (e.g., HIV/AIDS) and indicates disseminated infection

C = colonizer; C* = skin contaminant; NP = non-pathogen at site; P = pathogen at site; (IV/PO) = IV or PO. See p. 1 for all other abbreviations

Table 4. Clinical Significance of YEAST/FUNGI Pending Susceptibility Testing (cont'd)

YEAST/FUNGI

Isolate	Isolate Significance	Preferred Therapy	Alternate Therapy	Comments
Histoplasma capsulatum	• CSF = P (from disseminated infection, pneumonia) • Blood = P (1° fungemia, rarely SBE) • Sputum = P (pneumonia, mediastinitis) • Urine = NP • Stool = NP • Wound = NP	Amphotericin B (IV) Itraconazole (IV/PO)	Fluconazole (IV/PO) Ketoconazole (PO) Voriconazole (IV/PO) Amphotericin B lipid formulation (IV)	Histoplasma recovered from CSF/blood cultures indicates dissemination. Disseminated histoplasmosis is most common in compromised hosts (e.g., HIV/AIDS). Itraconazole is ineffective for meningeal histoplasmosis, but is preferred for chronic suppressive therapy
Malassezia furfur	• CSF = NP • Blood = P (from IV line infection) • Sputum = NP • Urine = NP • Stool = NP • Wound = P (eosinophilic folliculitis)	Amphotericin B (IV)	Itraconazole (IV/PO) Fluconazole (IV/PO) Miconazole (IV) Ketoconazole (PO)	M. furfur IV line infections are associated with IV lipid hyperalimentation emulsions. Fungemia usually resolves with IV line removal. Morphology in blood is blunt buds on a broad base yeast. M. furfur requires long chain fatty acids for growth (overlay agar with thin layer of olive oil, Tween 80, or oleic acid)
Penicillium marneffei	• CSF = NP • Blood = P (usually from dissemination) • Sputum = P (pneumonia) • Urine = NP • Stool = NP • Wound = NP	Amphotericin B (IV) Itraconazole (IV/PO)	Fluconazole (IV/PO) Voriconazole (IV/PO)	Histoplasma-like yeast forms seen in lymph nodes, liver, skin, bone marrow, blood. Characteristic red pigment diffuses into agar. Causes granulomatous tissue reaction ± necrosis. Skin lesions indicate dissemination. Rash may be papular, or resembles molluscum contagiosum with central umbilication. Hepatosplenomegaly is common. Dissemination is common in HIV

C = colonizer; C* = skin contaminant; P = pathogen at site; P* = non-pathogen at site; NP = non-pathogen; (IV/PO) = IV or PO. See p. 1 for all other abbreviations

Chapter 4

Parasites, Fungi, Unusual Organisms

Burke A. Cunha, M.D.

Parasites, Fungi, Unusual Organisms in Blood

Microfilaria in Blood

Subset	Pathogen	Preferred Therapy	Alternate Therapy
Filariasis	Brugia malayi	Diethylcarbamazine: day 1: 50 mg (PO) day 2: 50 mg (PO) q8h day 3: 100 mg (PO) q8h days 4-14: 2 mg/kg (PO) q8h	Ivermectin 400 mcg/kg (PO) x 1 dose ± albendazole 400 mg (PO) x 1 dose
	Wuchereria bancrofti	Diethylcarbamazine: day 1: 50 mg (PO) day 2: 50 mg (PO) q8h day 3: 100 mg (PO) q8h days 4-14: 2 mg/kg (PO) q8h	Ivermectin 400 mcg/kg (PO) x 1 dose ± albendazole 400 mg (PO) x 1 dose

Brugia malayi

Clinical Presentation: May present as an obscure febrile illness, chronic lymphedema, lymphangitis, or cutaneous abscess. "Filarial fevers" usually last 1 week and spontaneously remit

Diagnostic Considerations: Diagnosis by demonstrating microfilaria on Giemsa's stained thick blood smear or by using the concentration method; yield is increased by passing blood through a Millipore filter before staining. Several smears should be taken over 24 hours. Common infection in Southeast Asia (primarily China, Korea, India, Indonesia, Malaysia, Philippines, Sri Lanka). Most species have nocturnal periodicity (microfilaria in blood at night). Eosinophilia is most common during periods of acute inflammation

Pitfalls: Genital manifestations—scrotal edema, epididymitis, orchitis, hydrocele—are frequent with W. bancrofti, but rare with B. malayi

Prognosis: Related to state of health and extent of lymphatic obstruction. No satisfactory treatment is available. Single-dose ivermectin is effective treatment for microfilaremia, but does not kill the adult worm (although diethylcarbamazine kills some). If no microfilaria in blood, full-dose diethylcarbamazine (2 mg/kg q8h) can be started on day one. Antihistamines or corticosteroids may decrease allergic reactions from disintegration of microfilaria

Wuchereria bancrofti

Clinical Presentation: May present as an obscure febrile illness, chronic lymphedema, lymphangitis, or cutaneous abscess. Genital (scrotal) lymphatic edema, groin lesions, epididymitis, orchitis, hydroceles are characteristic. Chyluria may occur. "Filarial fevers" usually last 1 week and spontaneously remit

Diagnostic Considerations: Diagnosis by demonstrating microfilaria on Giemsa's stained thick blood smear or by using the concentration method; yield is increased by passing blood through a Millipore filter before staining. Several smears should to be taken over 24 hours. W. bancrofti is the most common human filarial infection, particularly in Asia (China, India, Indonesia, Japan, Malaysia, Philippines), Southeast Asia, Sri Lanka, Tropical Africa, Central/South America, and Pacific Islands. Most species have nocturnal periodicity (microfilaria in blood at night). Eosinophilia is common

Pitfalls: Differentiate from "hanging groins" of Loa Loa, which usually do not involve the scrotum

Prognosis: Related to state of health and extent of lymphatic obstruction. No satisfactory treatment is available. Single-dose ivermectin is effective treatment for microfilaremia, but does not kill the adult worm (although diethylcarbamazine kills some). If no microfilaria in blood, full-dose diethylcarbamazine (2 mg/kg q8h) can be started on day one. Antihistamines or corticosteroids decrease allergic reactions from disintegration of microfilaria

Trypanosomes in Blood

Subset	Pathogen	Preferred Therapy	Alternate Therapy
Chagas' disease (American trypanosomiasis)	Trypanosoma cruzi	Nifurtimox 8-10 mg/kg/day (PO) in 3-4 divided doses x 3-4 months	Benznidazole 2.5-3.5 mg/kg (PO) q12h x 2 months
Sleeping sickness *West African trypanosomiasis*	Trypanosoma brucei gambiense	<u>Hemolymphatic stage</u> Pentamidine 4 mg/kg (IM) q24h x 10 days <u>Late disease with CNS involvement</u> Melarsoprol 2–3.6 mg/kg (IV) q24h x 3 days. After 1 week, give 3.6 mg/kg (IV) q24h x 3 days; repeat again in 10-21 days	<u>Hemolymphatic stage</u> Suramin 200 mg test dose (IV), then 1 gm (IV) on days 1,3,7,14 and 21 **or** Eflornithine 100 mg/kg (IV) q6h x 2 weeks <u>Late disease with CNS involvement</u> None
East African trypanosomiasis	Trypanosoma brucei rhodesiense	<u>Hemolymphatic stage</u> Suramin 200 mg test dose (IV), then 1 gm (IV) on days 1,3,7,14 and 21 <u>Late disease with CNS involvement</u> Melarsoprol 2–3.6 mg/kg (IV) q24h x 3 days. After 1 week, give 3.6 mg/kg (IV) q24h x 3 days; repeat again in 10-21 days	<u>Hemolymphatic stage</u> Eflornithine, pentamidine (see doses above) variably effective <u>Late disease with CNS involvement</u> None

Chagas' Disease (Trypanosoma cruzi) American Trypanosomiasis

Clinical Presentation: Presents acutely after bite of infected reduviid bug with unilateral painless edema of the palpebrae/periocular tissues (Romaña's sign), or as an indurated area of erythema and swelling with local lymph node involvement (chagoma). Fever, malaise, and edema of the face and lower extremities may follow. Generalized lymphadenopathy and mild hepatosplenomegaly sometimes occur. Patients with chronic disease may develop cardiac involvement (cardiomyopathy with arrhythmias, heart block, heart failure, thromboembolism) or GI involvement (megaesophagus/megacolon)

Diagnostic Considerations: Common in Central and South America. Acquired from infected reduviid bug, which infests mud/clay parts of primitive dwellings. Diagnosis in acute disease by detecting parasites in wet prep of anticoagulated blood or buffy coat smear, Giemsa-stained smears, bone marrow or lymph node aspirates, or by xenodiagnosis. For chronic disease, serology is useful in non-endemic areas, but is of limited value (lacks specificity) in endemic areas

Pitfalls: Do not overlook the diagnosis in patients from endemic areas with unexplained heart block

Prognosis: Related to extent of cardiac/GI involvement

Sleeping Sickness (T. brucei gambiense/rhodesiense) West African/East African Trypanosomiasis

Clinical Presentation: Sleeping sickness from T. brucei gambiense is milder than sleeping sickness from T. brucei rhodesiense, which is usually a fulminant infection. A few days to weeks after bite of tsetse fly, patients progress through several clinical stages:

- *Chancre stage*: Trypanosomal chancre occurs at bite site and lasts several weeks
- *Blood/lymphatic stage*: Blood parasitemia is associated with intermittent high fevers, headaches and insomnia, followed by generalized adenopathy. Posterior cervical lymph node enlargement (Winterbottom's sign) is particularly prominent with T. brucei gambiense. Hepatosplenomegaly and transient edema/pruritus/irregular circinate rash are common. Myocarditis (tachycardia unrelated to fevers) occurs early (before CNS involvement) and is responsible for acute deaths from T. brucei rhodesiense
- *CNS stage*: Occurs after a few months of non-specific symptoms, and is characterized by increasing lethargy, somnolence (sleeping sickness), and many subtle CNS findings. Coma and death ensue without treatment. With melarsoprol, use prednisolone 1 mg/kg (PO) q24h

Diagnostic Considerations: Diagnosis by demonstrating trypanosomes in blood, chancre, or lymph nodes aspirates by Giemsa-stained thin and thick preparations, light microscopy, or buffy coat concentrates with acridine orange

Pitfalls: Do not miss other causes of prominent bilateral posterior cervical lymph node enlargement (e.g., lymphoma, EBV)

Prognosis: Related to extent of cardiac/CNS involvement. Relapse may occur

Spirochetes in Blood

Subset	Pathogen	Preferred Therapy	Alternate Therapy
Relapsing fever *Louse-borne (LBRF)* *Tick-borne (TBRF)*	Borrelia recurrentis. At least 15 Borrelia species (U.S.: B. hermsi; Africa: B. duttonii; Africa/Middle East: B. crocidurae)	<u>LBRF</u> Erythromycin 500 mg (IV or PO) q6h x 7 days <u>TBRF</u> Doxycycline 200 mg (PO) x 3 days, then 100 mg (PO) q12h x 7 days	<u>TBRF with CNS involvement</u> Penicillin G 2 mu (IV) q4h x 2 weeks **or** Ceftriaxone 1 gm (IV) q12h x 2 weeks **or** Cefotaxime 3 gm (IV) q6h x 2 weeks
Rat bite fever	Spirillum minus	Penicillin G 4 mu (IV) q4h. Can switch to amoxicillin 1 gm (PO) q8h for total therapy of 2 weeks **or** Doxycycline 200 mg (IV or PO) q12h x 3 days, then 100 mg (IV or PO) q12h x 11 days	Erythromycin 500 mg (IV or PO) q6h x 2 weeks **or** Chloramphenicol 500 mg (IV) q6h x 2 weeks

Relapsing Fever, Louse-Borne (LBRF) / Tick-Borne (TBRF)

Clinical Presentation: Abrupt onset of "flu-like" illness with high fever, rigors, headache, myalgias, arthralgias, tachycardia, dry cough, abdominal pain after exposure to infected louse or tick. Truncal petechial rash and conjunctival suffusion are common. Hepatosplenomegaly/DIC may occur. Bleeding complications are more common in LBRF. Fevers last ~ 1 week, remit for a week, and usually relapse only once in LBRF, but several times in TBRF. Relapses usually last 2-3 days. Fevers are often higher in TBRF

Diagnostic Considerations: Borreliae are found in > 70% of infected febrile patients when wet blood smears are examined by dark field, Giemsa, or Wright-stained thick and thin peripheral blood smears. LBRF is endemic in South American Andes, Central and East Africa, and is associated with crowded, unhygienic conditions. TBRF is seen throughout the world, and is endemic in Western U.S., British Columbia, Mexico, Central/South America, Mediterranean, Central Asia, and Africa

Pitfalls: Spirochetes are most likely to be seen during febrile periods. Some treatment failures occur in TBRF with single-dose therapy

Prognosis: Good if treated early. Usually no permanent sequelae

Rat Bite Fever (Spirillum minus)

Clinical Presentation: Infection develops 1-4 weeks following bite of wild rat. Healed rat bite becomes red, painful, swollen and ulcerated, with regional lymphangitis/adenopathy. Relapsing fever occurs in 2-4 day fever cycles. Fevers are usually accompanied by chills, headache, photophobia, nausea, vomiting. Rash on palms/soles develops in > 50%. Arthritis, myalgias, and SBE are rare

Diagnostic Considerations: Short thick spirochetes are seen in peripheral blood smears, exudate, or lymph node tissue examined by dark field, Giemsa, or Wright's stain. Mostly seen in Asia. Differential diagnosis includes Borrelia, malaria, and lymphoma. VDRL is positive

Pitfalls: May be confused with syphilis, due to rash on palms/soles and false-positive syphilis serology in 50%. SBE occurs with S. moniliformis, not S. minus (unless there is preexisting valvular disease). Bite wound ulcerates in S. minus, not S. moniliformis

Prognosis: Patients with arthritis have a protracted course

Intracellular Inclusion Bodies in Blood

Subset	Pathogen	Preferred Therapy	Alternate Therapy
Babesiosis	Babesia microti	Azithromycin 1 gm (PO) q24h x 3 days, then 500 mg (PO) q24h x 7 days **plus** Atovaquone (suspension) 750 mg (PO) q12h x 7-10 days	Clindamycin 600 mg (PO) q8h x 7 days **plus** Quinine 650 mg (PO) q8h x 7 days
Ehrlichiosis *Human monocytic (HME)* *Human granulocytic (HGE)*	Ehrlichia chaffeensis Ehrlichia phagocytophilia/ equi	Doxycycline 200 mg (IV or PO) q12h x 3 days, then 100 mg (IV or PO) q12h x 1-2 weeks total	Levofloxacin 500 mg (IV or PO) q24h x 1-2 weeks **or** Ciprofloxacin 400 mg (IV) or 750 mg (PO) q12h x 1-2 weeks **or** Chloramphenicol 500 mg (IV or PO) q6h x 1-2 weeks

Intracellular Inclusion Bodies in Blood (cont'd)

Subset	Pathogen	Preferred Therapy	Alternate Therapy

Malaria
  Benign
  tertian
 	
  Malignant
  tertian
 	
  Quartan
	Plasmodium ovale
	Plasmodium vivax
	
	Plasmodium
	falciparum
	
	Plasmodium
	malariae
		<u>Chloroquine-sensitive strains</u>
		Chloroquine phosphate
		1 gm (600 mg base) (PO) x 1
		dose, then 500 mg (300 mg
		base) (PO) at 6, 24, and 48
		hours
		<center>**or**</center>Quinidine gluconate
		10 mg/kg (maximum 600
		mg) (IV) over 1-2 hours,
		followed by continuous IV
		infusion of 0.02 mg/kg/min
		until parasitemia < 1% or for
		72 hours
		<center>**or**</center>Chloroquine phosphate
		10 mg (base)/kg (IV) over 4
		hours, then 5 mg (base)/kg
		(IV) over 2 hours q12h
		(total dose not to exceed
		25 mg/kg)
		
		<u>For P. vivax or P. ovale, add:</u>
		Primaquine phosphate
		26.3 mg (15 mg base) (PO)
		q24h x 2 weeks
			<u>Chloroquine-resistant strains</u>
			Mild/moderately ill
			Quinine sulfate
			650 mg (500 mg base) (PO)
			q8h x 7 days
			<center>**plus**</center>Doxycycline 200 mg (PO)
			q12h x 3 days, then
			100 mg (PO) q12h x 7 days
			<center>**or monotherapy**
			with</center>Atovaquone/proguanil
			(250/100 mg tab) 4 tabs
			as a single dose (PO) q24h
			x 3 days
			
			Critically ill
			Quinidine gluconate
			15 mg/kg (IV) over 1-2 hours,
			followed by either 7.5 mg/kg
			(IV) over 1-2 hours q8h or
			1-1.5 mg/kg/hr constant (IV)
			infusion until parasitemia
			< 1%. Then complete 7 days
			of total therapy with an oral
			agent(s), listed above
			<center>**or**</center>Quinine dihydrochloride
			20 mg (salt)/kg (IV) over
			4 hours (in D_5W), then 10 mg
			(salt)/kg (IV) over 2 hours
			q8h until able to take oral
			medication. Then use oral
			agent(s) listed above to
			complete 7 days total therapy

Babesiosis (Babesia microti)

Clinical Presentation: "Malarial-like illness" with malaise, fever, shaking chills, myalgias, arthralgias, headaches, abdominal pain, relative bradycardia, and splenomegaly. Laboratory abnormalities include anemia, atypical lymphocytes in peripheral smear, lymphopenia, thrombocytopenia, mildly elevated LFTs, ↑ LDH, proteinuria, and hemoglobinuria. Transmitted by infected Ixodes ticks

Diagnostic Considerations: Characteristic "tetrad" when examined by Giemsa or Wright-stained thick and thin peripheral blood smears. IFA serology ≥ 1:256 is diagnostic of acute infection. Hyposplenic patients may have profound hemolytic anemia and life-threatening infection

Pitfalls: Co-infection with Lyme disease may occur. No serological cross-reactivity between Babesia and Borrelia (Lyme disease)

Prognosis: Severe/fatal in patients with decreased or absent splenic function. Exchange transfusions may be life-saving

Ehrlichiosis, Human Monocytic (HME) / Human Granulocytic (HGE)

Clinical Presentation: Acute febrile illness with chills, headache, malaise, myalgias, leukopenia, thrombocytopenia, ↑ LFTs. No vasculitis. Resembles Rocky Mountain spotted fever (RMSF), but rash much less frequent

Diagnostic Considerations: Characteristic "morulae" (spherical, basophilic, Mulberry-shaped, cytoplasmic inclusion bodies) seen in peripheral blood neutrophils in HGE. PCR from blood is 86% sensitive and highly specific for early diagnosis. Obtain acute and convalescent IFA serology. Vector is I. scapularis tick. Co-infection with B. burgdorferi (Lyme Disease) is uncommon, but may occur

Pitfalls: Morulae are not seen in HME, so blood smears are unhelpful. Rash occurs in > 90% in Rocky Mountain spotted fever, but is uncommon in HME and rare in HGE

Prognosis: Excellent if treated early

Malaria (Plasmodium ovale/vivax/falciparum/malariae)

Clinical Presentation: Presents acutely with fever/chills, severe headaches, cough, nausea/vomiting, diarrhea, abdominal/back pain. Typical "malarial paroxysm" consists of chills, fever and profuse sweating, followed by extreme prostration. There are a paucity of physical findings, but most have tender hepatomegaly/splenomegaly and relative bradycardia. Anemia, thrombocytopenia, atypical lymphocytes, and ↑ LDH/LFTs are common

Diagnostic Considerations: Diagnosis by demonstrating Plasmodium on thick and thin Giemsa or Wright-stained smears

Pitfalls: Be wary of diagnosing malaria without headache/anemia. Assume all P. falciparum are chloroquine-resistant. Chloroquine-resistant P. vivax are now seen in South America, New Guinea, and Oceania (Indonesia). Chloroquine-sensitive strains are acquired in Central America (north of Panama Canal), Haiti, and parts of the Middle East (although chloroquine-resistant strains have been reported in Yemen, Oman, Saudi Arabia, and Iran)

Prognosis: Related to species. P. falciparum with high-grade parasitemia is most severe, and may be complicated by coma, hypoglycemia, renal failure, or non-cardiogenic pulmonary edema. If parasitemia exceeds 15%, consider exchange transfusions

Fungi/Mycobacterium in Blood

See histoplasmosis (pp. 219, 226), Mycobacterium tuberculosis (treat as pulmonary TB, pp. 216, 222), Mycobacterium avium-intracellulare (pp. 219, 225)

Parasites, Fungi, Unusual Organisms in CSF/Brain

Cysts/Mass Lesions in CSF/Brain

Subset	Pathogens	Preferred Therapy	PO Therapy
Cerebral nocardiosis	Nocardia sp.	Amikacin 500 mg (IV) q12h x 2 weeks *plus either* Imipenem 500 (IV) q6h x 2 weeks *or* Cefotaxime 1 gm (IV) q6h x 2 weeks. Then switch to PO therapy for 6 months total therapy	Preferred PO Therapy TMP-SMX 1 DS tablet (PO) q12h x 6 months Alternate PO Therapy Minocycline 200 mg (IV or PO) q12h x 6 months

Cysts/Mass Lesions in CSF/Brain (cont'd)

Subset	Pathogens	Preferred Therapy	Alternate Therapy
Cerebral amebiasis	Entamoeba histolytica	Metronidazole 750 mg (PO) q8h x 10 days **or** Tinidazole 600 mg (PO) q12h x 5 days	
Primary amebic meningo-encephalitis	Naegleria fowleri	See p. 19	
Granulomatous amebic encephalitis	Acanthamoeba	See p. 20	
Cerebral echinococcosis (hydatid cyst disease)	Echinococcus granulosus	Surgical resection plus albendazole 400 mg* (PO) q12h until cured	Surgical resection plus mebendazole 50 mg/kg (PO) q24h until cured
	Echinococcus multilocularis	Surgical resection plus albendazole 400 mg* (PO) q12h until cured	Surgical resection plus mebendazole 50 mg/kg (PO) q24h until cured
Cerebral gnathostomiasis	Gnathostoma spinigerum	Surgical resection	Albendazole 400 mg (PO) q12h x 3 weeks
Cerebral coenurosis	Taenia multiceps	Surgical resection	
Neuro-cysticercosis	Taenia solium	Praziquantel 17 mg/kg (PO) q8h x 3 weeks	Albendazole 400 mg* (PO) q12h x 3 weeks
Cerebral paragonimiasis (lung fluke)	Paragonimus westermani	Praziquantel 25 mg/kg (PO) q8h x 2 days	Bithionol 50 mg/kg (PO) q48h x 10 days
Cerebral toxoplasmosis	Toxoplasmosis gondii	See p. 217	
Cryptococcomas/ meningitis	Cryptococcus neoformans	See p. 217	
Chagas' disease (American trypanosomiasis)	Trypanosoma cruzi	Nifurtimox 2 mg/kg (PO) q6h x 4 months	Benznidazole 3.5 mg/kg (PO) q12h x 2 months

* If < 60 kg, give albendazole 7.5 mg/kg

Cerebral Nocardiosis

Clinical Presentation: CNS mass lesion resembling brain tumor/abscess. Symptoms are highly variable, and result from local effects of granulomas/abscesses on CNS. Up to 40% of patients with systemic nocardiosis have associated mass lesions in CNS

Diagnostic Considerations: Diagnosis by demonstrating Nocardia in brain biopsy specimens. Notify laboratory for AFB specimen staining/aerobic cultures if suspect Nocardia. Nocardia are weakly acid-fast and aerobic

Pitfalls: Usually not limited to brain. Look for Nocardia in lungs or liver. Use in-vitro susceptibility data to guide therapy for refractory cases. IV regimens are recommended for critically ill patients. HIV/AIDS patients require life-long suppression with TMP-SMX

Prognosis: Related to health of host, degree of immunosuppression, and extent of lesions

Cerebral Amebiasis (Entamoeba histolytica)

Clinical Presentation: Rare cause of brain abscess. Onset is frequently abrupt with rapid progression. Suspect in patients with a history of amebiasis and altered mental status/focal neurologic signs. If present, meningeal involvement resembles acute bacterial meningitis. CT/MRI shows focal lesions. CSF eosinophilia is not a feature of CNS involvement

Diagnostic Considerations: Diagnosis by demonstrating E. histolytica trophozoites from aspirated brain lesions under CT guidance. Worldwide distribution. Mass lesions may be single or multiple, and more commonly involve the left hemisphere. Most patients have concomitant liver ± lung abscesses

Pitfalls: Trophozoites/eggs in stool are not diagnostic of CNS disease. E. histolytica is serology often positive, but is nonspecific. E. histolytica trophozoites are not present in CSF

Prognosis: Related to size/location of CNS lesions

Primary Amebic Meningoencephalitis (Naegleria fowleri) (see p. 21)

Granulomatous Amebic Encephalitis (Acanthamoeba) (see p. 21)

Cerebral Echinococcosis (Echinococcus granulosus) Hydatid Cyst Disease

Clinical Presentation: Most cysts are asymptomatic. Mass lesions may cause seizures, cranial nerve abnormalities, other focal neurologic symptoms

Diagnostic Considerations: CT/MRI typically shows a single large cyst without edema or enhancement. Multiple cysts are rare. Diagnosis by demonstrating protoscolices in "hydatid sand" in cysts. Usually associated with liver/lung hydatid cysts

Pitfalls: E. granulosus serology lacks specificity

Prognosis: Related to size/location of CNS cysts. Treatment consists of surgical removal of total cyst after instilling cysticidal agent (hypertonic saline, iodophor, ethanol) into cyst plus albendazole

Cerebral Echinococcosis (Echinococcus multilocularis) Hydatid Cyst Disease

Clinical Presentation: Frequently associated with hydatid bone cysts (may cause spinal cord compression), liver/lung cysts. Peripheral eosinophilia occurs in 50%, but eosinophils are not seen in the CSF

Diagnostic Considerations: E. multilocularis ELISA is sensitive and specific

Pitfalls: Praziquantel is ineffective for CNS hydatid cyst disease. Imaging studies suggest carcinoma/sarcoma. Diagnosis is frequently not made until brain biopsy

Prognosis: If treatment is effective, improvement of CNS lesions is evident in 8 weeks (2/3 improve). Brain/bone cysts are difficult to cure

Cerebral Gnathostomiasis (Gnathostoma spinigerum)

Clinical Presentation: Nausea, vomiting, increased salivation, skin flushing, pruritus, urticaria, and upper abdominal pain 1-6 days after exposure. Cerebral form presents as eosinophilic meningitis with radiculomyeloencephalitis, with headache and severe sharp/shooting pains in extremities often followed by paraplegia and coma. Any cranial nerve may be involved. The most characteristic feature is changing/migratory neurological findings. Intense peripheral eosinophilia occurs in 90% of patients. CSF has eosinophilic pleocytosis and may have RBCs

Diagnostic Considerations: In cases with ocular involvement, the worm may be seen in the anterior chamber of eye. Specific Gnathostoma serology of CSF is helpful in establishing the diagnosis. Acquired from infected cat/dog feces. Most cases occur in Southeast Asia. Few other CNS infections have both

RBCs and eosinophils in the CSF
Pitfalls: Do not miss associated eye involvement
Prognosis: Related to invasion of medulla/brainstem

Cerebral Coenurosis (Taenia multiceps)

Clinical Presentation: CNS mass lesion with seizures/cranial nerve abnormalities, often presenting as a posterior-fossa syndrome. Common sites of CNS involvement include paraventricular and basal subarachnoid spaces
Diagnostic Considerations: Diagnosis by demonstrating protoscolices in brain specimens. Worldwide distribution. Transmitted via dog feces
Pitfalls: Do not miss associated ocular lesions, which mimic intraocular neoplasms/granulomas
Prognosis: Related to size/extent of CNS lesions

Neurocysticercosis (Taenia solium)

Clinical Presentation: Chronic meningitis/mass lesions with seizures. Hydrocephalus is common. Spinal involvement may result in paraplegia. Cerebral cysts are usually multiple
Diagnostic Considerations: CT/MRI shows multiple enhancing and non-enhancing unilocular cysts. Diagnosis by specific T. solium serology of serum/CSF. Neurocysticercosis is the most common CNS parasite. Worldwide in distribution, but most common in Eastern Europe, Asia, and Latin America
Pitfalls: Cranial nerve abnormalities are uncommon
Prognosis: Related to extent/location of CNS lesions. Adjunctive therapy includes corticosteroids, anti-epileptics, and shunt for hydrocephalus

Cerebral Paragonimiasis (Paragonimus westermani) Lung Fluke

Clinical Presentation: Can resemble epilepsy, cerebral tumors, or brain embolism. Primary focus of infection is pulmonary, with pleuritic chest pain, cough, and night sweats. CNS findings are a manifestation of extrapulmonary (ectopic) organ involvement
Diagnostic Considerations: Diagnosis by demonstrating operculated eggs in sputum, pleural fluid, or feces. Multiple sputum samples are needed to demonstrate P. westermani eggs. Charcot-Leyden crystals are seen in sputum. Endemic in Far East, India, Africa, and Central/South America
Pitfalls: Extrapulmonary (ectopic) organ involvement (cerebral, subcutaneous, abdominal) is common. Up to 20% of patients have normal chest x-rays
Prognosis: Related to size/location of CNS cysts and extent of lung involvement

Cerebral Toxoplasmosis (T. gondii) (see p. 222)

Cerebral Cryptococcosis (C. neoformans) (see p. 223)

Chagas' Disease (Trypanosoma cruzi) American Trypanosomiasis

Clinical Presentation: Acute unilateral periorbital cellulitis (Romaña's sign) or regional adenopathy and edema of extremity at site of infected reduviid bug (Chagoma). Chronic disease manifests as myocarditis/heart block or megaesophagus/megacolon. Hepatosplenomegaly is common. Overt CNS signs are frequently absent. If meningoencephalitis develops, the prognosis is very poor. In immunosuppressed patients (especially AIDS), recrudescence of disease occurs with development of T. cruzi brain abscesses
Diagnostic Considerations: Diagnosis in acute disease by demonstrating parasite in wet prep of anticoagulated blood/Buffy coat smear, Giemsa-stained smear, bone marrow/lymph node aspirate, or by xenodiagnosis. Serology (mostly used for chronic disease) has limited value in endemic areas due to lack of specificity, but is useful in non-endemic areas. Common in Central/South America. Acquired from infected reduviid bugs, which infest mud/clay/stone parts of primitive dwellings. Infection in humans occurs only in areas containing reduviids that defecate during or immediately after a blood

meal
Pitfalls: Do not overlook diagnosis in persons from endemic areas with unexplained heart block. For children ages 11-16 years, use nifurtimox 3.5 mg/kg (PO) q6h x 3 months. For children < 11 years, use nifurtimox 5 mg/kg (PO) q6h x 3 months
Prognosis: Related to extent of GI/cardiac involvement

Parasites, Fungi, Unusual Organisms in Lungs

Pulmonary Cystic Lesions/Masses

Subset	Pathogens	Preferred Therapy	Alternate Therapy
Alveolar echinococcosis	Echinococcus multilocularis	Operable cases Wide surgical resection plus albendazole 400 mg* (PO) q12h or mebendazole 50 mg/kg (PO) q24h until cured	Inoperable cases Albendazole 400 mg* (PO) q12h x 1 month, then repeat therapy after 2 weeks x 3 cycles (i.e., 4 total months of albendazole)
Pulmonary amebiasis	Entamoeba histolytica	Metronidazole 750 mg (PO) q8h x 10 days	Tinidazole 600 mg (PO) q12h x 5 days
Pulmonary paragonimiasis (lung fluke)	Paragonimus westermani	Praziquantel 25 mg/kg (PO) q8h x 2 days	Bithionol 50 mg/kg (PO) q48h x 4 weeks (14 doses)

* If < 60 kg, give albendazole 7.5 mg/kg

Alveolar Echinococcosis (Echinococcus multilocularis)
Clinical Presentation: Slowly growing cysts remain asymptomatic for 5-20 years, until space-occupying effect elicits symptoms. Rupture or leak into bronchial tree can cause cough, chest pain, and hemoptysis
Diagnostic Considerations: Diagnosis is suggested by typical "Swiss cheese calcification" findings on chest x-ray, and confirmed by specific E. multilocularis serology (which does not cross react with E. granulosus). Most common in Northern forest areas of Europe, Asia, North America, and Arctic. Acquired by ingestion of viable parasite eggs in food. Tapeworm-infected canines/cats or wild rodents are common vectors. Less common than infection with E. granulosus
Pitfalls: Do not confuse central cavitary lesions with squamous cell carcinoma
Prognosis: Related to severity/extent of cysts

Pulmonary Amebiasis (Entamoeba histolytica)
Clinical Presentation: Cough, pelvic pain, fever, and right lung/pleural mass mimicking pneumonia or lung abscess. Bronchopleural fistulas may occur. Sputum has "liver-like" taste if cyst ruptures into bronchus. Bacterial co-infection is rare. Amebic lung lesions are associated with hepatic liver abscesses, and invariably involve the right lobe of lung/diaphragm
Diagnostic Considerations: Diagnosis by aspiration of lungs cysts, which may be massive. Amebic serology is sensitive and specific. Worldwide distribution. Acquired by ingesting amebic cysts. Key to diagnosis is concomitant liver involvement; liver abscess presents years after initial diarrheal episode
Pitfalls: Lung involvement is rarely the sole manifestation of amebic infection, and is usually due to direct extension of amebic liver abscess (10-20% of amebic liver abscesses penetrate through the diaphragm and into the lungs). Follow metronidazole with paromomycin 500 mg (PO) q8h x 7 days to eliminate intestinal focus
Prognosis: Related to severity/extent of cysts

Pulmonary Paragonimiasis (Paragonimus westermani) Lung Fluke

Clinical Presentation: Mild infection; may be asymptomatic. Acute phase of infection is accompanied by abdominal pain, diarrhea and urticaria, followed by pleuritic chest pain. Chronic symptoms occur within 6 months after exposure, with dyspnea/dry cough leading to productive cough ± hemoptysis. Complications include pleural effusion, lung abscess, bronchiectasis, cough, and night sweats. Eosinophilia may be evident acutely

Diagnostic Considerations: Oriental lung fluke acquired by ingestion of freshwater crayfish/crabs. After penetration of the gut/peritoneal cavity, the fluke migrates through the diaphragm/pleural space and invades lung parenchyma. Incubation period is 2-20 days. Diagnosis by demonstrating operculated eggs in sputum, pleural fluid, or feces. Multiple sputum samples are needed to demonstrate P. westermani eggs. Charcot-Leyden crystals are seen in sputum, and characteristic chest x-ray findings of ring-shaped/crescent infiltrates with "thin-walled" cavities are evident in ~ 60%. Endemic in Asia, Africa, and Latin America. Chest x-ray findings take months to resolve

Pitfalls: May have extrapulmonary (ectopic) organ involvement (e.g., cerebral, subcutaneous, abdominal). Up to 20% have normal chest x-rays

Prognosis: Related to degree of lung damage (e.g., bronchiectasis) and extrapulmonary organ involvement, especially CNS

Pulmonary Coin Lesions

Subset	Pathogens	Preferred Therapy	Alternate Therapy
Dog heartworm	Dirofilaria immitis	No therapy necessary	
Aspergilloma	Aspergillus	No therapy if asymptomatic. Surgery for massive hemoptysis	Itraconazole 200 mg (PO) q24h x 3-6 months (role unclear)

Dog Heartworm (Dirofilaria immitis)

Clinical Presentation: Asymptomatic "coin lesion" after bite of infected mosquito transmits parasite from dogs to humans. Differential diagnosis includes granulomas and malignancy

Diagnostic Considerations: Diagnosis by specific serology or pathological demonstration of organism in granuloma, usually when a coin lesion is biopsied to rule out malignancy. Worldwide distribution. Acquired from pet dogs. Dirofilariasis causes dog heartworm in carrier, but presents as a solitary lung nodule in humans

Pitfalls: Often confused with malignancy

Prognosis: Excellent

Pulmonary Aspergilloma

Clinical Presentation: Coin lesion(s) ± productive cough, hemoptysis, wheezing. May be asymptomatic. Usually occurs in pre-existing cavitary lung lesions, especially TB with cavity > 2 cm

Diagnostic Considerations: Diagnosis by chest x-ray appearance of fungus ball in cavity and Aspergillus precipitins/biopsy. May present with "crescent sign" on chest x-ray (white fungus ball silhouetted against black crescent of the cavity)

Pitfalls: Role of itraconazole as therapy is unclear

Prognosis: Related to degree of hemoptysis

Pulmonary Infiltrates/Mass Lesions

Subset	Pathogens	Preferred Therapy	Alternate Therapy
Pulmonary blastomycosis	Blastomyces dermatitidis	Itraconazole 200 mg (PO)* q12h until cured <u>Severely ill</u> Amphotericin B 0.5 mg/kg (IV) q24h until 1-2 grams given	Fluconazole 400-800 mg (PO) q24h until cured
Pulmonary histoplasmosis	Histoplasma capsulatum	<u>Immunocompetent</u> Itraconazole 200 mg (PO)* q24h until cured <u>Immunocompromised or severely ill</u> Amphotericin B 1 mg/kg (IV) q24h x 7 days, then 0.8 mg/kg q48h until 2-2.5 grams given	<u>Immunocompetant</u> Fluconazole 1600 mg (PO) x 1 dose, then 800 mg (PO) q24h until cured <u>Immunocompromised or severely ill</u> Itraconazole 200 mg (IV) q12h x 2 days, then 200 mg (PO) q12h until cured
Pulmonary paracoccidioido-mycosis (South American blastomycosis)	Paracoccidioides brasiliensis	Itraconazole 200 mg (PO) q24h x 6 months **or** Ketoconazole 400 mg (PO) q24h x 6 months	Amphotericin B 0.5 mg/kg (IV) q24h until 1.5-2.5 grams given
Pulmonary actinomycosis	Actinomyces israelii	Amoxicillin 1 gm (PO) q8h x 6 months **or** Doxycycline 100 mg (PO) q12h x 6 months	Clindamycin 300 mg (PO) q8h x 6 months
Pulmonary aspergillosis *Broncho-pulmonary aspergillosis*	Aspergillus	Systemic oral steroids	None
Acute invasive aspergillus pneumonia	Aspergillus	See p. 217	
Chronic aspergillus pneumonia	Aspergillus	Amphotericin B 1 mg/kg (IV) q24h until 2-3 grams given **or** Itraconazole 200 mg (PO)* q12h until cured	Voriconazole 400 mg (IV or PO) x 1 dose, then 200 mg (PO) q12h until cured **or** Caspofungin 70 mg (IV) x 1 dose, then 50 mg (IV) q24h until improved. Follow with itraconazole 200 mg (PO) q12h until cured

* Consider initiating therapy with itraconazole 200 mg (IV) q12h x 2 days

Pulmonary Infiltrates/Mass Lesions (cont'd)

Subset	Pathogens	Preferred Therapy	Alternate Therapy
Pulmonary sporotrichosis	Sporothrix schenckii	Itraconazole 200 mg (PO)* q12h until cured **or** Voriconazole 400 mg (IV or PO) x 1 dose, then 200 mg (PO) q12h until cured	Amphotericin B 0.5 mg/kg (IV) q24h until 1-2 grams given **or** Amphotericin B lipid formulation 5 mg/kg (IV) q24h x 3 weeks **or** Fluconazole 800 mg (IV or PO) x 1 dose, then 400 mg (PO) q24h x 6 months, then 200 mg (PO) q12h until cured
Pulmonary coccidioido-mycosis	Coccidioides immitis	Fluconazole 800 mg (IV or PO) x 1 dose, then 400 mg (PO) q24h until cured **or** Itraconazole 200 mg (PO)* q12h until cured	Amphotericin B 1 mg/kg (IV) q24h x 7 days, then 0.8 mg/kg (IV) q48h until 2-3 grams given
Pulmonary nocardiosis	Nocardia asteroides	TMP-SMX 1 DS tablet (PO) q12h until cured	Minocycline 100 mg (PO) q12h until cured
Pulmonary cryptococcosis	Cryptococcus neoformans	Amphotericin B 0.5 mg/kg (IV) q24h until 1-2 grams given **or** Amphotericin B lipid formulation 5 mg/kg (IV) q24h x 3 weeks	Fluconazole 800 mg (IV or PO) x 1 dose, then 400 mg (PO) q24h until cured **or** Voriconazole 400 mg (IV or PO) x 1 dose, then 200 mg (PO) q12h until cured
Pulmonary mucormycosis	Rhizopus/Mucor/Absidia	Amphotericin B 1-1.5 mg/kg (IV) q24h until 2-3 grams given	Itraconazole 200 mg (PO)* q12h until cured **or** Voriconazole 400 mg (IV or PO) x 1 dose, then 200 mg (PO) q12h until cured
Pulmonary pseudall-escheriasis	Pseudallescheria boydii/Scedosporium apiospermum	Itraconazole 200 mg (PO)* q12h until cured **or** Voriconazole 400 mg (IV or PO) x 1 dose, then 200 mg (PO) q12h until cured	Miconazole 600 mg (IV) q8h until cured

* Consider initiating therapy with itraconazole 200 mg (IV) q12h x 2 days

Pulmonary Blastomycosis (Blastomyces dermatitidis)

Clinical Presentation: Highly variable. May present as a chronic/non-resolving pneumonia with fever/cough and characteristic "right-sided perihilar infiltrate" ± small pleural effusion

Diagnostic Considerations: May be recovered from sputum or demonstrated in lung tissue

specimens. Usual sites of dissemination include skin, bones and prostate, not CNS or adrenals
Pitfalls: Dissemination to extra-pulmonary sites may occur years after pneumonia
Prognosis: Related to severity/extent of infection. One-third of cases are self-limited and do not require treatment

Pulmonary Histoplasmosis (Histoplasma capsulatum)
Clinical Presentation: Acute primary infection presents as self-limiting flu-like illness with fever, headache, nonproductive cough, chills, and chest pain. Minority of patients become overtly ill with complicated respiratory or progressive pulmonary infection. Can cause arthralgias, E. nodosum, E. multiforme, or pericarditis. May occur in outbreak. Chronic infection presents as chronic pneumonia resembling TB or chronic disseminated infection
Diagnostic Considerations: May be recovered from sputum or demonstrated in lung tissue specimens. Complement fixation (CF) titer ≥ 1:32 of yeast/mycelial phase of Histoplasma antigen is diagnostic. Worldwide distribution, but most common in Central/South Central United States. Acute disseminated histoplasmosis suggests HIV/AIDS
Pitfalls: Pleural effusion is uncommon. Do not treat old/inactive/minimal histoplasmosis, histoplasmosis pulmonary calcification, or histoplasmosis fibrosing mediastinitis. Differentiate from TB
Prognosis: Related to severity/extent of infection. No treatment is needed for self-limiting acute histoplasmosis presenting as flu-like illness. HIV/AIDS patients should receive life-long suppressive therapy with itraconazole

Pulmonary Paracoccidioidomycosis (South American Blastomycosis)
Clinical Presentation: Typically presents as a chronic pneumonia syndrome with productive cough, blood-tinged sputum, dyspnea, and chest pain. May also develop fever, malaise, weight loss, mucosal ulcerations in/around mouth and nose, dysphagia, changes in voice, cutaneous lesions on face/limbs, or cervical adenopathy. Can disseminate to prostate, epididymis, kidneys, or adrenals
Diagnostic Considerations: Characteristic "pilot wheel" shaped yeast in sputum. Diagnosis by culture and stain (Gomori) of organism from clinical specimen. Found only in Latin American. One-third of cases have only pulmonary involvement. Skin test is non-specific/non-diagnostic
Pitfalls: No distinguishing radiologic features. No clinical adrenal insufficiency, in contrast to TB or histoplasmosis. Hilar adenopathy/pleural effusions are uncommon
Prognosis: Related to severity/extent of infection. HIV/AIDS require life-long suppression with TMP-SMX 1 DS tablet (PO) q24h or itraconazole 200 mg (PO) q24h

Pulmonary Actinomycosis (Actinomyces israelii)
Clinical Presentation: Indolent, slowly progressive infiltrates involving the pulmonary parenchyma ± pleural space. Presents with fever, chest pain, weight loss. Cough/hemoptysis are less common. Chest wall sinuses frequently develop. Chest x-ray shows adjacent dense infiltrate. "Sulfur granules" are common in sinus drainage fluid
Diagnostic Considerations: Diagnosis by stain/culture of drainage from sinuses or lung/bone biopsy specimens. Actinomyces are non-acid fast and anaerobic
Pitfalls: No CNS lesions, but bone erosion is common with chest lesions. Prior antibiotic therapy may interfere with isolation of organism
Prognosis: Excellent when treated until lesions resolve. Use IV regimen in critically ill patients, then switch to oral regimen

Bronchopulmonary Aspergillosis (BPA / ABPA)
Clinical Presentation: Migratory pulmonary infiltrates in chronic asthmatics. Eosinophilia is common, and sputum shows Charcot-Leyden crystals/brown flecks containing Aspergillus
Diagnostic Considerations: Diagnosis by Aspergillus in sputum and high-titers of Aspergillus precipitins in serum. BPA is an allergic reaction in chronic asthmatics, *not* an infectious disease. Pulmonary infiltrates with peripheral eosinophilia in chronic asthmatics suggests the diagnosis

Pitfalls: Correct diagnosis is important since therapy is steroids, not antifungals
Prognosis: Related to severity/duration of asthma and promptness of steroid therapy

Acute Invasive Aspergillus Pneumonia (see p. 222)

Chronic Aspergillus Pneumonia
Clinical Presentation: Occurs in patients with AIDS, chronic granulomatous disease, alcoholism, diabetes, and those receiving steroids for chronic pulmonary disease. Usual features include chronic productive cough ± hemoptysis, low-grade fever, weight loss, and malaise. Chronic Aspergillus pneumonia resembles TB, histoplasmosis, melioidosis
Diagnostic Considerations: Diagnosis by lung biopsy demonstrating septate hyphae invading lung parenchyma. Aspergillus may be in sputum, but is not diagnostic of Aspergillus pneumonia
Pitfalls: May extend into chest wall, vertebral column, or brachial plexus
Prognosis: Related to severity/extent of infection

Pulmonary Sporotrichosis (Sporothrix schenckii)
Clinical Presentation: Occurs in normal hosts, alcoholics, and patients with concomitant medical illness (TB, diabetes, sarcoidosis, steroid use). Usually presents as productive cough, low-grade fever, and weight loss. Chest x-ray shows cavitary thin-walled lesions with associated infiltrate. Hemoptysis is unusual. Differential diagnosis includes other thin-walled cavitary lung lesions (e.g., histoplasmosis, coccidioidomycosis, TB, atypical TB, paragonimiasis)
Diagnostic Considerations: Diagnosis by lung biopsy demonstrating invasive lung disease, not broncho-alveolar lavage. Usually a history of puncture/traumatic wound involving an extremity. May be associated with septic arthritis/osteomyelitis
Pitfalls: Sporotrichosis in lungs implies disseminated disease. May need repeated attempts at culture
Prognosis: Related to extent of infection/degree of imunosuppression

Pulmonary Coccidioidomycosis (Coccidioides immitis)
Clinical Presentation: Usually presents as a solitary, peripheral, thin-walled cavitary lesion in early or later stage of primary infection. May present as a solitary pulmonary nodule. E. nodosum and bilateral hilar adenopathy are common (in contrast to sporotrichosis). Hemoptysis is unusual
Diagnostic Considerations: Diagnosis by biopsy/Coccidioides serology. Increased incidence of dissemination in Filipinos, Blacks, and American Indians. May be associated with chronic meningitis/osteomyelitis
Pitfalls: Dissemination is preceded by ↓ Coccidioides titers/disappearance of E. nodosum
Prognosis: Related to extent of infection/degree of immunosuppression

Pulmonary Nocardiosis (Nocardia asteroides)
Clinical Presentation: Usually presents as a dense lower lobe lung mass without cavitation. May have associated mass lesions in CNS. Chest wall sinuses are more common with Actinomycosis
Diagnostic Considerations: Diagnosis by demonstrating organisms by stain/culture of lung specimens. Nocardia are weakly acid-fast and aerobic
Pitfalls: Use IV regimens in critically ill patients. HIV/AIDS patients require life-long suppressive therapy with TMP-SMX or minocycline
Prognosis: Related to extent of infection/degree of immunosuppression

Pulmonary Cryptococcosis (Cryptococcus neoformans)
Clinical Presentation: Individual focus of infection is usually inapparent/minimal when patient presents with disseminated cryptococcal infection. Pneumonia is typically a minor part of disseminated disease; CNS manifestations usually predominate (e.g., headache, subtle cognitive changes, occasional meningeal signs, focal neurological deficits)

Diagnostic Considerations: Diagnosis by demonstrating organisms in sputum/lung specimens
Pitfalls: Clinical presentation of isolated cryptococcal pneumonia is rare. HIV/AIDS patients require life-long suppressive therapy with fluconazole
Prognosis: Related to extent of dissemination/degree of immunosuppression

Pulmonary Mucormycosis (Rhizopus/Mucor/Absidia)
Clinical Presentation: Progressive pneumonia with fever, dyspnea, and cough unresponsive to antibiotic therapy. Usually seen only in compromised hosts. Chest x-ray is not characteristic, but shows infiltrate with consolidation in > 50% of patients. Cavitation occurs in 40% as neutropenia resolves
Diagnostic Considerations: Diagnosis by demonstrating organisms in lung biopsy. Pleural effusion is not a feature of pulmonary mucormycosis
Pitfalls: Causes rhinocerebral mucormycosis in diabetics, pneumonia in leukopenic compromised hosts
Prognosis: Related to degree of immunosuppression and underlying disease

Pulmonary Pseudallescheriasis (P. boydii/S. apiospermum)
Clinical Presentation: Progressive pulmonary infiltrates indistinguishable from Aspergillosis or Mucor. Usually seen only in compromised hosts (e.g., prolonged neutropenia, high-dose steroids, bone marrow or solid organ transplants, AIDS). Manifests as cough, fever, pleuritic pain, and often hemoptysis. No characteristic chest x-ray appearance
Diagnostic Considerations: Diagnosis by demonstrating organism in lung biopsy. Hemoptysis is common in patients with cavitary lesions. CNS involvement is rare
Pitfalls: One of few invasive fungi unresponsive to amphotericin B. Cause of sinusitis in diabetics, and pneumonia in leukopenic compromised hosts
Prognosis: Related to severity/extent of infection and degree of immunosuppression. Cavitary lesions causing hemoptysis often require surgical excision. Disseminated infection is often fatal

Parasites, Fungi, Unusual Organisms in Liver

Liver Flukes

Subset	Pathogens	Preferred Therapy	Alternate Therapy
Fascioliasis	Fasciola hepatica Fasciola gigantica	Triclabendazole 10 mg/kg (PO) x 1 dose	Bithionol 30-50 mg/kg (PO) q48h x 10-15 doses
Clonorchiasis/ Opisthorchiasis	Clonorchis sinensis Opisthorchis viverrini	Praziquantel 25 mg/kg (PO) q8h x 3 doses	<u>C. sinensis</u> Albendazole 400 mg (PO) q12h x 7 days <u>O. viverrini</u> None

Hepatic Fascioliasis (F. hepatica/F. gigantica)
Clinical Presentation: Frequently asymptomatic, but may present acutely with fever, right upper quadrant pain, nausea, diarrhea, wheezing, urticaria, hepatomegaly, eosinophilia, anemia. Chronic disease is associated with gallstones, cholecystitis, cholangitis, liver abscess, generalized adenopathy. Subacute nodules, hydrocele, lung/brain abscess can be seen in ectopic forms. "Linear echogenic structures" are evident on liver ultrasound
Diagnostic Consideration: Diagnosis by F. hepatica/F. gigantica eggs in stool. Endemic in sheep-raising areas (sheep liver flukes). Acquired from freshwater plants (watercress). Not associated with cholangiocarcinoma

Pitfalls: May present as Katayama syndrome resembling schistosomiasis, with high fever, eosinophilia, and hepatosplenomegaly. Unlike other trematodes, praziquantel is ineffective

Prognosis: Related to extent/location of liver damage

Hepatic Clonorchiasis (C. sinensis) / Opisthorchiasis (O. viverrini)

Clinical Presentation: Frequently asymptomatic, but may present 2-4 weeks after ingestion of fluke with fever, tender hepatomegaly, rash, and eosinophilia. Chronically presents as recurrent cholangitis, chronic cholecystitis, or pancreatitis. Associated with cholangiocarcinoma (unlike fascioliasis)

Diagnostic Considerations: Diagnosis by demonstrating C. sinensis/O. viverrini eggs in stool. Clonorchiasis is acquired from ingesting raw/inadequately cooked infected freshwater (Cyprinoid) fish in Southeast Asia. Opisthorchiasis is acquired from ingesting raw/inadequately cooked infected freshwater fish/crayfish from Laos, Cambodia, or Thailand

Pitfalls: Cholecystitis with eosinophilia should suggest clonorchiasis

Prognosis: Related to extent/location of hepatic damage. Associated with cholangiocarcinoma

Cystic Masses in Liver

Subset	Pathogens	Preferred Therapy	Alternate Therapy
Hepatic amebiasis	Entamoeba histolytica	Metronidazole 750 mg (PO) q8h x 7-10 days	Tinidazole 2 gm/day (PO) in 3 divided doses x 3 days
Hepatic echinococcosis (hydatid cyst disease)	Echinococcus granulosus	Operable Surgical resection **plus** Albendazole 400 mg* (PO) q12h x 1-6 months	Inoperable Albendazole 400 mg* (PO) q12h x 1-6 months

* If < 60 kg, give albendazole 7.5 mg/kg

Hepatic Amebiasis (Entamoeba histolytica)

Clinical Presentation: Presents insidiously with weight loss and night sweats, or acutely ill with fever, nausea, vomiting, right upper quadrant pain. Typically, amebic liver abscesses are single, affect the posterior right lobe of liver, and do not show air/fluid levels. (In contrast, bacterial liver abscesses are usually multiple, distributed in all lobes of liver, and often show air/fluid levels.) Amebic liver abscesses do not calcify like hydatid cysts

Diagnostic Considerations: Diagnosis by E. histolytica serology/E. histolytica in cyst walls. Worldwide distribution. Acquired by ingesting amebic cysts. Amebic liver abscess usually presents years after initial mild amebic dysenteric episode

Pitfalls: Amebic abscess fluid ("Anchovy paste") contains no PMNs or amebas; amebas are found only in cyst walls. Eosinophilia is not a feature of amebiasis

Prognosis: Related to health of host/extrapulmonary spread

Hepatic Echinococcosis (Echinococcus granulosus) Hydatid Cyst Disease

Clinical Presentation: Right upper quadrant pain/mass when cysts enlarge enough to cause symptoms. Hepatic cysts are unilocular in 70%, multilocular in 30%

Diagnostic Considerations: Diagnosis by demonstrating E. granulosus in cyst. Serology is unreliable. Worldwide distribution in sheep/cattle raising areas. Acquired by ingestion of eggs from dogs

Pitfalls: Eosinophilia not a feature of hydatid cyst disease. Hydatid cysts are multifaceted, loculated, and calcified

Prognosis: Related to location/extent of extrahepatic cysts. Large cysts are best treated by surgical removal after injection with hypertonic saline, alcohol, or iodophor to kill germinal layer/daughter cysts. Percutaneous drainage under ultrasound guidance plus albendazole may be effective

Hepatomegaly

Subset	Pathogen	Preferred Therapy	Alternate Therapy
Visceral leishmaniasis (Kala-azar)	Leishmania donovani	Antimony stibogluconate or meglumine antimonate 10 mg/kg (IM) q12h x 20-28 days **or** Amphotericin B 0.5–1 mg/kg (IV) q24h or q48h up to 8 weeks **or** Amphotericin B lipid formulation 3 mg/kg (IV) on days 1-5,14, and 21. If immunocompromised, give 4 mg/kg (IV) on days 1-5,10,17, 24,31,38. Can repeat if needed	Pentamidine 4 mg/kg (IM or IV) q48h x 15 doses
Schistosomiasis	Schistosoma mansoni	Praziquantel 20 mg/kg (PO) q12h x 2 doses	Oxamniquine 15 mg/kg (PO) x 1 dose. In Africa, give 20 mg/kg (PO) q24h x 3 days
	Schistosoma japonicum	Praziquantel 20 mg/kg (PO) q8h x 3 doses	None

Visceral Leishmaniasis (Leishmania donovani) Kala-azar
Clinical Presentation: Subacute or chronic systemic cases manifest months to years after initial exposure to Leishmania, most often with fever, weight loss, anemia, hepatosplenomegaly ± generalized adenopathy. Laboratory abnormalities include leukopenia, anemia, and polyclonal gammopathy on SPEP. Incubation period is usually 3-8 months. May have atypical presentation in HIV/AIDS (e.g., no splenomegaly). Acutely can mimic malaria with chills/temperature spikes. Post–Kala-azar dermatitis may resemble leprosy, and is persistent/common on face
Diagnostic Considerations: Double quotidian fever (double daily temperature spike) in persons from endemic areas with hepatosplenomegaly suggests the diagnosis. Diagnosis by liver/bone marrow biopsy demonstrating Leishmania bodies or specific L. donovani serology. Most common in Southern Europe, Middle East, Asia, Africa, and South America. Facial lesion is a clue to the diagnosis
Pitfalls: In acute cases, can mimic malaria with chills and temperature spikes, but no thrombocytopenia or atypical lymphocytes. Antimony resistance is common in India
Prognosis: Related to degree of liver/spleen involvement

Hepatic Schistosomiasis (Schistosoma mansoni/japonicum)
Clinical Presentation: May present acutely with Katayama fever (serum sickness-like illness with wheezing and eosinophilia) 4-8 weeks after exposure. May be accompanied or followed by fever/chills, headache, cough, abdominal pain, diarrhea, generalized lymphadenopathy, or hepatosplenomegaly. Laboratory abnormalities include leukocytosis, eosinophilia, and polyclonal gammopathy on SPEP. Resolves spontaneously after 2-4 weeks. After 10-15 years, may present chronically as hepatosplenic schistosomiasis, with pre-sinusoidal portal hypertension, hepatomegaly (L > R lobe enlargement), no jaundice, and intact liver function
Diagnostic Considerations: Diagnosis by S. mansoni/S. japonicum eggs in stool/liver biopsy. Serology is good for acute (not chronic) schistosomiasis. CT/MRI of liver shows "turtle back" septal calcifications. Rare complications include cor pulmonale and protein-losing enteropathy. Increased incidence of hepatitis B/C and chronic Salmonella infections. Renal complications include glomerulonephritis and

nephrotic syndrome
Pitfalls: Chronic schistosomiasis is not associated with eosinophilia. S. hematobium does not infect the liver/spleen. Oxamniquine is contraindicated in pregnancy
Prognosis: Related to egg burden

Parasites, Fungi, Unusual Organisms in Stool/Intestines

Intestinal Protozoa

Subset	Pathogens	Preferred Therapy	Alternate Therapy
Amebiasis	E. histolytica	See p. 63	
Giardiasis	Giardia lamblia	See p. 63	
Isosporiasis	Isospora belli	TMP-SMX 1 SS tablet (PO) q6h x 10 days, then q12h x 3 weeks	Ciprofloxacin 500 mg (PO) q12h x 7 days **or** Pyrimethamine 75 mg (PO) q24h + folinic acid 10 mg (PO) q24h x 2 weeks
Dientamoebiasis	Dientamoeba fragilis	Doxycycline 100 mg (PO) q12h x 10 days	Iodoquinol 650 mg (PO) q8h x 20 days **or** Paromomycin 8-12 mg/kg (PO) q8h x 7 days
Blastocystis	Blastocystis hominis	Metronidazole 750 mg (PO) q8h x 10 days	Iodoquinol 650 mg (PO) q8h x 20 days
Cyclospora	Cyclospora	See p. 63	
Cryptosporidiosis	Cryptosporidia	See p. 63 (for HIV/AIDS, see p. 218)	
Balantidiasis	Balantidium coli	Doxycycline 100 (PO) q12h x 10 days	Iodoquinol 650 mg (PO) q8h x 20 days **or** Metronidazole 750 mg (PO) q8h x 5 days

Amebiasis (Entamoeba histolytica) (see p. 65)

Giardiasis (Giardia lamblia) (see p. 65)

Isosporiasis (Isospora belli)
Clinical Presentation: Acute/subacute onset of diarrhea. Isospora belli is the only protozoa to cause diarrhea with eosinophils in stool
Diagnostic Considerations: Diagnosis by demonstrating organism in stool/intestinal biopsy specimen. Associated with HIV, immigration from Latin America, daycare centers, and mental institutions. If stool

exam is negative, "string test"/duodenal aspirate and biopsy may be helpful
Pitfalls: Difficult to eradicate; may last months. Multiple stool samples may be needed for diagnosis. Add folinic acid 10 mg (PO) q24 if pyrimethamine is used. In HIV/AIDS, may need life-long suppressive therapy with TMP-SMX 1-2 DS tablet (PO) q24h (pp. 219, 225)
Prognosis: Related to adequacy of treatment/degree of immunosuppression

Dientamoebiasis (Dientamoeba fragilis)
Clinical Presentation: Acute/subacute onset of diarrhea. No cyst stage. Lives only as trophozoite
Diagnostic Considerations: Diagnosis by demonstrating organism in stool/intestinal biopsy specimen. Mucus in diarrheal stools, not blood. May have abdominal pain. Diarrhea may last for months/years
Pitfalls: Frequently associated with pinworm (Enterobius vermicularis) infection
Prognosis: Related to adequacy of fluid replacement/underlying health of host

Blastocystis (Blastocystis hominis)
Clinical Presentation: Acute/subacute onset of diarrhea
Diagnostic Considerations: Diagnosis by demonstrating organism in stool/intestinal biopsy specimen. Trichrome stain reveals characteristic "halo" (slime capsule) in stool specimens
Pitfalls: Uncommon GI pathogen. Consider as cause of diarrhea only after other pathogens excluded
Prognosis: Related to adequacy of fluid replacement/underlying health of host

Cyclospora (see p. 65)

Cryptosporidiosis (see p. 65; for HIV/AIDS, see p. 225)

Balantidiasis (Balantidium coli)
Clinical Presentation: Acute/subacute onset of diarrhea. Fecal WBCs only with mucosal invasion. Largest intestinal protozoa and only ciliated protozoa to infect humans
Diagnostic Considerations: Diagnosis by demonstrating organism in stool/intestinal biopsy specimen. Identifying features include darkly staining "kidney shaped" nucleus and large size. Fulminant dysentery seen only in debilitated/compromised hosts
Pitfalls: Stools not bloody. Diarrhea may be intermittent
Prognosis: Related to adequacy of fluid replacement/underlying health of host

Intestinal Nematodes (Roundworms)

Subset	Pathogens	Preferred Therapy	Alternate Therapy
Capillariasis	Capillaria philippinensis	Mebendazole 200 mg (PO) q12h x 20 days	Albendazole 400 mg (PO) q24h x 10 days
Angiostrongyliasis (rodent lung/ intestinal worm)	Angiostrongylus costaricensis	Mebendazole 200-400 mg (PO) q8h x 10 days	Thiabendazole 25 mg/kg (PO) x q8h x 3 days (max. 3 gm/day)
Hookworm	Necator americanus/ Ancylostoma duodenale	Albendazole 400 mg (PO) x 1 dose **or** Mebendazole 100 mg (PO) q12h x 3 days or 500 mg (PO) x 1 dose	Pyrantel pamoate 11 mg/kg (PO) q24h x 3 days (max. 1 gm/day)

Intestinal Nematodes (Roundworms) (cont'd)

Subset	Pathogens	Preferred Therapy	Alternate Therapy
Strongyloidiasis	Strongyloides stercoralis	Ivermectin 200 mcg/kg (PO) q24h x 2 days **or** Thiabendazole 25 mg/kg (PO) q12h x 2 days (max. 3 gm/day)	Albendazole 400 mg (PO) q24h x 3 days
Ascariasis	Ascaris lumbricoides	Albendazole 400 mg (PO) x 1 dose **or** Mebendazole 100 mg (PO) q12h x 3 days or 500 mg (PO) x 1 dose	Pyrantel pamoate 11 mg/kg (PO) x 1 dose (max. 1 gm)
Trichostrongyliasis	Trichostrongylus orientalis	Pyrantel pamoate 11 mg/kg (PO) x 1 dose (max. 1 gm)	Albendazole 400 mg (PO) x 1 dose **or** Mebendazole 100 mg (PO) q12h x 3 days
Pinworm	Enterobius vermicularis	Pyrantel pamoate 11 mg/kg (PO) x 1 dose (max. 1 gm); repeat in 2 weeks **or** Albendazole 400 mg (PO) x 1 dose; repeat in 2 weeks	Mebendazole 100 mg (PO) x 1 dose; repeat in 2 weeks
Whipworm	Trichuris trichiura	Mebendazole 100 mg (PO) q12h x 3 days, or 500 mg (PO) x 1 dose	Albendazole 400 mg (PO) x 1 dose

Capillariasis (Capillaria philippinensis)
Clinical Presentation: Intermittent voluminous watery diarrhea ± malabsorption. Fever is uncommon
Diagnostic Considerations: Diagnosis by demonstrating ova or parasite in stools. Resembles Trichuris, but C. philippinensis ova are larger and have a "pitted shell" with prominent polar plugs. Peripheral eosinophilia is uncommon until after therapy
Pitfalls: Serology is positive in 85%, but cross-reacts with other parasites
Prognosis: Related to severity of malabsorption/extra-intestinal disease

Angiostrongyliasis (A. contaricensis) Rodent Lung/Intestinal Worm
Clinical Presentation: Presents as appendicitis (worm resides and deposits eggs in arteries/arterioles around ileocecum/appendix)
Diagnostic Considerations: Diagnosis by demonstrating organism in biopsied/excised tissue. May involve proximal small bowel, liver, CNS
Pitfalls: Can present as RLQ mass/fever resembling regional enteritis (Crohn's disease), but with eosinophilia and leukocytosis
Prognosis: Related to severity of malabsorption and extra-intestinal disease

Hookworm (Necator americanus/Ancylostoma duodenale)

Clinical Presentation: Pruritic, vesicular eruptions at site of filariform larval entry ("ground itch"). Pulmonary symptoms and transient eosinophilia may occur during migratory phase to intestines. Later, abdominal pain, diarrhea, weight loss, hypoalbuminemia, and anemia develop

Diagnostic Considerations: Diagnosis by demonstrating eggs/larvae in stool specimens. N. americanus can ingest 0.3 ml of blood/worm/day, much greater than A. duodenale. Anemia may be severe with heavy infestation (up to 100 mL/day)

Pitfalls: Eggs in fresh stool, not rhabditiform larvae

Prognosis: Related to severity of anemia/malabsorption

Strongyloidiasis (Strongyloides stercoralis)

Clinical Presentation: Pruritic, papular, erythematous rash. Pulmonary symptoms (cough, asthma) may occur during lung migration phase. May develop Loeffler's syndrome (pulmonary infiltrates with eosinophilia) or ARDS in heavy infections. Intestinal phase associated with colicky abdominal pain, diarrhea, and malabsorption

Diagnostic Considerations: Diagnosis by demonstrating larvae in stool specimens/duodenal fluid. Usually asymptomatic in normal hosts, but causes "hyperinfection syndrome" in compromised hosts. CNS strongyloides (part of hyperinfection syndrome) should suggest diagnosis of HIV in non-immunosuppressed patients. Diarrhea/abdominal pain mimics regional enteritis (Crohn's disease) or ulcerative colitis. Malabsorption is common and mimics tropical sprue. Anemia is usually mild

Pitfalls: Usually rhabditiform larvae (not eggs) in stools

Prognosis: Related to severity of malabsorption

Ascariasis (Ascaris lumbricoides)

Clinical Presentation: Pulmonary symptoms (cough, asthma) may occur during lung migration phase. May develop Loeffler's syndrome (pulmonary infiltrates with eosinophilia), as with hookworm/Strongyloides. Intestinal symptoms develop late. Usually asymptomatic until intestinal/biliary obstruction occurs. Can obstruct the appendix/pancreatic duct

Diagnostic Considerations: Diagnosis by demonstrating eggs in stool specimens. Abdominal ultrasound can detect obstruction from adult worms. Most infections are asymptomatic; symptoms are related to "worm burden"/ectopic migration. Each female worm may produce up to 250,000 eggs/day

Pitfalls: Lung involvement (bronchospasm, bronchopneumonia, lung abscess) is prominent in HIV/AIDS

Prognosis: Related to worm burden/extra-intestinal organ invasion

Trichostrongyliasis (Trichostrongylus orientalis)

Clinical Presentation: Mild intestinal symptoms with persistent eosinophilia

Diagnostic Considerations: Diagnosis by demonstrating eggs in stool specimens. Most prevalent in the Middle East and Asia. Mild anemia. Eosinophilia is usually > 10%

Pitfalls: Must differentiate eggs from hookworm, and rhabditiform larvae from Strongyloides. T. orientalis eggs have "pointed ends"

Prognosis: Related to extent of disease/underlying health of host

Pinworm (Enterobius vermicularis)

Clinical Presentation: Primarily affects children. Perianal pruritus is the main symptom. Worm lives in the cecum, but patients do not have intestinal symptoms

Diagnostic Considerations: Scotch tape of anus at night can be used to detect eggs left by migrating female worms (Scotch tape test). Number of E. vermicularis in stool is low

Pitfalls: Abdominal pain and diarrhea should prompt search for Dientamoeba fragilis, since co-infection is common

Prognosis: Excellent

Whipworm (Trichuris trichiura)

Clinical Presentation: May present as "chronic appendicitis." Severe infestation may cause bloody diarrhea/abdominal pain ("Trichuris dysentery syndrome"), rectal prolapse

Diagnostic Considerations: Diagnosis by demonstrating large eggs with bile-stained, triple-layered eggshell walls and doubly operculated transparent plugs. Most patients are asymptomatic or mildly anemic

Pitfalls: Commonly co-exists with Ascaris, hookworm, or E. histolytica

Prognosis: Related to severity/extent of dysentery

Intestinal Cestodes (Tapeworms)

Subset	Pathogens	Preferred Therapy	Alternate Therapy
Beef tapeworm	Taenia saginata	Praziquantel 5-10 mg/kg (PO) x 1 dose	Niclosamide 2 gm (PO) x 1 dose
Pork tapeworm	Taenia solium	Praziquantel 5-10 mg/kg (PO) x 1 dose	Niclosamide 2 gm (PO) x 1 dose
Dwarf tapeworm	Hymenolepis nana	Praziquantel 25 mg/kg (PO) x 1 dose	None
Fish tapeworm	Diphyllobothrium latum	Praziquantel 10 mg/kg (PO) x 1 dose	Niclosamide 2 gm (PO) x 1 dose

Beef Tapeworm (Taenia saginata) / Pork Tapeworm (Taenia solium)

Clinical Presentation: Usually mild symptoms (weight loss, anemia), since most infections are caused by a single tapeworm

Diagnostic Considerations: Diagnosis by demonstrating tapeworm in stool. Taenia eggs in stool cannot be speciated; all are brown and spherical with a radially-striated inner shell. T. saginata may survive for 10 years, T. solium for 25 years

Pitfalls: Severe cases may cause appendicitis, intestinal obstruction/perforation

Prognosis: Related to severity of malabsorption/intestinal obstruction

Dwarf Tapeworm (Hymenolepis nana)

Clinical Presentation: Usually asymptomatic

Diagnostic Considerations: Diagnosis by demonstrating typical eggs in stool, with two shells enclosing inner oncosphere with hooklets. ELISA is positive in 85%, but cross-reacts with Taenia/Cysticercosis. GI symptoms develop with stool egg counts > 15,000/gm

Pitfalls: Abdominal pain and diarrhea in heavy infestations

Prognosis: Related to severity of malabsorption/underlying health of host

Fish Tapeworm (Diphyllobothrium latum)

Clinical Presentation: Symptoms secondary to macrocytic anemia from vitamin B_{12} deficiency. Most infestations are asymptomatic

Diagnostic Considerations: Diagnosis by demonstrating eggs/proglottids in stool

Pitfalls: Vitamin B_{12} deficiency anemia requires prolonged infection (> 3 years)

Prognosis: Related to severity of B_{12} deficiency anemia/underlying health of host

Intestinal Trematodes (Flukes/Flatworms)

Subset	Pathogens	Preferred Therapy
Fasciolopsiasis	Fasciolopsis buski	Praziquantel 25 mg/kg (PO) q8h x 3 doses
Heterophyiasis	Heterophyes heterophyes Metagonimus yokogawai	Praziquantel 25 mg/kg (PO) q8h x 3 doses

Fasciolopsiasis (Fasciolopsis buski)
Clinical Presentation: Diarrhea with copious mucus in stool. Most cases are asymptomatic
Diagnostic Considerations: Diagnosis by demonstrating eggs in stool. May have eosinophilia, low-grade fever ± malabsorption. Intestinal obstruction is the most serious complication
Pitfalls: Mimics peptic ulcer disease with upper abdominal pain relieved by food
Prognosis: Related to severity/extent of malabsorption/intestinal obstruction

Heterophyiasis (Heterophyes heterophyes / Metagonimus yokogawai)
Clinical Presentation: Usually asymptomatic or mild intestinal symptoms. Embolization of eggs may result in myocarditis, myocardial fibrosis, or cerebral hemorrhage. Eosinophilia may be present
Diagnostic Considerations: Diagnosis by demonstrating eggs in stool. Small intestinal fluke
Pitfalls: Difficult to differentiate from Clonorchis sinensis
Prognosis: Related to extent/severity of extra-intestinal dissemination to heart, lungs, CNS

Other Intestinal Infections

Subset	Pathogen	Preferred Therapy
Whipple's disease	Tropheryma whippelii	Ceftriaxone 2 gm (IV) q12h x 2 weeks + streptomycin 1 gm (IM) q24h x 2 weeks. Follow with TMP-SMX 1 DS tablet (PO) q12h x 1 year

Whipple's Disease (Tropheryma whippelii)
Clinical Presentation: Diarrhea, fever, encephalopathy/dementia, weight loss, polyarthritis, myocarditis, pericarditis, general lymphadenopathy ± malabsorption
Diagnostic Considerations: Diagnosis by demonstrating organism by stain/culture from macrophages in small bowel biopsy specimens
Pitfalls: May present with dementia mimicking Alzheimer's disease, or FUO mimicking celiac disease or lymphoma. Optimum length of treatment is unknown. Relapses occur
Prognosis: Related to severity/extent of extra-intestinal disease

Parasites, Fungi, Unusual Organisms in Skin/Muscle

Infiltrative Skin/Subcutaneous Lesions

Subset	Pathogens	Preferred Therapy
Cutaneous leishmaniasis *Old World*	Leishmania major Leishmania tropica	Antimony stibogluconate or meglumine antimonate 10 mg/kg (IM or IV) q12h x 4 weeks **or** Pentamidine 4 mg/kg (IV) q48h x 4 doses
New World	Leishmania mexicana Leishmania braziliense	Antimony stibogluconate or meglumine antimonate 10 mg/kg (IM or IV) q12h x 4 weeks **or** Pentamidine 4 mg/kg (IV) q48h x 4 doses
Leprosy *Lepromatous*	Mycobacterium leprae	Dapsone 100 mg (PO) q24h x 1-2 years + clofazimine 50 mg (PO) q24h x 1-2 years + rifampin 600 mg (PO) monthly x 1-2 years
Non-lepromatous	Mycobacterium leprae	Dapsone 100 mg (PO) q24h x 6 months + rifampin 600 mg (PO) monthly x 6 months
Erythrasma	Corynebacterium minutissimum	Erythromycin 250 mg (PO) q6h x 2 weeks

Cutaneous Leishmaniasis (Old World/New World)
Clinical Presentation: Variable presentation. Typically, a nodule develops then ulcerates, with a raised/erythematous outer border and a central area of granulation tissue. May be single or multiple. Usually non-pruritic/non-painful. Occurs weeks after travel to endemic areas (New World leishmaniasis: Latin America; Old World leishmaniasis: Central Asia)

Diagnostic Considerations: Diagnosis by demonstrating Leishmania amastigotes or promastigotes in biopsy specimen

Pitfalls: Most skin lesions undergo spontaneous resolution. However, treatment is advisable for lesions caused by L. braziliensis or related species causing mucosal leishmaniasis

Prognosis: Excellent

Lepromatous Leprosy (Mycobacterium leprae)
Clinical Presentation: Diffuse, symmetrical, red or brown skin lesions presenting as macules, papules, plaques, or nodules. May also present as diffuse thickening of skin, especially involving ear lobes, face, and extremities. Loss of eyebrows/body hair may occur

Diagnostic Considerations: Diagnosis by demonstrating organism in tissue specimens. Afebrile bacteremia is frequent, with blood culture buffy coat smears positive for M. leprae. E. nodosum and polyclonal gammopathy on SPEP are common, and lepromin skin test/PPD are negative (anergic). When present, peripheral neuropathy is often symmetrical and acral in distribution

Pitfalls: Differential diagnosis is large. Consider leprosy in patients with unexplained skin diseases

Prognosis: Good if treated early

Non-Lepromatous Leprosy (Mycobacterium leprae)
Clinical Presentation: Small number of asymmetrical, hypopigmented skin lesions, which are often scaly with sharp borders and associated anesthesia. Asymmetric peripheral nerve trunk involvement is common
Diagnostic Considerations: Diagnosis by demonstrating granulomas with few acid-fast bacilli. Differentiate from cutaneous leishmaniasis by skin biopsy. Lepromin skin test/PPD are positive and SPEP is normal (in contrast to lepromatous leprosy)
Pitfalls: Wide spectrum of presentations depending on immune status and duration of disease. Differential diagnosis is large. Consider leprosy in patients with unexplained skin diseases
Prognosis: Good if treated early

Erythrasma (Corynebacterium minutissimum)
Clinical Presentation: Reddened/raised skin lesions on face/trunk. Not hot or pruritic
Diagnostic Considerations: Differentiated from Tinea versicolor by culture. C. minutissimum skin lesions fluoresce red under UV light
Pitfalls: Resembles Tinea versicolor, but lesions primarily involve the face, not trunk
Prognosis: Excellent

Infiltrative Skin Lesions ± Ulcers/Sinus Tracts/Abscesses

Subset	Pathogens	Preferred Therapy
Cutaneous histoplasmosis	Histoplasma capsulatum	Amphotericin B 0.5-1 mg/kg (IV) q24h x 7 days, then 0.8 mg/kg (IV) q48h or 3x/week until total of 10-15 mg/kg. Follow with suppressive therapy with itraconazole 200 mg (PO) q24h x 6-24 months (or indefinitely if HIV/AIDS) <u>Mild or moderate symptoms, no need for hospitalization</u> Itraconazole 200 mg (PO) q12h x 2 days, then 200 mg (PO) q24h x 9 months
Cutaneous blastomycosis	Blastomyces dermatitidis	Treat the same as pulmonary infection (p. 168)
Cutaneous coccidioidomycosis	Coccidioides immitis	Treat the same as pulmonary infection (p. 169)
Cutaneous actinomycosis	Actinomyces israelii	Treat the same as pulmonary infection (p. 168)
Cutaneous nocardiosis	Nocardia sp.	Treat the same as pulmonary infection (p. 169)
Cutaneous amebiasis	Entamoeba histolytica	Treat the same as pulmonary infection (p. 166)

Infiltrative Skin Lesions ± Ulcers/Sinus Tracts/Abscesses (cont'd)

Subset	Pathogens	Preferred Therapy
Cutaneous mycobacteria *Scrofula*	Mycobacterium tuberculosis	INH 300 mg (PO) q24h + rifampin 600 mg (PO) q24h x 6 months
	Mycobacterium scrofulaceum	Surgical excision is curative
M. fortuitum-chelonae	Mycobacterium fortuitum-chelonae	Surgical excision + clarithromycin 500 mg (PO) q12h x 6 months
Swimming pool granuloma	Mycobacterium marinum	TMP-SMX 1 DS tablet (PO) q12h + ethambutol 15 mg/kg (PO) q24h x 6-12 weeks **or** Minocycline or doxycycline 100 mg (PO) q12h x 6-12 weeks
Buruli ulcer	Mycobacterium ulcerans	TMP-SMX 1 DS tablet (PO) q12h + ethambutol 15 mg/kg (PO) q24h x 6 weeks
Cutaneous MAI	Mycobacterium avium-intracellulare	Ethambutol 15 mg/kg (PO) q24h + azithromycin 1200 mg (PO) weekly x 6 months

Cutaneous Histoplasmosis (Histoplasma capsulatum)
Clinical Presentation: Chronic, raised, verrucous lesions
Diagnostic Considerations: Diagnosis by demonstrating organism by culture/tissue staining
Pitfalls: Skin nodules represent disseminated histoplasmosis, not isolated skin infection. Look for histoplasmosis elsewhere (e.g., lung, liver, bone marrow)
Prognosis: Related to extent of infection/degree of immunosuppression

Cutaneous Blastomyces (Blastomyces dermatitidis)
Clinical Presentation: Painless, erythematous, well-circumscribed, hyperkeratotic, crusted nodules or plaques that enlarge over time. Some may ulcerate and leave an undermined edge
Diagnostic Considerations: Diagnosis by demonstrating organism by culture/tissue staining. Blastomyces dermatitidis affects many organs
Pitfalls: When found in skin, look for Blastomyces elsewhere (e.g., lungs, prostate)
Prognosis: Related to extent of infection/degree of immunosuppression

Cutaneous Coccidioidomycosis (Coccidioides immitis)
Clinical Presentation: Skin lesions take many forms, including raised verrucous lesions, cold subcutaneous abscesses, indolent ulcers, or small papules
Diagnostic Considerations: Diagnosis by demonstrating organism by culture/tissue staining
Pitfalls: Skin nodules represent disseminated coccidioidomycosis, not isolated skin infection. Look for Coccidioides elsewhere (e.g., CNS, bone, lungs)
Prognosis: Related to extent of infection/degree of immunosuppression

Cutaneous Actinomycosis (Actinomyces israelii)
Clinical Presentation: Erythematous, uneven, indurated, woody, hard, cervicofacial tumor. Localized single/multiple sinus tracts in chest wall, abdominal wall, or inguinal/pelvic area may be present
Diagnostic Considerations: Diagnosis by demonstrating organism by culture/tissue staining

Pitfalls: Look for underlying bone involvement
Prognosis: Good with early/prolonged treatment

Cutaneous Nocardia (Nocardia brasiliensis)

Clinical Presentation: Subcutaneous abscesses may rupture to form chronically draining fistulas
Diagnostic Considerations: Diagnosis by demonstrating organism by culture/tissue staining. May present as "Madura foot"
Pitfalls: Look for underlying immunosuppressive disorder
Prognosis: Related to extent of infection/degree of immunosuppression

Cutaneous Amebiasis (Entamoeba histolytica)

Clinical Presentation: Ulcers with ragged edges, sinus tracts, amebomas, and strictures may develop around the anus/rectum or abdominal wall
Diagnostic Considerations: Diagnosis by demonstrating organism by culture/tissue staining
Pitfalls: If abdominal sinus tract is present, look for underlying ameboma and evidence of infection in other organs (e.g., CNS, lung, liver)
Prognosis: Related to extent of infection/degree of organ damage

Scrofula (Mycobacterium tuberculosis)

Clinical Presentation: Cold, chronic, anterior cervical adenopathy ± sinus tracts. Usually in children
Diagnostic Considerations: Diagnosis by culture of node/drainage for speciation
Pitfalls: Cured by antibiotic therapy alone. No need for surgical excision
Prognosis: Excellent with treatment

Scrofula (Mycobacterium scrofulaceum)

Clinical Presentation: Cold, chronic, anterior cervical adenopathy ± sinus tracts. Usually in adults
Diagnostic Considerations: Diagnosis by culture of node/drainage for speciation
Pitfalls: Highly resistant to anti-TB therapy
Prognosis: Excellent with surgical excision

Cutaneous Mycobacterium fortuitum-chelonae

Clinical Presentation: Usually associated with chronic foreign body infection, especially infected breast implants. May present as cold abscess
Diagnostic Considerations: Diagnosis by demonstrating organism by acid fast smear or culture of drainage/infected prosthetic material
Pitfalls: Highly resistant to anti-TB therapy, but sensitive to clarithromycin and azithromycin
Prognosis: Good with surgical excision/treatment with clarithromycin or azithromycin

Swimming Pool Granuloma (Mycobacterium marinum)

Clinical Presentation: Begins as erythema with tenderness at inoculation site, followed by a papule or violaceous nodule that ulcerates and drains pus. May have sporotrichoid spread. Presents as a skin lesion unresponsive to antibiotics after abrasive water exposure (e.g., cutting finger or scraping knee in swimming pool/lake)
Diagnostic Considerations: Diagnosis by demonstrating organism by acid-fast smear/culture
Pitfalls: Resistant to INH/pyrazinamide. Surgical excision is an option
Prognosis: Good with prolonged therapy

Buruli Ulcer (Mycobacterium ulcerans)

Clinical Presentation: Begin as a firm, painless, movable, subcutaneous nodule. In 1-2 months, nodule becomes fluctuant, ulcerates, and develops an undermined edge. May have edema around lesion and in extremity (if involved)

Diagnostic Considerations: Diagnosis by acid-fast culture of punch biopsy of ulcer rim. Patient is usually from Africa, but M. ulcerans also exists in Asia, Australia, and Central/South America
Pitfalls: Steroids/skin grafting sometimes needed
Prognosis: Good with surgical excision

Cutaneous MAI (Mycobacterium avium-intracellulare)
Clinical Presentation: Nodules, abscesses, ulcers, plaques, ecthyma and draining sinuses can occur, but are uncommon in normal hosts and usually only seen in immunosuppressed patients
Diagnostic Considerations: Diagnosis by demonstrating organism by acid-fast staining of tissue biopsy specimens
Pitfalls: Usually represents disseminated infection. Look for non-cutaneous evidence of infection (e.g., lungs, bone marrow, liver/spleen)
Prognosis: Related to extent of organ damage/degree of immunosuppression

Skin Vesicles/Bullae

Subset	Pathogens	Preferred Therapy
Herpes simplex	Herpes simplex virus (HSV)	See p. 102 (for HIV/AIDS, see pp. 220, 226)
Herpes zoster	Varicella zoster virus (VZV)	See pp. 102-103 (for HIV/AIDS, see pp. 220, 226)

Subcutaneous Serpiginous Lesions

Subset	Pathogens	Preferred Therapy
Cutaneous larva migrans (creeping eruption)	Ancylostoma braziliense	Ivermectin 150 mcg/kg (PO) q24h x 2 days **or** Albendazole 200 mg (PO) q12h x 3 days
Guinea worm	Dracunculus medinensis	Surgical removal of worm near skin surface. Metronidazole 250 mg (PO) q8h x 10 days facilitates worm removal
Cutaneous gnathostomiasis	Gnathostoma spinigerum	Surgical removal or albendazole 400 mg (PO) q24h x 1-3 weeks

Cutaneous Larva Migrans (Ancylostoma braziliense) Creeping Eruption
Clinical Presentation: Intensely pruritic, migratory, subcutaneous, raised serpiginous lesions
Diagnostic Considerations: Diagnosis by clinical appearance
Pitfalls: Must be differentiated from "swimmer's itch" caused by schistosomal cercariae
Prognosis: Excellent with treatment

Guinea Worm (Dracunculus medinensis)
Clinical Presentation: Serpiginous, raised, subcutaneous tract overlying worm
Diagnostic Considerations: Diagnosis by demonstrating Dracunculus worm when surgically removed
Pitfalls: Resembles cutaneous larva migrans, but worm is visible below the skin and lesions are serpiginous with Dracunculus
Prognosis: Excellent with treatment. Soaking extremity in warm water promotes emergence/removal of worm. Metronidazole can also be used to decrease inflammation and facilitate worm removal. Mebendazole 200-400 mg (PO) q12h x 6 days may kill worms directly

Cutaneous Gnathostomiasis (Gnathostoma spinigerum)

Clinical Presentation: Painful, intermittent, subcutaneous swelling with local edema, intense pruritus, and leukocytosis with eosinophilia. Acquired by eating undercooked fish, frogs, and other intermediate larvae-containing hosts

Diagnostic Considerations: Diagnosis by demonstrating Gnathostoma in tissue specimens. Relatively common infection in Thailand and parts of Japan, South America, and Southeast Asia

Prognosis: Good if limited to the skin and surgically removed. Poor with CNS involvement

Skin Papules/Nodules/Abscesses

Subset	Pathogens	Preferred Therapy
Bacillary angiomatosis (peliosis hepatis)	Bartonella henselae Bartonella quintana	Doxycycline 100 mg (PO) q12h until cured **or** Azithromycin 250 mg (PO) q24h until cured **or** Ciprofloxacin 500 mg (PO) q12h until cured **or** Levofloxacin 500 mg (PO) q24h until cured
Cutaneous Alternaria	Alternaria alternata	Amphotericin B 1.5 mg/kg (IV) q24h x 2-3 grams*
Entomophthoromycosis	E. basidiobolus E. conidiobolus	Amphotericin B 1.5 mg/kg (IV) q24h x 1-2 grams **or** TMP-SMX 1 DS tablet (PO) q24h until cured
Chromomycosis	Fonsecaea pedrosoi, compactum Phialophora verrucosa, others	<u>Few small lesions:</u> Wide/deep surgical excision or cryosurgery with liquid nitrogen <u>Larger lesions:</u> Itraconazole 200 mg (PO) q24h until lesions regress ± cryosurgery
Cutaneous Fusarium	Fusarium solani	Amphotericin B 1.5 mg/kg (IV) q24h x 2-3 grams **or** Voriconazole 400 mg (IV or PO) x 1 dose, then 200 mg (PO) q12h until cured
Cutaneous Penicillium	Penicillium marneffei	Amphotericin B 0.6 mg/kg (IV) q24h x 14 days, then itraconazole 200 mg (IV) q12 x 2 days then 200 mg (PO) q12h x 10 weeks. For HIV/AIDS, continue with itraconazole 200 mg (PO) q24h indefinitely
Cutaneous Prototheca	Prototheca wikermanii	Surgical excision. If excision is incomplete, add either: Amphotericin B 1.5 mg/kg (IV) q24h x 2-3 grams **or** Itraconazole 200 mg (PO)† q12h until cured
Cutaneous Trichosporon	Trichosporon beigelii	Amphotericin B 1.5 mg/kg (IV) q24h x 2-3 grams*
Cutaneous aspergillosis	Aspergillus fumigatus	Itraconazole 200 mg (IV) q12h x 2 days then 200 mg (PO) q12h until cured **or** Caspofungin 70 mg (IV) x 1 dose, then 50 mg (IV) q24h until improved, then give itraconazole 200 mg (PO) q12h until cured

Skin Papules/Nodules/Abscesses (cont'd)

Subset	Pathogens	Preferred Therapy
Cutaneous mucormycosis	Mucor/Rhizopus/ Absidia	Amphotericin B 1-1.5 mg/kg (IV) q24h x 2-3 grams <u>Alternate therapy</u> Itraconazole 200 mg (PO)† q12h until cured **or** Voriconazole 400 mg (IV or PO) x 1 dose, then 200 mg (PO) q12h until cured
Cutaneous coccidioido- mycosis	Coccidioides immitis	Fluconazole 800 mg (PO) x 1 dose, then 400 mg (PO) q24h until cured **or** Itraconazole 200 mg (PO)† q12h until cured <u>Alternate therapy</u> Amphotericin B 1 mg/kg (IV) q24h x 7 days, then 0.8 mg/kg (IV) q48h x 2-3 grams total dose
Cutaneous histoplasmosis	Histoplasmosis capsulatum	See p. 182
Cutaneous cryptococcosis	Cryptococcus neoformans	Amphotericin B 0.5 mg/kg (IV) q24h x 1-2 grams **or** Amphotericin B lipid formulation 5 mg/kg (IV) q24h x 3 weeks, **then follow with** Fluconazole 800 mg (PO) x 1 dose, then 400 mg (PO) q24h x 8-10 weeks
Cutaneous sporotrichosis	Sporothrix schenckii	Itraconazole 200 mg (PO) q24h x 6 months. If HIV/AIDS, follow with 200 mg (PO) q24h until cured
Papular candidiasis	Candida sp.	Treat as disseminated infection (see Candida sepsis, p. 112)
Cutaneous onchocerciasis	Onchocerca volvulus	Ivermectin 150 mcg/kg (PO) x 1 dose **plus** Doxycycline 100 mg (PO) q12h x 6 weeks

* Given the refractory nature of this infection, if unresponsive to amphotericin, it is not unreasonable to attempt treatment with voriconazole 400 mg (IV or PO) x 1 dose, then 200 mg (IV or PO) q12h until cured (experience is limited)
† Initiate treatment with itraconazole 200 mg (IV) q12h x 2 days

Bacillary Angiomatosis (Bartonella henselae/quintana) Peliosis Hepatis
Clinical Presentation: Skin lesions resemble Kaposi's sarcoma. Liver lesions resemble CMV hepatitis in HIV/AIDS patients
Diagnostic Considerations: Diagnosis by demonstrating organism by stain/culture of skin lesions or by blood culture after lysis-centrifugation
Pitfalls: Requires life-long suppressive therapy
Prognosis: Related to extent of infection/degree of immunosuppression

Cutaneous Alternaria (Alternaria alternata)
Clinical Presentation: Bluish/purple papules that are often painful and non-pruritic. Usually seen only in leukopenic compromised hosts

Diagnostic Considerations: Diagnosis by demonstrating organism by stain/culture in tissue specimen
Pitfalls: Skin lesions usually represent disseminated disease in compromised hosts, not local infection
Prognosis: Poor/fair. Related to degree of immunosuppression

Cutaneous Entomophthoromycosis (E. basidiobolus / E. conidiobolus)

Clinical Presentation: E. conidiobolus infection presents as swelling of nose, paranasal tissues and mouth, accompanied by nasal stuffiness, drainage, and sinus pain. Begins as swelling of inferior nasal turbinates and extends until generalized facial swelling occurs. Subcutaneous nodules can be palpated in tissue. E. basidiobolus infection presents as a non-painful, firm, slowly progressive, subcutaneous nodule of the trunk, arms, legs, or buttocks
Diagnostic Considerations: Diagnosis by demonstrating organism by stain/culture in tissue specimen. Skin lesions usually represent disseminated disease in compromised hosts, not localized infection
Pitfalls: Unlike Mucor, E. basidiobolus does not usually invade blood vessels, although tissue infarction/necrosis is occasionally seen in diabetics and immunocompromised patients
Prognosis: May spontaneously resolve. Surgical removal of accessible nodules and reconstructive surgery may be helpful for disfigurement

Cutaneous Chromomycosis (F. pedrosoi/compactum, P. verrucosa, others)

Clinical Presentation: Warty papule/nodule that enlarges slowly to form a scarred, verrucous plaque. May also begin as a pustule, plaque, or ulcer. Over time, typical papule/nodule ulcerates, and the center becomes dry/crusted with raised margins. Lesions can be pedunculated/cauliflower-like
Diagnostic Considerations: Diagnosis by demonstrating organism by stain/culture in tissue specimen. Chromomycosis remains localized within cutaneous/subcutaneous tissues
Pitfalls: May resemble other fungal diseases. Sclerotic bodies in tissue and exudate distinguish chromomycosis from other related fugal diseases
Prognosis: Related to degree of organ damage

Cutaneous Fusarium (Fusarium solani)

Clinical Presentation: Presents in compromised hosts as multiple papules or painful nodules, initially macular with central pallor, which become raised, erythematous, and necrotic. Seen mostly in leukopenic compromised hosts (especially acute leukemia and bone marrow transplants). Also a cause of mycetoma/onchomycosis
Diagnostic Considerations: Diagnosis by demonstrating organism by stain/culture from blood/tissue
Pitfalls: Skin lesions usually represent disseminated disease, not localized infection
Prognosis: Poor/fair. Related to degree of immunosuppression. Amphotericin B lipid formulation, colony-stimulating granulocyte factor, and granulocyte transfusions may be useful

Cutaneous Penicillium (Penicillium marneffei)

Clinical Presentation: Papules, pustules, nodules, ulcers, or abscesses. Mostly seen in HIV/AIDS (requires life-long suppressive therapy with itraconazole)
Diagnostic Considerations: Diagnosis by demonstrating organism by stain/culture in tissue specimen. Affects residents/visitors of Southeast Asia/Southern China
Pitfalls: Lesions commonly become umbilicated and resemble molluscum contagiosum
Prognosis: Poor/fair. Related to degree of immunosuppression

Cutaneous Prototheca (Prototheca wikermanii)

Clinical Presentation: Most common presentation is a single plaque or papulonodular lesion of the skin or subcutaneous tissue. Lesions are usually painless, slowly progressive (enlarge over weeks to months without healing), well-circumscribed, and may become eczematoid/ulcerated
Diagnostic Considerations: Diagnosis by demonstrating organism by stain/culture in tissue specimen. Skin lesions in HIV/AIDS are not different from normal hosts

Pitfalls: Lesions are usually painless and may resemble eczema
Prognosis: Poor/fair. Related to degree of immunosuppression. Surgical excision has been successful

Cutaneous Trichosporon (Trichosporon beigelii)
Clinical Presentation: Seen mostly in leukopenic compromised hosts (especially in acute leukemia, but also in HIV/AIDS, burn wounds, and organ transplants). Usually presents as multiple red-bluish/purple papules, which are often painful and non-pruritic
Diagnostic Considerations: Diagnosis by demonstrating organism by stain/culture in tissue specimen
Pitfalls: Skin lesions usually represent disseminated disease, not localized infection
Prognosis: Related to extent of infection/degree of immunosuppression

Cutaneous Aspergillosis (Aspergillus fumigatus)
Clinical Presentation: Seen at site of IV catheter insertion or adhesive dressing applied to skin in leukopenic, compromised hosts. Lesion is similar to pyoderma gangrenosum. May also invade burn wounds and cause rapidly progressive necrotic lesions
Diagnostic Considerations: Diagnosis by demonstrating organism by stain/culture in tissue specimen
Pitfalls: Infiltrative/ulcerative skin lesions usually represent disseminated disease in compromised hosts, not localized infection. May cause invasive dermatitis/skin lesions in HIV/AIDS
Prognosis: Related to extent of infection/degree of immunosuppression

Cutaneous Mucormycosis/Rhizopus/Absidia
Clinical Presentation: Necrotic skin lesion secondary to vascular invasion. Involves epidermis and dermis. Black eschars are evident
Diagnostic Considerations: Diagnosis by demonstrating broad, non-septate hyphae with branches at right angles by stain/culture in tissue specimen
Pitfalls: Skin lesions usually represent disseminated disease in compromised hosts, not localized infection. Contaminated elastic bandages have been associated with cutaneous Mucor
Prognosis: Related to extent of infection/degree of immunosuppression

Cutaneous Coccidioidomycosis (Coccidioides immitis)
Clinical Presentation: Skin lesions may take many forms, including verrucous granulomas, cold subcutaneous abscesses, indolent ulcers, or small papules
Diagnostic Considerations: Diagnosis by demonstrating organism by stain/culture in tissue specimen
Pitfalls: Skin lesions usually represent disseminated disease in compromised hosts, not local infection
Prognosis: Related to extent of infection/degree of immunosuppression

Cutaneous Histoplasmosis (Histoplasma capsulatum)
Clinical Presentation: Common cutaneous findings include maculopapular eruption, petechiae, and ecchymosis. Histopathology reveals necrosis around superficial dermal vessels
Diagnostic Considerations: Diagnosis by demonstrating organism by stain/culture in tissue specimen
Pitfalls: Skin lesions usually represent disseminated disease in compromised hosts, not local infection
Prognosis: Related to extent of infection/degree of immunosuppression

Cutaneous Cryptococcosis (Cryptococcus neoformans)
Clinical Presentation: May present as single or multiple papules, pustules, erythematous indurated plaques, soft subcutaneous masses, draining sinus tracts, or ulcers with undermined edges
Diagnostic Considerations: Diagnosis by demonstrating organism by stain/culture in tissue specimen
Pitfalls: Skin lesions usually represent disseminated disease in compromised hosts, not localized infection. In AIDS patients, umbilicated papules resemble molluscom contagiosum. In organ transplants, cellulitis with necrotizing vasculitis may occur
Prognosis: Related to extent of infection/degree of immunosuppression

Cutaneous Sporotrichosis (Sporothrix schenckii)

Clinical Presentation: Primary cutaneous lymphatic sporotrichosis starts as a small, firm, movable, subcutaneous nodule, which then becomes soft and breaks down to form a persistent, friable ulcer. Secondary lesions usually develop proximally along lymphatic channels, but do not involve lymph nodes. Plaque form does not spread locally

Diagnostic Considerations: Diagnosis by demonstrating organism by stain/culture in tissue specimen. Cutaneous disease arises at sites of minor trauma with inoculation of fungus into skin. Skin lesions usually represent disseminated disease in compromised hosts, not localized infection

Pitfalls: HIV/AIDS patients with CD_4 < 200 may have widespread lymphocutaneous disease that ulcerates and is associated with arthritis. Unusual in axilla due to increased temperature

Prognosis: Related to extent of infection/degree of immunosuppression

Papular/Disseminated Candidiasis (see sepsis in chronic steroids, p. 114)

Cutaneous Onchocerciasis (Onchocerca volvulus)

Clinical Presentation: Early manifestation is pruritic, papular rash with altered pigmentation. Later, papules, scaling, edema, and depigmentaiton may develop. Nodules develop in deep dermis/subcutaneous tissue (especially over bony prominences) or in deeper sites near joints, muscles, bones

Diagnostic Considerations: Diagnosis by serology/demonstration of microfilaria in tissue specimens. Intradermal edema produces "peau d'orange" effect with pitting around hair follicles/sebaceous glands

Pitfalls: Ivermectin is effective against microfilaria, not adult worms

Prognosis: Related to location/extent of organ damage

Rickettsias (Fever/Petechial Skin Rash)

Subset	Pathogens	Preferred Therapy	Alternate Therapy
Rocky Mountain spotted fever (RMSF)	Rickettsia rickettsii	Doxycycline 200 mg (IV or PO) q12h x 3 days, then 100 mg (IV or PO) x 4 days	Any quinolone (IV or PO) x 7 days **or** Chloramphenicol 500 mg (IV or PO) q6h x 7 days
Epidemic (louse-borne) typhus, flying squirrel typhus	Rickettsia prowazekii	Same as RMSF	Same as RMSF
Murine (flea-borne) typhus	Rickettsia typhi	Same as RMSF	Same as RMSF
Scrub (chigger mite-borne) typhus (Tsutsugamushi fever)	Rickettsia tsutsugamushi	Same as RMSF	Rifampin 600-900 mg (PO) q24h x 7 days
Rickettsialpox	Rickettsia akari	Same as RMSF	Same as RMSF
Tick typhus fevers (Mediterranean spotted fever, Boutonneuse fever, Israeli spotted fever)	Rickettsia conorii	Same as RMSF	Same as RMSF
African tick bite fever	Rickettsia africae	Same as RMSF	Same as RMSF

Rocky Mountain Spotted Fever (Rickettsia rickettsia) RMSF

Clinical Presentation: Fever with relative bradycardia, severe frontal headache, severe myalgias of abdomen/back/legs 3-12 days after tick bite. Rash begins as erythematous macules on wrists and ankles 3-5 days after tick bite, and progresses to petechiae/palpable purpura with confluent areas of ecchymosis. Periorbital edema, conjunctival suffusion, acute deafness, and edema of the dorsum of the hands/feet are important early signs. Abdominal pain can mimic acute abdomen, and meningismus and headache can mimic meningitis. Hepatosplenomegaly, cough, and coma may develop late. Laboratory findings include normal leukocyte count, thrombocytopenia, ↑ LFTs, and pre-renal azotemia. Hypotension/shock may occur secondary to myocarditis, which is the most common cause of death. Primary vector in United States is the Dermacentor tick; primary animal reservoir is small wild animals

Diagnosis: Primarily a clinical diagnosis requiring a high index of suspicion and early empiric therapy. Early/rapid diagnosis can be made by DFA of biopsy specimen of rash. Specific R. rickettsii IFA, complement fixation, ELISA antibody titers are confirmatory. Include RMSF in differential diagnosis of any patient with fever and potential tick exposure, especially during the summer months

Pitfalls: Most cases occur in eastern and southeastern United States, not Rocky Mountain area. Many cases go unrecognized due to nonspecific early findings. Early antibiotic therapy may blunt/eliminate serologic response. Patients with signs/symptoms of RMSF but without a rash should be considered as having ehrlichiosis ("spotless RMSF") until proven otherwise. Early therapy is essential; begin empiric therapy as soon as RMSF is suspected. Other adjunctive measures may be required

Prognosis: Late (after day 5) initiation of treatment increases the risk of death by 5-fold. Adverse prognostic factors include myocarditis and severe encephalitis

Epidemic (Louse-Borne) Typhus (Rickettsia prowazekii)

Clinical Presentation: High fever with relative bradycardia, chills, headache, conjunctival suffusion, and myalgias. A macular, rubella-like, truncal rash develops in most on the fifth febrile day, which may become petechial and involve the extremities, but spares the palms/soles. Facial swelling/flushing occurs at end of first week, along with CNS symptoms (e.g., tinnitus, vertigo, delirium) and GI complaints (diarrhea, constipation, nausea, vomiting, abdominal pain). Hypotension, pneumonia, renal failure, gangrene, cerebral infarction may develop late. Laboratory findings include normal leukocyte count, thrombocytopenia, and ↑ serum creatinine/LFTs. Primary vector is the human body louse; primary reservoir is humans

Diagnosis: Primarily a clinical diagnosis requiring a high index of suspicion and early empiric therapy. Specific R. prowazekii antibody titers are confirmatory. Consider epidemic (louse-borne) typhus in febrile impoverished persons infested with lice, especially in Africa and parts of Latin America. Rarely seen in the United States. Milder recrudescent form (Brill-Zinsser disease) is also rare

Pitfalls: Many cases go unrecognized due to nonspecific early findings. Early therapy is essential

Prognosis: Gangrene of nose, ear lobes, genitalia, toes, and fingers may develop in severe cases. Death occurs in 10-50% of untreated patients

Murine (Flea-Borne) Typhus (Rickettsia typhi)

Clinical Presentation: Similar to epidemic typhus but less severe, with fever in most, and headache, myalgias, and a macular rash in half. Laboratory findings include a normal leukocyte count, mild thrombocytopenia, and mildly ↑ LFTs. Primary vector is the Asian rat flea (Xenopsylla cheopis); primary reservoir is the commensal rat (Rattus genus). Uncommon in United States; most cases from Texas, California, Florida, Hawaii

Diagnosis: Primarily a clinical diagnosis requiring a high index of suspicion. More common during summer and fall. Specific R. typhi antibody titers are confirmatory

Pitfalls: Many cases go unrecognized due to nonspecific findings. Rash becomes maculopapular, compared to epidemic typhus, which remains macular

Prognosis: Good if treated early. Death occurs in < 1%

Scrub Typhus (Rickettsia tsutsugamushi) Tsutsugamushi Fever

Clinical Presentation: Fever, chills, headache, myalgias, arthralgias, GI symptoms, other nonspecific complaints. Eschar at mite bite site (tache noire) ± regional adenopathy. A macular, truncal rash develops in most, usually in the first week, and may progress to involve the extremities and face, but spares the palms/soles. Vasculitis may lead to cardiopulmonary, CNS, hematologic abnormalities during the second week. Hepatosplenomegaly is common. Primary vector/reservoir is the larval (chigger) trombiculid mite. Endemic areas include northern Australia, southeastern Asia, Indian subcontinent
Diagnosis: Presumptive diagnosis is clinical. Specific R. tsutsugamushi serology is confirmatory
Pitfalls: Incomplete therapy frequently results in relapse
Prognosis: Excellent if treated early

Rickettsialpox (Rickettsia akari)

Clinical Presentation: Milder illness than other rickettsioses, with initial eschar at bite site, high fever, and generalized rash (usually erythematous papules which become vesicular and spares the palms/soles). Fever peak is usually < 104°F, occurs 1-3 weeks after mite bite, and lasts ~ 1 week without therapy. Headache, photophobia, marked diaphoresis, sore throat, GI complaints (nausea/vomiting following initial headache) may occur. Most labs are normal, although leukopenia may be present. Primary vector is the mouse mite; primary animal reservoir is the house mouse. Rare in the United States
Diagnosis: Presumptive diagnosis by clinical presentation. Specific R. akari serology is confirmatory
Pitfalls: Do not confuse with African tick-bite fever, which may also have a vesicular rash
Prognosis: Excellent even without therapy

Tick Typhus Fevers (Rickettsia conorii) Mediterranean Spotted Fever, Boutonneuse Fever, Israeli Fever

Clinical Presentation: Similar to RMSF with fever, chills, myalgias, but less severe. Unlike RMSF, an eschar is usually present at the site of the tick bite ± regional adenopathy. Leukocyte count is normal and thrombocytopenia is common. Transmitted by the brown dog tick, Rhipicephalus sanguineus
Diagnosis: Presumptive diagnosis by clinical presentation. Specific R. conorii serology is confirmatory
Pitfalls: Suspect in travelers from endemic areas with a RMSF-like illness. Consider different diagnosis in absence of an eschar
Prognosis: Good with early treatment. Prostration may be prolonged even with proper therapy

African Tick Bite Fever (Rickettsia africae)

Clinical Presentation: Similar to murine typhus with fever, chills, myalgias, but regional adenopathy and multiple eschars are common. Incubation period ~ 6 days. Amblyomma hebraeum/variegatum tick vectors frequently bite humans multiple times
Diagnosis: Presumptive diagnosis by clinical presentation. Specific R. africae serology is confirmatory
Pitfalls: Rash is transient, and may be vesicular or absent
Prognosis: Good even without therapy; excellent with therapy

Other Skin Lesions

Subset	Pathogens	Topical Therapy	PO Therapy
Tinea versicolor (pityriasis)	Malassezia furfur (Pityrosporum orbiculare)	Clotrimazole cream (1%) *or* miconazole cream (2%) *or* ketoconazole cream (2%) daily x 7 days	Ketoconazole 200 mg (PO) q24h x 7 days **or** Itraconazole 200 mg (PO) q24h x 7 days **or** Fluconazole 400 mg (PO) x 1 dose

Other Skin Lesions (cont'd)

Subset	Pathogens	Preferred Therapy
Eosinophilic folliculitis	Malassezia furfur (Pityrosporum orbiculare)	Ketoconazole cream (2%) topically x 2-3 weeks ± ketoconazole 200 mg (PO) q24h x 2-3 weeks

Tinea Versicolor/Pityriasis (Malassezia furfur)
Clinical Presentation: Hyper– or hypopigmented scaling papules (0.5-1 cm), which may coalesce into larger plaques. Most commonly affects the upper trunk and arms. May be asymptomatic or pruritic
Diagnostic Considerations: M. furfur also causes eosinophilic folliculitis in HIV/AIDS, and catheter-acquired sepsis mostly in neonates or immunosuppressed patients. Diagnosis is clinical
Pitfalls: Skin pigmentation may take months to return to normal after adequate therapy
Prognosis: Excellent

Eosinophilic Folliculitis (Malassezia furfur)
Clinical Presentation: Intensely pruritic folliculitis, usually on lower extremities
Diagnostic Considerations: Tissue biopsy shows eosinophilic folliculitis. Diagnosis by demonstrating organism by culture on Sabouraud's agar overlaid with olive oil
Pitfalls: Resembles folliculitis, but lesions are concentrated on lower extremities (not on trunk as with cutaneous candidiasis)
Prognosis: Related to degree of immunosuppression. Use oral therapy if topical therapy fails

Myositis

Subset	Pathogens	Preferred Therapy
Chromomycosis	Cladosporium/Fonsecaea	Itraconazole 200 mg (PO) q24h until cured **or** Terbinafine 250 mg (PO) q24h until cured
Trichinosis	Trichinella spiralis	Albendazole 400 mg (PO) q12h x 8-14 days **or** Mebendazole 5 mg/kg (PO) q12h x 2 weeks

Chromomycosis (Cladosporium/Fonsecaea)
Clinical Presentation: Subcutaneous/soft tissue nodules or verrucous lesions
Diagnostic Considerations: Diagnosis by demonstrating organism by culture/tissue biopsy specimen
Pitfalls: May resemble Madura foot or cause ulcerative lesions in muscle
Prognosis: Related to degree of immunosuppression

Trichinosis (Trichinella spiralis)
Clinical Presentation: Muscle tenderness, low-grade fevers, peripheral eosinophilia, conjunctival suffusion
Diagnostic Considerations: Diagnosis by Trichinella serology or by demonstrating larvae in muscle biopsy
Pitfalls: ESR is very low (near zero), unlike other causes of myositis, which have elevated ESRs
Prognosis: Excellent with early treatment. Short-term steroids may be useful during acute phase. Therapy is ineffective against calcified larvae in muscle

Chapter 5

HIV Infection

Paul E. Sax, M.D.

HIV Infection

Paul E. Sax, M.D.

Infection with Human Immunodeficiency Virus (HIV-1) leads to a chronic and usually fatal infection characterized by progressive immunodeficiency, a long clinical latency period, and opportunistic infections. The hallmark of HIV disease is infection and viral replication within T-lymphocytes expressing the CD_4 antigen (helper-inducer lymphocytes), a critical component of normal cell-mediated immunity. Qualitative defects in CD_4 responsiveness and progressive depletion in CD_4 cell counts increase the risk for opportunistic infections such as Pneumocystis carinii pneumonia, and neoplasms such as lymphoma and Kaposi's sarcoma. HIV infection can also disrupt blood monocyte, tissue macrophage, and B-lymphocyte (humoral immunity) function, predisposing to infection with encapsulated bacteria. Direct attack of CD_4-positive cells in the central and peripheral nervous system can cause HIV meningitis, peripheral neuropathy, and dementia. Nearly 1 million people in the United States and 36 million people worldwide are infected with HIV. Without treatment, the average time from acquisition of HIV to an AIDS-defining opportunistic infection is about 10 years; survival then averages 1-2 years. There is tremendous individual variability in these time intervals, with some patients progressing from acute HIV infection to death within 1-2 years, and others not manifesting HIV-related immunosuppression for > 20 years after HIV acquisition. Antiretroviral therapy and prophylaxis against opportunistic infections has markedly improved the overall prognosis of HIV disease. The approach to HIV infection is shown in Figure 1.

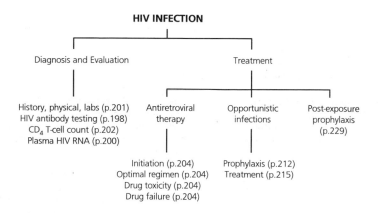

Figure 1. Diagnosis, Evaluation, and Treatment of HIV Infection

STAGES OF HIV INFECTION

A. Viral Transmission. HIV infection is acquired primarily by sexual intercourse (anal, vaginal, infrequently oral), exposure to contaminated blood (primarily needle transmission), or maternal-fetus (perinatal) transmission. Sexual practices with the highest risk of transmission include unprotected receptive anal intercourse (especially with mucosal tearing), unprotected receptive vaginal intercourse (especially during menses), and unprotected rectal/vaginal intercourse in the presence of genital ulcers (e.g., primary syphilis, genital herpes, chancroid). Lower risk sexual practices include insertive anal/vaginal intercourse and oral-genital contact. The risk of transmission after a single encounter with an HIV source has been estimated to be 1 in 150 with needle sharing, 1 in 300 with occupational percutaneous exposure, 1 in 300-1000 with receptive anal intercourse, 1 in 500-1250 with receptive vaginal intercourse, 1 in 1000-3000 with insertive vaginal intercourse, and 1 in 3000 with insertive anal intercourse. Transmission risk increases with the number of encounters. The mode of transmission does not affect the natural history of HIV disease.

B. Acute (Primary) HIV Infection (p. 197). Acute HIV occurs 1-4 weeks after transmission, and is accompanied by a burst of viral replication with a decline in CD_4 cell count. Most patients manifest a symptomatic flu-like syndrome, which is often overlooked. Acute HIV infection is confirmed by demonstrating a high viral load in the absence of HIV antibody. Antiretroviral therapy is indicated, although the optimal duration of therapy and role of intermittent treatment await definition.

C. Seroconversion. Development of a positive HIV antibody test usually occurs within 4 weeks of acute infection, and invariably (with few exceptions) by 6 months.

D. Asymptomatic HIV Infection lasts a variable amount of time (average 8-10 years), and is accompanied by a gradual decline in CD_4 cell counts and a relatively stable HIV RNA level (sometimes referred to as the viral "set point").

E. Symptomatic HIV Infection. Previously referred to as "AIDS Related Complex (ARC)," findings include thrush or vaginal candidiasis (persistent, frequent, or poorly responsive to treatment), cervical dysplasia/carcinoma in-situ, herpes zoster (recurrent episodes or involving multiple dermatomes), oral hairy leukoplakia, peripheral neuropathy, diarrhea, or constitutional symptoms (e.g., low-grade fevers, weight loss).

F. AIDS is defined by a CD_4 cell count < 200/mm^3, a CD_4 cell percentage of total lymphocytes <14%, or one of several AIDS-related opportunistic infections. Common opportunistic infections include Pneumocystis carinii pneumonia, cryptococcal meningitis, recurrent bacterial pneumonia, Candida esophagitis, CNS toxoplasmosis, tuberculosis, and non-Hodgkin's lymphoma. Other AIDS indicators in HIV-infected patients include candidiasis of the bronchi, trachea, or lungs; disseminated/extrapulmonary coccidiomycosis, cryptococcosis, or histoplasmosis; chronic (>1 month) intestinal cryptosporidiosis or isosporiasis; Kaposi's sarcoma; lymphoid interstitial pneumonia/pulmonary lymphoid hyperplasia; disseminated/extrapulmonary Mycobacterium (avium-intracellular, kansasii, other species) infection; progressive multifocal leukoencephalopathy (PML); recurrent Salmonella septicemia; or HIV wasting syndrome.

G. Advanced HIV Disease is diagnosed when the CD_4 cell count is < $50/mm^3$. Most AIDS-related deaths occur at this point. Common late stage opportunistic infections are caused by CMV disease (retinitis, colitis) or disseminated Mycobacterium avium-intracellulare (MAI).

ACUTE (PRIMARY) HIV INFECTION

A. Description. Acute clinical illness associated with primary acquisition of HIV, occurring 1-4 weeks after viral transmission (range: 6 days to 6 weeks). Symptoms develop in 50-90%, but are often mistaken for the flu. More severe symptoms may correlate with more rapid HIV disease progression. Even without therapy, most patients recover, reflecting development of an effective immune response and depletion of susceptible CD_4 cells.

B. Differential Diagnosis includes **EBV, CMV**, viral hepatitis, enteroviral infection, 2° syphilis, toxoplasmosis, HSV with erythema multiforme, drug reaction, Behcet's disease, acute lupus.

C. Signs and Symptoms usually reflect hematogenous dissemination of virus to lymphoreticular and neurologic sites:
- Fever (97%)
- Pharyngitis (73%). Typically non-exudative (unlike EBV, which is usually exudative)
- Rash (77%). Maculopapular viral exanthem of the face and trunk is most common, but can involve the extremities, palms and soles
- Arthralgia/myalgia (58%)
- Neurologic symptoms (12%). Headache is most common. Neuropathy, Bell's palsy, and meningoencephalitis are rare, but may predict worse outcome
- Oral/genital ulcerations, thrush, nausea, vomiting, diarrhea, weight loss

D. Laboratory Findings
1. **CBC.** Lymphopenia followed by lymphocytosis (common. Atypical lymphocytosis is absent/mild (unlike EBV, where atypical lymphocytosis may be 20-30% or higher). Thrombocytopenia occurs in some
2. **Elevated transaminases**
3. **Depressed CD_4 cell count.** Can rarely be low enough to induce opportunistic infections
4. **HIV antibody.** Usually negative, although persons with prolonged symptoms of acute HIV may have positive antibody tests if diagnosed late during the course of illness

E. Confirming the Diagnosis of Acute HIV Infection
1. **Obtain HIV antibody** after informed consent to exclude prior disease
2. **Order viral load test (HIV RNA PCR)**, preferably RT-PCR (lower limit 400 copies/mL).

HIV RNA confirms acute HIV infection prior to seroconversion. Most individuals will have very high viral loads (>100,000 copies/mL). Be suspicious of a false-positive test if the viral load is low (< 20,000 copies/mL). For any positive test, follow-up antibody testing at 1, 3, and 6 months is mandatory to confirm HIV infection. p24 antigen can also be used to establish the diagnosis, but is less sensitive than HIV RNA PCR

3. **Order other tests/serologies if viral load test is negative.** Order throat cultures for bacterial/viral respiratory pathogens, EBV VCA IgM/IgG, CMV IgM/IgG, HHV-6 IgM/IgG, and hepatitis serologies as appropriate to establish a diagnosis for patient's symptoms

4. **Repeat HIV serology** is recommended at 1, 3, and 6 months to document seroconversion in patients who are viral load positive but HIV antibody negative

F. Management of Acute HIV Infection

1. **Initiate antiretroviral therapy.** Patients with acute HIV infection should be enrolled into clinical studies. Otherwise, initiate therapy with antiretroviral therapy as recommended in Table 4 (p. 209) to suppress viral replication below the level of detection (viral load < 50 copies/mL). The optimal duration of therapy and role of intermittent treatment are under investigation.

2. **Obtain HIV resistance genotype (p. 207)** because of a rising background prevalence of transmission of antiretroviral therapy-resistant virus

3. **Refer to an HIV specialist** (highly recommended)

4. **Rationale for treatment of acute HIV infection.** Hastens resolution of symptoms (possibly); reduces dissemination of virus to other organs (unlikely); reduces viral transmission (sometimes); lowers virologic "set point" (possibly); preserves virus-specific CD_4 response to slow disease progression (likely); eradicates HIV (extremely unlikely)

APPROACH TO HIV TESTING (Figure 2)

A. **HIV Antibody Tests.** Most patients produce antibody to HIV within 6-8 weeks of exposure; half will have a positive antibody test in 3-4 weeks, and nearly 100% will have detectable antibody by 6 months

1. **ELISA.** Usual screening test. All positives must be confirmed with Western blot or other more specific tests

2. **Western blot.** CDC criteria for interpretation:
   a. **Positive:** At least two of the following bands: p24, gp41, gp160/120
   b. **Negative:** No bands
   c. **Indeterminate:** Any HIV band, but does not meet criteria for positivity

3. **Test performance.** Standard method is ELISA screen with Western blot confirmation
   a. **ELISA negative:** Western blot is not required (ELISA sensitivity 99.7%, specificity 98.5%). Obtain HIV RNA if acute HIV infection is suspected
   b. **ELISA positive:** Confirm with Western blot. Probability that ELISA and Western blot are both false-positives is extremely low (< 1 per 140,000). Absence of p31 band could be a clue to a false positive Western blot
   c. **Unexpected ELISA/Western blot:** Repeat test to exclude clerical/computer error

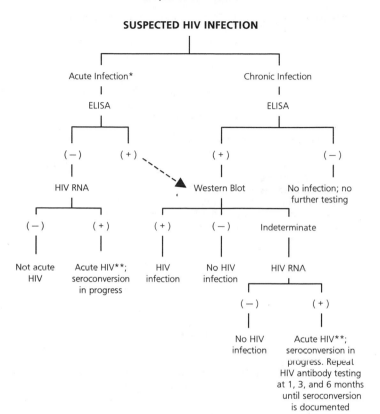

Figure 2. Approach to HIV Testing

(−) = negative test; (+) = positive test
*   Occurs 1-4 weeks after viral transmission. Most patients manifest a viral syndrome (fever, pharyngitis ± rash/arthralgias), which is often mistaken for the flu and therefore overlooked
** HIV RNA in acute HIV infection should be very high (> 50,000 copies/mL; usually > 100,000 copies/mL)

4. **Indeterminate Western Blot.** Common clinical problem, affecting 4-20% of reactive ELISAs. Usually due to a single p24 band or weak other bands. Causes include seroconversion in progress, advanced HIV disease with loss of antibody response, cross-reacting antibody from pregnancy, blood transfusions, organ transplantation, autoantibodies from collagen vascular disease, infection with HIV-2, influenza vaccination, or recipient of HIV vaccine. In low-risk patients, an indeterminate result almost never represents true HIV infection; options include repeating the test in 2-3 and 6 months (if still indeterminate, reassure) or ordering a viral load test (if negative, reassure; if viral load is high, seroconversion is in progress).

B. **Quantitative Plasma HIV RNA (HIV Viral Load Assays)**

1. **Description.** Measures amount of HIV RNA in plasma. High sensitivity of assays allows detection of virus in most patients not on antiviral therapy. Used to diagnosis HIV infection and guide antiretroviral therapy.

2. **Uses of Viral Load Assay**
   a. **Confirms diagnosis of acute HIV infection.** A high viral load with a negative HIV antibody test confirms acute HIV infection prior to seroconversion.
   b. **Helpful in initial evaluation of HIV infection.** Establishes baseline viral load and helps determine whether to initiate or defer therapy.
   c. **Identifies potential "long-term non-progressors"** (i.e., 10 or more years of HIV infection without immunologic decline even without antiretroviral therapy). Such patients almost invariably have viral load assays consistently < 5000 (usually < 1000).
   d. **Monitors response to antiviral therapy.** Viral load changes rapidly decline 2-4 weeks after starting or changing effective antiretroviral therapy, with slower decline thereafter. Patients with the greatest viral load response have the best clinical outcome. "No change" in viral load suggests therapy will be ineffective.
   e. **Estimates risk for opportunistic infection.** For patients with similar CD_4 cell counts, the risk of opportunistic infections is higher with higher viral loads.

3. **Assays and Interpretation**
   a. **Tests, sensitivities, and dynamic range**. Three main assays, each with advantages and disadvantages. Any assay can be used to diagnose acute HIV infection and guide/monitor therapy, but the same test should be used to follow patients longitudinally.
      1. **RT-PCR Amplicor** (Roche): Sensitivity = 400 copies/mL; dynamic range = 400-750,000 copies/mL
      2. **RT-PCR Ultrasensitive** (Roche): Sensitivity = 50 copies/mL; dynamic range = 50-50,000 copies/mL
      3. **bDNA Quantiplex 3.0** (Chiron): Sensitivity = 50 copies/mL; dynamic range = 50-500,000 copies/mL
   b. **Correlation between viral load and CD_4.** Viral load assays correlate inversely with CD_4 cell counts, but do so imperfectly (e.g., some patients with high CD_4 counts have relatively high viral loads, and vice versa.) For any given CD_4, higher viral loads correlate with more rapid disease progression. In response to antiretroviral therapy, changes in viral load generally precede changes in CD_4 cell count.
   c. **Significant change in viral load assay** is defined by at least a 2-fold (0.3 log)

change in viral RNA (accounts for normal variation in clinically stable patients), or a 3-fold (0.5 log) change in response to new antiretroviral therapy (accounts for intra-laboratory and patient variability). For example, if a viral load result = 50,000 copies/mL, then the range of possible actual values = 25,000-100,000 copies/mL, and the value needed to demonstrate antiretroviral activity = 17,000 copies/mL or less.

4. **Indications for Viral Load Testing**. Usually performed in conjunction with CD_4 cell counts. Indicated for the diagnosis of acute HIV infection, and for initial evaluation of newly diagnosed HIV. Also recommended 2-8 weeks after initiation of antiretroviral therapy and every 3-4 months in all HIV patients.

5. **When to Avoid Viral Load Testing**
   a. **During acute illnesses and immunizations.** Patients with acute opportunistic infections may experience significant (> 5-fold) rises in viral load, which return to baseline 1-2 months after recovery; similar patterns have been reported for bacterial pneumonia and HSV recurrences. Although data are conflicting, many studies show at least a transient increase in viral loads following influenza and other immunizations, which return to baseline after 2 months
   b. **When results of test would not influence therapy.** Frequent scenario in patients with advanced disease who have no antiretroviral options or cannot tolerate therapy
   c. **To diagnose HIV infection**, except if acute (primary) HIV disease is suspected during the HIV antibody window (i.e., first 3-6 weeks after viral transmission)

INITIAL ASSESSMENT OF HIV-INFECTED PATIENTS

A. **Clinical Evaluation.** History and physical exam should focus on diagnoses associated with HIV infection. Compared to patients without HIV, the severity, frequency, and duration of these conditions are usually increased in HIV disease.

1. **Dermatologic:** Severe herpes simplex (oral/anogenital); herpes zoster (especially recurrent, cranial nerve, or disseminated); molluscum contagiosum; staphylococcal abscesses; tinea nail infections; Kaposi's sarcoma (from HHV-8 infection); petechiae (from ITP); seborrheic dermatitis; new or worsening psoriasis; eosinophilic pustular folliculitis; severe cutaneous drug eruptions (especially sulfonamides)
2. **Oropharyngeal:** Oral candidiasis; oral hairy leukoplakia (from EBV); Kaposi's sarcoma (frequently on palate/gums); gingivitis/periodontitis; warts; aphthous ulcers (especially esophageal/perianal)
3. **Constitutional symptoms:** Fatigue, fevers, chronic diarrhea, weight loss
4. **Lymphatic:** Persistent, generalized lymphadenopathy
5. **Others:** Active TB (especially extrapulmonary); non-Hodgkin's lymphoma (especially CNS); unexplained leukopenia, anemia, thrombocytopenia (especially ITP); myopathy; miscellaneous neurologic conditions (cranial/peripheral neuropathies, Guillain-Barre syndrome, mononeuritis multiplex, aseptic meningitis, cognitive impairment)

B. **Baseline Laboratory Testing (Table 1)**

C. CD$_4$ Cell Count (lymphocyte subset analysis)

1. **Overview.** Acute HIV infection is characterized by a marked decline in CD$_4$ cell count, followed by a gradual rise associated with clinical recovery. Chronic HIV infection shows progressive declines (~ 50-80 cells/year) in CD$_4$ cell count without treatment, followed by more rapid decline 1-2 years prior to opportunistic infection (AIDS-defining diagnosis). Cell counts remain stable over 5-10 years in 5% of patients, while others may show rapid declines (> 300 cells/year). Since variability exists within individual patients and between laboratories, it is useful to *repeat any value before making management decisions.*

2. **Uses of CD$_4$ Cell Count**

   a. **Gives context of degree of immunosuppression** for interpretation of symptoms/signs (Table 2)

   b. **Used to guide therapy.** Most guidelines support CD$_4$ < 350/mm^3 as a threshold for initiating treatment, regardless of viral load. For prophylaxis against PCP, toxoplasmosis, and MAI/CMV infection, CD$_4$ cell counts of 200/mm^3, < 100/mm^3, and < 50/mm^3 are used as threshold levels, respectively

   c. **Provides estimate of risk of death.** CD$_4$ cell counts < 50/mm^3 are associated with a markedly increased risk of death (median survival 1 year), although some patients with low counts survive > 3 years even without antiretroviral therapy. Prognosis is heavily influenced by viral load, presence/history of opportunistic infections or neoplasms, and the immune reconstitution response to antiretroviral therapy

D. Viral Load Assay (HIV RNA PCR) (p. 200)

Table 1. Baseline Laboratory Testing for HIV-Infected Patients

Test	Rationale
Repeat HIV serology (ELISA/confirmatory Western blot)	Indicated for patients unable to document a prior positive test, and for "low risk" individuals with a positive test (to detect computer/clerical error). Repeat serology is now less important since viral load testing provides an additional means of confirming HIV infection
CBC with differential, platelets	Detects cytopenias (e.g., ITP) seen in HIV. Needed to calculate CD$_4$ cell count
Chemistry panel ("SMA 20")	Detects renal dysfunction and electrolyte/LFT abnormalities, which may accompany HIV and associated infections (e.g., HIV nephropathy, HCV)
CD$_4$ cell count	Determines the need for antiretroviral therapy and opportunistic infection (OI) prophylaxis. Best test for defining risk of OIs and prognosis
"Viral load" assay (plasma HIV RNA)	Provides a marker for the pace of HIV disease progression. Determines indication for and response to antiretroviral therapy
Tuberculin skin test (standard 5 TU of PPD)	Detects latent TB infection and targets patients for preventive therapy. Anergy skin tests are no longer indicated due to poor predictive value. HIV is the most powerful co-factor for the development of active TB
PAP smear	Risk of cervical cancer is nearly twice as high in HIV-positive women compared to uninfected controls

Table 1. Baseline Laboratory Testing for HIV-Infected Patients

Test	Rationale
Toxoplasmosis serology (IgG)	Identifies patients at risk for subsequent cerebral/systemic toxoplasmosis and the need for prophylaxis. Those with negative tests should be counseled on how to avoid infection
Syphilis serology (VDRL or RPR)	Identifies co-infection with syphilis, which is epidemiologically-linked to HIV. Disease may have accelerated course in HIV patients
Hepatitis C serology (anti-HCV)	Identifies HCV infection and usually chronic carriage. If positive, follow with HCV genotype and HCV viral load assay
Hepatitis B serologies (HBsAb, HBcAb, HBsAg)	Identifies patients who are immune to hepatitis B (HBsAb) or chronic carriers (HBsAg). HBcAb alone usually indicates low-level chronic carrier state. If all three are negative, hepatitis B vaccine is indicated
G6PD screen	Identifies patients at risk for dapsone/primaquine-associated hemolysis
CMV serology (IgG)	Identifies patients who should receive CMV-negative or leukocyte-depleted blood if transfused
VZV serology (IgG)	Identifies patients at risk for varicella (chickenpox), and those who should avoid contact with active varicella or herpes zoster patients. Serology-negative patients exposed to chickenpox should receive varicella-zoster immune globulin (VZIG)
Chest x-ray	Sometimes ordered as a baseline test for future comparisons. May detect healed granulomatous diseases/other processes. Indicated in all tuberculin skin test positive patients

Table 2. Use of CD_4 Cell Count for Interpretation of Patient Signs/Symptoms

CD_4 Cell Count (cells/mm^3)	Associated Conditions
> 500	Most illnesses are similar to those in HIV-negative patients. Some increased risk of bacterial infections (pneumococcal pneumonia, sinusitis), herpes zoster, tuberculosis, skin conditions
200-500*	Bacterial infections (especially pneumococcal pneumonia, sinusitis), cutaneous Kaposi's sarcoma, vaginal candidiasis, ITP
50-200*	Thrush, oral hairy leukoplakia, classic HIV-associated opportunistic infections (e.g., P. carinii pneumonia, cryptococcal meningitis, toxoplasmosis). For patients receiving prophylaxis, most opportunistic infection do not occur until CD_4 cell counts fall significantly below 100/mm^3
< 50*	"Final common pathway" opportunistic infections (disseminated M. avium-intracellulare, CMV retinitis), HIV-associated wasting, neurologic disease (neuropathy, encephalopathy)

* Patients remain at risk for all processes noted in earlier stages

ANTIRETROVIRAL THERAPY

A. Initiation of Antiretroviral Therapy (Figure 3). Advances in antiretroviral therapy have led to dramatic reductions in HIV-related morbidity and mortality for patients with severe immunosuppression ($CD_4 < 200$) or a prior AIDS-defining illness. Treatment of asymptomatic patients is far more controversial, many of whom live years before developing any HIV-related symptom. Potential benefits of early antiretroviral therapy include control of viral replication, reduction in viral load, prevention of immunodeficiency, delayed time to onset of AIDS, and decreased risk of drug toxicity, viral transmission, and selecting resistant virus. Potential risks of early antiretroviral therapy include reduced quality of life (from side effects/inconvenience), earlier development of drug resistance (with consequent transmission of resistant virus and limitation in future antiretroviral choices), unknown long-term toxicity of antiretroviral drugs, and unknown duration of effectiveness. The primary goals of therapy are prolonged suppression of viral replication to undetectable levels (viral load < 50 copies/mL), restoration/preservation of immune function, and improved clinical outcome. Once initiated, antiretroviral therapy is usually continued indefinitely.

B. Choice of Initial Antiretroviral Therapy (Tables 3-5, Figure 4). Specific regimens are chosen to improve the length and quality of life by reducing the viral load to undetectable levels. No single regimen is ideal for all patients. At least 3 active agents are required.
   1. **Protease inhibitor + 2 NRTIs** (e.g., lopinavir + ritonavir [Kaletra] plus lamivudine + zidovudine [Combivir]): Advantages: Most clinical data and longest follow-up for viral suppression. Disadvantages: Complexity, high pill burden, long-term toxicity, compromises future protease inhibitor regimens.
   2. **2 Protease inhibitors + 2 NRTIs:** Advantages: High potency, convenient dosing. Disadvantages: High pill burden, long-term toxicity, compromises future protease inhibitor regimens.
   3. **NNRTI + 2 NRTIs** (e.g., efavirenz [Sustiva] plus lamivudine + zidovudine [Combivir]). Advantages: Defers protease inhibitor, low pill burden. Disadvantages: Compromises future NNRTI regimen.
   4. **3 NRTIs** (e.g, zidovudine + lamivudine + abacavir [Trizivir]). Advantages: Defers protease inhibitor/NNRTI regimens, lowest pill burden (1 pill q12h). Disadvantages: Limited long-term data, abacavir hypersensitivity in 3%.

C. Antiretroviral Treatment Failure (Figure 4). There are several overlapping definitions of drug failure, including virologic failure, immunologic failure, and clinical failure. Virologic failure generally precedes immunologic failure, and immunologic failure generally precedes clinical failure. Before changing therapy, it is important to distinguish drug toxicity from drug failure. For drug toxicity, single drug substitutions from the same drug class may be appropriate. For drug failure, most cases require ≥ 2 new drugs or a new drug regimen. It is also important to determine the cause of drug failure (e.g, viral resistance, drug interactions, malabsorption, poor patient compliance). Treatment of mental health disorders and measures to improve compliance may obviate the need to change therapy.

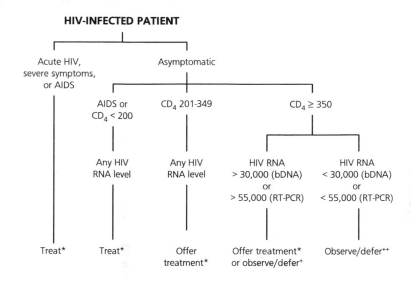

Figure 3. Indications for Initiating Antiretroviral Therapy

*   See Table 4 (p. 209), Figure 4 (p. 206)
+   Some experts would initiate therapy, given the high (>30%) 3-year risk of AIDS in untreated patients. In the absence of very high plasma HIV RNA levels, some would defer therapy and monitor CD_4 cell counts and HIV RNA levels frequently
++   Many experts would defer therapy and observe, given the relatively lower (<15%) 3-year risk of AIDS in untreated patients

Adapted from: Guidelines on the Use of Antiretroviral Therapy from the Panel on Clinical Practices for Treatment of HIV Infection, Dept. of Health and Human Services, April 23, 2001 (www.hivatis.org)

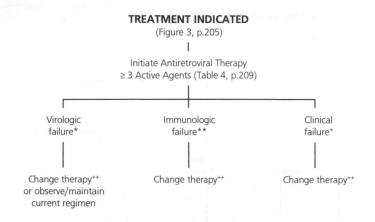

TREATMENT INDICATED
(Figure 3, p.205)

Initiate Antiretroviral Therapy
≥ 3 Active Agents (Table 4, p.209)

Virologic failure*	Immunologic failure**	Clinical failure+
Change therapy++ or observe/maintain current regimen	Change therapy++	Change therapy++

Figure 4. Approach to Antiretroviral Therapy

*   See below for criteria
** 30% decline in CD$_4$ cell count or 3% decline in CD$_4$ % from baseline, confirmed on repeat testing
+   Disease progression (constitutional symptoms, opportunistic infection, recurrent bacterial pneumonia)
++ Based on resistance testing and previous antiretroviral regimen

1. **Virologic failure.** Viral load fails to reach undetectable levels or rebounds. Drug failure is confirmed by significant increases in viremia on repeat testing not caused by a transient stimulus (e.g., acute illness, immunization), regardless of CD$_4$ cell counts.
    a. **Criteria for virologic failure** are based on demonstrating either a suboptimal reduction in viremia after starting therapy, re-emergence of viremia after suppression to undetectable levels, or a significant increase in viremia from the nadir of suppression.
        1. **Less than a 0.5-0.75 log reduction in plasma HIV RNA by 4 weeks** after starting therapy, or < 1 log reduction by 8 weeks
        2. **Failure to suppress plasma HIV RNA to undetectable levels within 4-6 months of starting therapy.** The degree of initial decrease in plasma HIV RNA and overall trend in decreasing viremia should be considered before changing therapy. For example, a patient with a viral load >750,000 copies/mL before therapy who stabilizes after 6 months of therapy at a level that is detectable but <10,000 copies/mL may not warrant an immediate change in therapy, so long as the trend is still downward
        3. **Repeated detection of virus in plasma after initial suppression to undetectable levels**, suggesting the development of resistance. The degree of plasma HIV RNA increase should be considered. For example, it may be reasonable to consider close, short-term observation in a patient whose plasma HIV RNA increases from undetectable to low-level detectability (50-5000

copies/mL) at 4 months. Most patients who fall into this category, however, will likely show progressive increases in plasma viremia and require a change in therapy

    4. Any reproducible significant (≥ 3-fold) increase from the nadir of plasma HIV RNA not caused by intercurrent infection, vaccination, or test methodology

  b. Risk factors for virologic failure include low drug levels (due to poor adherence, enhanced metabolism, or diminished absorption), high baseline viral load or low baseline CD_4 cell counts (patients with advanced disease are at greater risk of failing therapy), slow viral load response, genetic factors (heterozygotes for mutant CCR5 are more likely to respond), baseline viral resistance (due to prior antiretroviral therapy [common] or primary acquisition of a highly drug-resistant strain [uncommon]), and double nucleoside therapy.

  c. Management of virologic failure in patients who are otherwise doing well is not well established. One approach is to change therapy as soon as virologic failure is evident, since continued treatment with "non-suppressive" regimens selects for additional resistance mutations. Another approach is to change therapy only for immunologic or clinical failure, given the discordance between virologic failure and clinical failure ("CD_4/viral load disconnect"), increased pill burden/side effects associated with subsequent regimens, the perception that changing treatment too soon may exhaust future options, and lack of guarantee that changing regimens improves prognosis.

2. Immunologic Failure. Progressive decline in CD_4 cell count. Change in therapy is recommended based on results of resistance testing and previous antiretroviral regimen.

3. Clinical Failure. HIV disease progression (e.g., constitutional symptoms, opportunistic infections, recurrent bacterial pneumonia) or death. Change in therapy is recommended based on results of resistance testing and previous antiretroviral regimen.

4. Resistance Testing and Selection of New Antiretroviral Therapy. Genotypic assays characterize nucleotide sequences of the reverse transcriptase/protease portions of the virus, and identify resistance mutations associated with various drugs. Phenotypic assays attempt to grow the virus in the presence of drugs, providing a more intuitively applicable measurement of resistance (similar to that done with bacteria). Compared to phenotypic assays, genotypic assays are faster (2-3 weeks vs. 3-4 weeks for results), less expensive ($500 vs. $1000), and have less inter-laboratory variability; however, mutations do not always correlate with resistance and results are difficult to interpret.

D. Body Shape Changes and Metabolic Abnormalities Associated with HIV Therapy

  1. Lipodystrophy Syndrome. Prevalence varies widely (5%-75%), depending on the definition used. Features are similar to Syndrome X, with truncal obesity, insulin resistance, and hyperlipidemia (especially in patients on protease inhibitors). Other features include peripheral fat wasting from the face and limbs, breast enlargement in women (sometimes gynecomastia in men), and dorsocervical fat pad. Frank diabetes mellitus and diabetic ketoacidosis have been reported; close monitoring of patients with pre-existing diabetes is recommended, especially if protease inhibitors are used. Risk factors include total duration of antiretroviral therapy and treatment with protease inhibitors or nucleoside reverse transcriptase inhibitors (NRTIs). Optimal treatment awaits definition. Options include liposuction, anabolic steroids, growth hormone, metformin, or aggressive treatment of hyperlipidemia. Since hypertriglyceridemia is often marked, initial use of a fibrate (gemfibrozil 600 mg q12h or fenofibrate 67 mg q24h) is recommended, followed if necessary by a statin. A recent study found that protease inhibitors increased levels of atorvastatin by 4.5-fold and simvastatin by 31.6-fold, and decreased levels of pravastatin by 50% (Fichtenbaum C. 7th CROI, San Francisco, 2000. Abstract LB6). Therefore, pravastatin (at a starting dose of 20 mg q24h) is the preferred statin for patients on protease inhibitors.

2. **Lactic Acidosis/Hepatomegaly with Fatty Degeneration (Hepatic Steatosis)** is a rare but potentially fatal complication, most often associated with prolonged use of NRTIs. Clinical presentation includes nonspecific GI complaints (abdominal distension/pain, nausea, vomiting), weakness, weight loss, and sometimes dyspnea. In addition to elevated serum lactate levels, patients may have an anion gap metabolic acidosis, and elevated liver transaminases, CPK, LDH, lipase, and amylase. Treatment includes hemodialysis, discontinuation of antiretroviral therapy, and possibly bicarbonate infusions.

3. **Osteopenia/Osteoporosis.** Avascular necrosis of the hip and compression fractures of the spine have occurred during antiretroviral therapy, but the relationship is unclear.

4. **Increased Bleeding in Hemophilia.** Spontaneous bleeding is increased in hemophilia patients on protease inhibitors. Joint/soft tissue bleeding is most common, but intracranial and GI bleeding have occurred.

5. **Rash.** Mild rashes are relatively common with NNRTIs. Severe rashes (including Stevens-Johnson syndrome) may rarely develop in a small percentage of patients.

Table 3. Antiretroviral Agents for HIV Infection

Drug Class	Drugs
Nucleoside analogue reverse transcriptase inhibitors (NRTIs)	Zidovudine (AZT, ZDV, Retrovir) Didanosine (ddI, Videx) Zalcitabine (ddC, Hivid) Stavudine (d4T, Zerit) Lamivudine (3TC, Epivir) Abacavir (Ziagen) Zidovudine + lamivudine (Combivir) Zidovudine + lamivudine + abacavir (Trizivir)
Non-nucleoside reverse transcriptase inhibitors (NNRTIs)	Nevirapine (Viramune) Delavirdine (Rescriptor) Efavirenz (Sustiva)
Protease inhibitors (PIs)	Saquinavir (hard-gel [Invirase]; soft-gel [Fortovase]) Ritonavir (Norvir) Indinavir (Crixivan) Nelfinavir (Viracept) Amprenavir (Agenerase) Lopinavir + ritonavir (Kaletra)
Nucleotide analogue	Tenofovir (available through expanded access programs only)

Table 4. Recommended Antiretroviral Therapy for HIV Infection[†]

| | One Choice Each from Columns A and B[††] | |
	Column A	Column B
Strongly recommended	Efavirenz Indinavir Nelfinavir Ritonavir + indinavir Ritonavir + lopinavir (Kaletra) Ritonavir + saquinavir (SGC or HGC)	Stavudine + didanosine* Stavudine + lamivudine Zidovudine + didanosine Zidovudine + lamivudine
Recommended as alternatives	Abacavir Amprenavir Delavirdine Nelfinavir + saquinavir-SGC Nevirapine Ritonavir Saquinavir-SGC	Didanosine + lamivudine Zidovudine + zalcitabine
No recommendation (insufficient data)	Hydroxyurea + antiretroviral drugs Ritonavir + amprenavir Ritonavir + nelfinavir	
Not recommended	Monotherapy**	Stavudine + zidovudine Zalcitabine + didanosine Zalcitabine + lamivudine Zalcitabine + stavudine

HGC = saquinavir hard-gel capsule (Invirase), SGC = saquinavir soft-gel capsule (Fortovase)

See Chapter 7 for individual drug summaries

† Based on clinical trial data, pill burden, dosing frequency, food requirements, convenience, toxicity, and drug interaction profile compared with other regimens. From: Panel on Clinical Practices for Treatment of HIV Infection. Guidelines for the Use of Antiretroviral Agents in HIV-Infected Adults and Adolescents. Department of Health and Human Services. April 23, 2001. www.hivatis.org

†† Drugs are listed in alphabetical order, not by priority

* Increased risk of lactic acidosis/liver damage in pregnant women. Use only when potential benefit outweighs potential risk

** Zidovudine monotherapy may be considered for prophylaxis in pregnant women with low viral loads and high CD_4 counts to prevent perinatal transmission

Table 5. Advantages and Disadvantages of Common Antiretroviral Therapy

Agent/Combination	Advantages	Disadvantages
NRTI COMBINATIONS		
AZT (zidovudine, Retrovir) 300 mg (PO) q12h + 3TC (lamivudine, Epivir) 150 mg (PO) q12h	Fixed-dose combination tablet (Combivir) reduces pill burden. Lowest mitochondrial toxicity in in-vitro systems. AZT especially effective in treating ITP	AZT has highest rate of subjective side effects (nausea, GI disturbance, headache) in NRTI class, and is the most marrow suppressive
d4T (stavudine, Zerit) 40 mg (PO) q12h + ddI (didanosine, Videx) 400 mg (PO) q24h	Virologic failure on this combination is least likely to produce broad NRTI resistance based on genotypic studies	Highest mitochondrial toxicity in in-vitro systems, with possible increased risk of neuropathy, pancreatitis, possible lipodystrophy
d4T (stavudine, Zerit) 40 mg (PO) q12h + 3TC (lamivudine, Epivir) 150 mg (PO) q12h	Low pill burden. Best tolerated initially of any combination	d4T associated with neuropathy. Possible highest risk of lipodystrophy in NRTI class
AZT (zidovudine, Retrovir) 300 mg (PO) q12h + 3TC (lamivudine, Epivir) 150 mg (PO) q12h + abacavir (Ziagen) 300 mg (PO) q12h	Defers protease inhibitor and NNRTI regimens. Fixed-dose combination tablet (Trizivir) has lowest pill burden (1 pill q12h)	Limited long-term data. Abacavir hypersensitivity in 3%
PROTEASE INHIBITORS		
Lopinavir + ritonavir (Kaletra) 3 caps (400 mg/100 mg) (PO) q12h	More effective than nelfinavir when combined with d4T and 3TC in randomized, double-blind trial (Walmsley, ICAAC 2000, abstract 693). Relatively low pill burden for a protease inhibitor (q12h therapy). Generally well-tolerated	More likely to cause elevations in cholesterol and triglycerides than nelfinavir. Associated with diarrhea
Indinavir (Crixivan) 800 mg (PO) q8h	Longest follow-up data showing viral suppression (MK-035 study)	Q8h dosing on empty stomach required. Variable between-person metabolism, with marginal trough levels potentially allowing viral escape. Nephrolithiasis, paronychia, dry skin are unique side effects to this agent
Nelfinavir (Viracept) 1250 mg (PO) q12h	Generally well-tolerated. Early virologic failure often associated with unique D30N mutation, allowing effective "salvage" with other protease inhibitors	Diarrhea may be incapacitating for some patients. High pill burden (5 pills q12h)

Table 5. Advantages and Disadvantages of Common Antiretroviral Therapy

Agent/Combination	Advantages	Disadvantages
PROTEASE INHIBITORS (cont.)		
Ritonavir (Norvir) 400 mg (PO) q12h + saquinavir (Fortovase or Invirase) 400 mg (PO) q12h	Pharmacokinetic enhancement of saquinavir ensures adequate blood levels to inhibit virus. Some studies show this combination to be more effective than single protease inhibitors	High pill burden (6 large caps q12h). Ritonavir associated with relatively high rates of GI toxicity. Most likely to produce elevations in triglycerides and cholesterol
NNRTIs		
Efavirenz (Sustiva) 600 mg (PO) q24h	Long half-life (60 hours) allows once-daily dosing. Superior to indinavir in open label head-to-head trial (Staszewski, NEJM 1999;341:1865)	Near-universal CNS disturbances (vivid dreams, daytime somnolence, dizziness) at outset of therapy (usually abates with time). Rash in ~ 20% (can generally can treat through). Not to be used in pregnancy (teratogenic in monkeys). Single mutation leads to high-level resistance
Nevirapine (Viramune) 200 mg (PO) q24h x 14 days, then 200 mg (PO) q12h	Low pill-burden. Can be taken with or without food. Appears safe during pregnancy	Relatively high rate of severe hepatotoxicity and dermatologic/systemic reactions (rate of Stevens-Johnson syndrome ~ 1%). Single mutation leads to high-level resistance
Delavirdine (Rescriptor) 400 mg (PO) q8h	Can be taken with or without food. Inhibits p450 enzymes and can act as a pharmacokinetic booster for some protease inhibitors, most notably indinavir	Highest pill burden and most frequent dosing in drug class. Rash in 18%, though usually mild

OPPORTUNISTIC INFECTIONS IN HIV DISEASE

Patients with HIV disease are at risk for infectious complications not otherwise seen in immunocompetent patients. Such opportunistic infections occur in proportion to the severity of immune system dysfunction (reflected by CD_4 cell count depletion). While community acquired infections (e.g., pneumococcal pneumonia) can occur at any CD_4 cell count, "classic" HIV-related opportunistic infections (PCP, toxoplasmosis, cryptococcus, disseminated M. avium-intracellulare, CMV) do not occur until CD_4 cell counts are dramatically reduced. Specifically, it is rare to encounter PCP in HIV patients with $CD_4 > 200/mm^3$, and CMV and disseminated MAI occur at median CD_4 cell counts $< 50/mm^3$. The U.S. Public Health Service/Infectious Diseases Society of America 2001 guidelines for the prevention of opportunistic infections in persons infected with HIV can be found at www.hivatis.org/trtgdlns.html#Opportunistic

PROPHYLAXIS OF OPPORTUNISTIC INFECTIONS (Tables 6, 7)

Table 6. Overview of Prophylaxis (See Table 7 [pp. 213-215] for details)

Infection	Indication	Intervention
PCP	$CD_4 < 200/mm^3$	TMP-SMX
TB	PPD > 5 mm (current or past) or contact with active case	INH
Toxoplasma	IgG Ab (+) and $CD_4 < 100/mm^3$	TMP-SMX
MAI	$CD_4 < 50/mm^3$	Azithromycin or clarithromycin
S. pneumoniae	All patients	Pneumococcal vaccine
Hepatitis B	Susceptible patients	Hepatitis B vaccine
Influenza	All patients	Annual flu vaccine
Hepatitis A	HCV (+) and HA Ab (–); HCV (–) and HA Ab (–) gay men and travelers to endemic areas	Hepatitis A vaccine
VZV	Exposure to chickenpox or shingles; no prior history	VZIG

Ab = antibody; HA = Hepatitis A; HCV = Hepatitis C virus; MAI = M. avium-intracellulare; TB = M. tuberculosis; PCP = Pneumocystis carinii pneumonia; VZIG = varicella-zoster immune globulin; VZV = varicella- zoster virus

Table 7. Prophylaxis of Opportunistic Infections in HIV

Infection	Indications and Prophylaxis	Comments
P. carinii pneumonia (PCP)	Indications: CD_4 < 200/mm³, oral thrush, constitutional symptoms, or previous history of PCP Preferred prophylaxis: TMP-SMX 1 DS tablet (PO) q24h or 1 SS tablet (PO) q24h. 1 DS tablet (PO) 3x/week is also effective, but daily dosing results in fewer missed doses Alternate prophylaxis: Dapsone 100 mg (PO) q24h (preferred as second-line by most; more effective than aerosolized pentamidine when CD_4 cell count < 100; may also protect against toxoplasmosis) **or** Atovaquone 1500 mg (PO) q24h (comparably effective to dapsone and aerosolized pentamidine; more GI toxicity vs. dapsone, but less rash) **or** Aerosolized pentamidine 300 mg via Respirgard II nebulizer once monthly (exclude active pulmonary TB first to avoid nosocomial transmission)	Without prophylaxis, 80% of AIDS patients develop PCP, and 60-70% relapse within one year after the first episode. Prophylaxis also reduces the risk for bacterial infections and cerebral toxoplasmosis. Among patients with prior non-life-threatening reactions to TMP-SMX, 55% can be successfully rechallenged with 1 SS tablet daily, and 80% can be rechallenged with gradual dose escalation using TMP-SMX elixir (8 mg TMP + 40 mg SMX/mL) given as 1 mL x 3 days, then 2 mL x 3 days, then 5 mL x 3 days, then 1 SS tablet (PO) q24h. Macrolide-regimens for MAI (azithromycin, clarithromycin) add to efficacy of PCP prophylaxis. Primary and secondary prophylaxis may be discontinued if CD_4 cell counts increase to > 200 cells/mm³ for 3 months or longer in response to antiretroviral therapy (i.e., immune reconstitution). Prophylaxis should be resumed if the CD_4 cell count decreases to < 200/mm³
Toxoplasmosis	Indications: CD_4 < 100/mm³ with positive toxoplasmosis serology (IgG) Preferred prophylaxis: TMP-SMX 1 DS tablet (PO) q24h Alternate prophylaxis: Dapsone 50 mg (PO) q24h + pyrimethamine 50 mg (PO) weekly + folinic acid 25 mg (PO) weekly **or** Dapsone 100 mg/pyrimethamine 50 mg twice weekly (no folinic acid) **or** Atovaquone 1500 mg (PO) q24h	Incidence of toxoplasmosis in seronegative patients is too low to warrant chemoprophylaxis. Primary prophylaxis can be discontinued if CD_4 cell counts increase to > 200/mm³ for at least 3 months in response to antiretroviral therapy. Secondary prophylaxis (chronic maintenance therapy) may be discontinued in patients who responded to initial therapy, remain asymptomatic, and whose CD_4 counts increase to > 200/mm³ for 6 months or longer in response to antiretroviral therapy. Secondary prophylaxis should be restarted if the CD_4 count decreases to < 200/mm³. Some experts would obtain an MRI of the brain as part of the evaluation

Table 7. Prophylaxis of Opportunistic Infections in HIV (cont'd)

Infection	Indications and Prophylaxis	Comments
Tuberculosis (M. tuberculosis)	Indications: Any CD₄ cell count with PPD induration ≥ 5 mm, history of positive PPD without prior treatment, or close contact with active case of TB. Must exclude active disease (chest x-ray mandatory) Preferred prophylaxis: INH 300 mg (PO) q24h x 9 months + pyridoxine 50 mg (PO) q24h x 9 months Alternate prophylaxis: Rifampin 600 mg (PO) q24h x 2 months + pyrazinamide 20 mg/kg (PO) q24h x 2 months. Rifampin should not be given to patients receiving amprenavir, indinavir, lopinavir + ritonavir, nelfinavir, saquinavir, or delavirdine	Consider prophylaxis for skin test negative patients when the probability of prior TB exposure is > 10% (e.g., patients from developing countries, IV drug abusers in some cities, prisoners). However, a trial testing this strategy in the U.S. did not find a benefit for empiric prophylaxis. INH prophylaxis delayed progression to AIDS and prolonged life in Haitian cohort with positive PPD treated x 6 months. Rifampin plus pyrazinamide x 2 months was effective in a multinational clinical trial. Rifabutin may be substituted for rifampin in rifampin-containing regimens (see p. 216 for dosing)
M. avium intracellulare (MAI), atypical mycobacterium	Indications: CD₄ < 50/mm³ Preferred prophylaxis: Azithromycin 1200 mg (PO) once a week (fewest number of pills; fewest drug interactions; may add to efficacy of PCP prophylaxis) **or** Clarithromycin 500 mg (PO) q12h (more effective than rifabutin; associated with survival advantage; resistance detected in some breakthrough cases) Alternate prophylaxis: Rifabutin (less effective). See TB (p. 216) for dosing	Macrolide options (azithromycin, clarithromycin) preferable to rifabutin. Azithromycin is preferred for patients on protease inhibitors. Primary prophylaxis may be discontinued if CD₄ cell counts increase to > 100/mm³ and viral load suppresses for 3-6 months or longer in response to antiretroviral therapy. Secondary prophylaxis may be discontinued for CD₄ cell counts that increase to > 100/mm³ x 6 months or longer in response to antiretroviral therapy if patients have completed 12 months of MAI therapy and have no evidence of disease. Resume MAI prophylaxis for CD₄ < 100/mm³
Pneumococcus (S. pneumoniae)	Indications: Generally recommended for all patients Preferred prophylaxis: Pneumococcal polysaccharide (23 valent) vaccine.* Re-vaccinate at 5 years	Incidence of invasive pneumococcal disease is > 100-fold higher in HIV patients. Re-immunize if initial vaccine is given when CD₄ < 200/mm³, but is now > 200/mm³ due to antiretroviral therapy
Influenza	Indications: Generally recommended for all patients Preferred prophylaxis: Influenza vaccine (inactivated whole virus and split virus vaccine)*	Give annually (optimally between October and January). Some experts do not administer vaccine if CD₄ is < 100/mm³, since antibody response is poor

Table 7. Prophylaxis of Opportunistic Infections in HIV (cont'd)

Infection	Indications and Prophylaxis	Comments
Hepatitis B	Indications: All susceptible (anti-HBcAb negative and anti-HBsAg negative) patients Preferred prophylaxis: Hepatitis B recombinant DNA vaccine*	Response rate is lower than in HIV-negative controls. Repeat series if no response, especially if CD_4 was low during initial series and is now increased
Hepatitis A	Indications: All susceptible patients who are also infected with hepatitis C; HAV-susceptible seronegative gay men or travelers to endemic areas Preferred prophylaxis: Hepatitis A vaccine*	Response rate is lower than in HIV-negative controls
Measles, mumps, rubella	Indications: Patients born after 1957 and never vaccinated; patients vaccinated between 1963-1967 Preferred prophylaxis: MMR (measles, mumps, rubella) vaccine*	Single case of vaccine-strain measles pneumonia in severely immunocompromised adult who received MMR suggests vaccine may be contraindicated in patients with severe immunodeficiency (CD_4 < 200)
H. influenzae	Indications: Not generally recommended for adults Preferred prophylaxis: H. influenzae type B polysaccharide vaccine*	Incidence of H. influenzae disease is increased in HIV patients, but 2/3 are caused by non-type B strains. Unclear whether vaccine offers protection
Travel vaccines*	Indications: Travel to endemic areas	All considered safe except oral polio, yellow fever, and live oral typhoid

* Same dose as for normal hosts (see pp. 245-246). If possible, give vaccines early in course of HIV infection, while immune system may still respond. Alternatively, to increase the likelihood of response in patients with advanced HIV disease, vaccines may be administered after 6-12 months of effective antiretroviral therapy. Vaccines should be given when patients are clinically stable, not acutely ill (e.g., give during a routine office visit, rather than during hospitalization for an opportunistic infection). Live vaccines (e.g., oral polio, oral typhoid, Yellow fever) are generally contraindicated, but measles vaccine is well-tolerated in children, and MMR vaccine is recommended for adults as described above

---

TREATMENT OF OPPORTUNISTIC INFECTIONS (Table 8)

Antiretroviral therapy (ART) and specific antimicrobial prophylaxis regimens have led to a dramatic decline in HIV-related opportunistic infections. Today, opportunistic infections occur predominantly in patients not receiving ART (due to undiagnosed HIV infection or nonacceptance of therapy), in the period after starting ART (due to lack of immune reconstitution or from eliciting a previously absent inflammatory host response), or because of failed ART (due to viral resistance). The incidence and ultimate control of opportunistic infections is dramatically improved by effective ART, which restores immune function.

Table 8. Treatment of Opportunistic Infections in HIV (see comments, pp. 221-227)

RESPIRATORY TRACT OPPORTUNISTIC INFECTIONS IN HIV		
Infection	**Preferred Therapy**	**Alternate Therapy**
Pneumocystis carinii pneumonia (PCP) *Mild disease (p0$_2$ > 70 mmHg, A-a gradient < 35)*	TMP-SMX 2 DS tablets (PO) q6-8h x 3 weeks	TMP 300 mg (PO) q8h + dapsone 100 mg (PO) q24h x 3 weeks (less leukopenia/hepatitis vs. TMP-SMX) **or** Clindamycin 450 mg (PO) q6h (or 600 mg q8h) + primaquine 30 mg (PO) q24h x 3 weeks **or** Atovaquone suspension 750 mg (PO) q12h with food x 3 weeks **or** Aerosolized pentamidine 600 mg q24h x 3 weeks (least effective)
Moderate/severe disease (p0$_2$ < 70 mmHg, A-a gradient > 35)	TMP-SMX (5 mg/kg TMP) (IV) q6h x 3 weeks **plus** Prednisone 40 mg (PO) q12h x 5 days, then 40 mg (PO) q24h x 5 days, then 20 mg (PO) q24h until end of therapy	Pentamidine 4 mg/kg (IV) q24h x 3 weeks + prednisone (see preferred therapy) **or** Trimetrexate 45 mg/m^2 (IV) q24h + folinic acid 20 mg/m^2 (PO or IV) q6h x 3 weeks, plus prednisone (see preferred therapy)
Bacterial pneumonia	See p. 43	
Tuberculosis (M. tuberculosis)	Patients **NOT** on protease inhibitors (PIs) or NNRTIs INH 300 mg (PO) q24h + rifampin 600 mg (PO) q24h + pyrazinamide 25 mg/kg (PO) q24h + ethambutol 15-20 mg/kg (PO) q24h x 8 weeks. Then continue INH + rifampin at same daily doses x 18 weeks. May substitute streptomycin 15 mg/kg (IM) q24h for ethambutol during 8-week induction	Patients **ON** PIs or NNRTIs INH 300 mg (PO) q24h + rifabutin*† + pyrazinamide 25 mg/kg (PO) q24h + ethambutol 15-20 mg/kg (PO) q24h x 8 weeks. Then continue INH + rifabutin at same daily doses x 18 weeks Intolerant to rifabutin† INH 300 mg (PO) q24h + streptomycin 15 mg/kg (IM) q24h + ethambutol 15-20 mg/kg (PO) q24h + pyrazinamide 25 mg/kg (PO) q24h x 8 weeks. Then continue INH + SM + PZA at same doses 2-3x/week x 30 weeks

* *Rifabutin is contraindicated in patients receiving delavirdine or hard-gel saquinavir. For concurrent use with nelfinavir, indinavir, or amprenavir, decrease rifabutin to 150 mg (PO) q24h. For concurrent use with ritonavir, decrease rifabutin to 150 mg (PO) q48h or 3x/week. For concurrent use with efavirenz, increase rifabutin to 450-600 mg (PO) q24h. (The dose of PIs or NNRTIs may need to be increased by 20-25%.) Monitor carefully for rifabutin drug toxicity (arthralgia, uveitis, leukopenia)*
† *Rifampin can be used with ritonavir, ritonavir + saquinavir, efavirenz, and possibly nevirapine*

Table 8. Treatment of Opportunistic Infections (cont'd) (see comments, pp. 221-227)

RESPIRATORY TRACT OPPORTUNISTIC INFECTIONS IN HIV		
Infection	Preferred Therapy	Alternate Therapy
Invasive pulmonary aspergillosis	Amphotericin B 1-1.5 mg/kg (IV) q24h until 2-3 gm total dose given (duration of therapy poorly defined)	Itraconazole 200 mg (IV) q12h x 2 days, then itraconazole suspension 200 mg (PO) q12h x 6-12 months **or** Caspofungin 70 mg (IV) x 1 dose, then 50 mg (IV) q24h x 6-12 months **or** Amphotericin B lipid formulation 5 mg/kg (IV) q24h x 6-12 months

CNS OPPORTUNISTIC INFECTIONS IN HIV		
Infection	Preferred Therapy	Alternate Therapy
Toxoplasma encephalitis (T. gondii)	Sulfadiazine 1.5-2 gm (PO) q6h + pyrimethamine 200 mg (PO) x 1 dose then 50 mg (PO) q6h + folinic acid 10 mg (PO) q24h x 6-8 weeks until good clinical response. Follow with life-long suppressive therapy* with sulfadiazine 1 gm (PO) q12h + pyrimethamine 50 mg (PO) q24h + folinic acid 10 mg (PO) q24h	Clindamycin 600 mg (IV or PO) q6h + pyrimethamine 200 mg (PO) x 1 dose then 50 mg (PO) q6h + folinic acid 10 mg (PO) q24h x 6-8 weeks until good clinical response. Follow with life-long suppressive therapy* with sulfadiazine 1 gm (PO) q12h + pyrimethamine 50 mg (PO) q24h + folinic acid 10 mg (PO) q24h
Cryptococcal meningitis (C. neoformans)	Amphotericin B 0.7-1 mg/kg (IV) q24h x 2-3 weeks + 5-FC (optional) 25 mg/kg (PO) q6h x 2-3 weeks. Follow with fluconazole 800 mg (IV or PO) x 1 dose followed by 400 mg (PO) q24h indefinitely*	Fluconazole 800 mg (IV or PO) q24h x 6-8 weeks, then 400 mg (PO) q24h indefinitely* **or** Amphotericin B lipid formulation 5 mg/kg (IV) q24h x 2-3 weeks, then fluconazole 800 mg (IV or PO) x 1 dose followed by 400 mg (PO) q24h indefinitely*
CMV encephalitis or polyradiculitis	Ganciclovir 5 mg/kg (IV) q12h x 3 weeks, followed by valganciclovir 900 mg (PO) q24h indefinitely†. For severe cases, consider ganciclovir + foscarnet	Foscarnet 60 mg/kg (IV) q8h or 90 mg/kg (IV) q12h x 3 weeks ± ganciclovir 5 mg/kg (IV) q12h x 3 weeks. Follow with valganciclovir 900 mg (PO) q24h indefinitely†
Progressive multifocal leukoencephalopathy (PML)	Antiretroviral therapy with immune reconstitution	May attempt treatment with cidofovir 5 mg/kg (IV) once weekly x 2, then every 2 weeks for total of 24 weeks. Give probenecid 2 gm (PO) 3 hours before and 1 gm (PO) 2 and 8 hours after cidofovir

* Consider discontinuation of therapy if CD_4 > 200 for ≥ 6 months in response to antiretroviral therapy
† Consider discontinuation of therapy if CD_4 > 100-150 for ≥ 6 months in response to antiretroviral therapy

Table 8. Treatment of Opportunistic Infections (cont'd) (see comments, pp. 221-227)

GI TRACT OPPORTUNISTIC INFECTIONS IN HIV		
Infection	**Preferred Therapy**	**Alternate Therapy**
Oral thrush (Candida) *Acute infection*	Fluconazole 200 mg (PO) x 1 dose, then 100 mg (PO) q24h until symptoms resolve (usually 1-2 weeks)	Clotrimazole oral troches 10 mg 5x/day until symptoms resolve Refractory to other oral therapy Itraconazole 200 mg (IV) q12h x 2 days, then 200 mg tablet (PO) or 100 mg oral suspension (PO) q24h until symptoms resolve
Maintenance therapy (severe immuno-suppression)	Fluconazole 100 mg (PO) q24h or 200 mg 3x/week indefinitely*	Itraconazole 200 mg tablet (PO) q24h or 100 mg oral suspension (PO) q24h indefinitely* **or** Ketoconazole 200 mg (PO) q24h indefinitely*
Candida esophagitis *Initial infection*	Fluconazole 400-800 mg (PO) x 1 dose, then 200-400 mg (PO) x 1-3 weeks	Itraconazole 200 mg (IV) q12h x 2 days, then 100-200 mg tab (PO) q12h or 100-200 mg oral suspension (PO) q12h for 1-3 week total course **or** Amphotericin B 0.3-0.5 mg/kg (IV) q24h x 5-7 days
Frequent relapses	Fluconazole 100-200 mg (PO) q24h indefinitely*	Itraconazole 200 mg tab (PO) q12h or 100 mg oral suspension (PO) q12h indefinitely*
CMV esophagitis/ colitis	Ganciclovir 5 mg/kg (IV) q12h x 3-6 weeks Ganciclovir failure Foscarnet 60 mg/kg (IV) q8h or 90 mg/kg (IV) q12h x 3-6 weeks Foscarnet failure Ganciclovir + foscarnet x 3-6 weeks	Relapsing disease Ganciclovir 1 gm (PO) q8h or 5-6 mg/kg (IV) q24h indefinitely* **or** Foscarnet 90-120 mg/kg (IV) q24h indefinitely*
Salmonella enteritis	See p. 63	
Cryptosporidia enteritis	Paromomycin 1 gm (PO) q12h x 2-4 weeks, then 500 mg (PO) q12h indefinitely*	Paromomycin 1 gm (PO) q12h + azithromycin 600 mg (PO) q24h x 4 weeks, then paromomycin 500 mg (PO) q12h indefinitely*

* *Consider discontinuation of therapy if CD_4 > 200 for ≥ 6 months in response to antiretroviral therapy*

Table 8. Treatment of Opportunistic Infections (cont'd) (see comments, pp. 221-227)

GI TRACT OPPORTUNISTIC INFECTIONS IN HIV		
Infection	**Preferred Therapy**	**Alternate Therapy**
Microsporidia enteritis	Albendazole 400-800 mg (PO) q12h x 2-4 weeks. Patients with low CD_4 cell counts prone to relapsing disease may require treatment indefinitely*	Metronidazole 500 mg (PO) q8h x 2-4 weeks; some may require treatment indefinitely* **or** Atovaquone 750 mg (PO) q8h x 2-4 weeks; some may require treatment indefinitely*
Isospora enteritis	TMP-SMX 2 DS tablets (PO) q12h or 1 DS tablet (PO) q8h x 2-4 weeks. Follow with TMP-SMX 1-2 DS tablet(s) (PO) q24h indefinitely*	Ciprofloxacin 500 mg (PO) q12h x 2-4 weeks, or combination therapy with pyrimethamine 50-75 mg (PO) q24h + folinic acid 5-10 mg (PO) q24h x 2-4 weeks. Follow with pyrimethamine 25 mg (PO) q24h + folinic acid 5 mg (PO) q24h indefinitely*
Antibiotic-associated diarrhea/colitis (C. difficile)	See p. 63	

OTHER OPPORTUNISTIC INFECTIONS IN HIV		
Infection	**Preferred Therapy**	**Alternate Therapy**
Disseminated M. avium-intracellulare (MAI)	<u>Life-long therapy with:</u> Clarithromycin 500 mg (PO) q12h + ethambutol 15-25 mg/kg (PO) q24h (usually 800 or 1200 mg daily) ± rifabutin 300 mg (PO) q24h. (See pulmonary TB [p. 216] for rifabutin dosing with antiretroviral therapy.) No guidelines for discontinuation	Preferred therapy **plus either** Amikacin 15 mg/kg (IV) q24h x 1-2 months **or** Ciprofloxacin 500-750 mg (PO) q24h indefinitely
Extrapulmonary TB (M. tuberculosis)	Treat the same as pulmonary TB (p. 216). May require longer duration of therapy based on clinical response	
Non-meningeal cryptococcosis	For cutaneous disease, see pp. 187,189. For pulmonary disease, see pp. 169,171. For pulmonary or disseminated disease, consider maintenance fluconazole 200 mg (PO) q24h indefinitely	
Histoplasmosis, disseminated *Initial therapy*	<u>Severe disease</u> Amphotericin B 0.5-1 mg/kg (IV) x 7-14 days <u>Mild disease</u> Itraconazole 200 mg oral suspension (PO) q12h x 3 days	<u>Severe disease</u> Amphotericin B lipid formulation 5 mg/kg (IV) q24h x 7-14 days

* *Consider discontinuation of therapy if CD_4 > 200 for ≥ 6 months in response to antiretroviral therapy*

Table 8. Treatment of Opportunistic Infections (cont'd) (see comments, pp. 221-227)

OTHER OPPORTUNISTIC INFECTIONS IN HIV		
Infection	**Preferred Therapy**	**Alternate Therapy**
Histoplasmosis, disseminated *Maintenance therapy* *(all patients)*	Itraconazole 100 mg oral suspension (PO) q12h indefinitely.** Give loading dose of 200 mg (IV) q12h x 2 days if treated initially with amphotericin B	Amphotericin B 1 mg/kg (IV) once a week indefinitely** **or** Fluconazole 800 mg (IV or PO) x 1 dose, then 400 mg (PO) q24h indefinitely**
Herpes simplex (genital/oral) *Mild infection*	Acyclovir 400 mg (PO) q8h x 7-10 days **or** Famciclovir 250 mg (PO) q8h x 7-10 days **or** Valacyclovir 1 gm (PO) q12h x 7-10 days	<u>Failure to respond</u> Famciclovir 500 mg (PO) q8h x 7 days **or** Valacyclovir 1 gm (PO) q8h x 7 days
Severe or refractory infection	Acyclovir 5 mg/kg (IV) q8h x 2-7 days. If improvement, switch to acyclovir 400 mg (PO) q8h to complete 7-10 days	<u>Failure to respond</u> Acyclovir 15 mg/kg (IV) q8h x 3 weeks **or** Foscarnet 60 mg/kg (IV) q12h x 3 weeks
Frequent recurrences (≥ 6/year)	Acyclovir 400 mg (PO) q12h indefinitely*	Famciclovir 125-250 mg (PO) q12h indefinitely* **or** Valacyclovir 500 mg (PO) q12h or 1 gm (PO) q24h indefinitely*
Herpes zoster (VZV) *Localized*	Acyclovir 800 mg (PO) 5x/day x 7 days or until lesions crust **or** Famciclovir 500 mg (PO) q8h x 7 days or until lesions crust **or** Valacyclovir 1 gm (PO) q8h x 7 days or until lesions crust	Acyclovir 10 mg/kg (IV) q8h, with transition to oral therapy when clinical improvement is evident **or** Foscarnet 60 mg/kg (IV) q12, with transition to oral therapy when clinical improvement is evident
Disseminated, ophthalmic nerve or visceral involvement	Acyclovir 10-12 mg/kg (IV) q8h x 7 days or longer	Foscarnet 60 mg/kg (IV) q12h x 7 days or longer
Acyclovir-resistant strains	Foscarnet 60 mg/kg (IV) q12h x 7 days or longer	Not applicable

* Consider discontinuation of therapy if CD₄ > 200 for ≥ 6 months in response to antiretroviral therapy
** Consider discontinuation of therapy if CD₄ > 100 for ≥ 6 months in response to antiretroviral therapy

Table 8. Treatment of Opportunistic Infections (cont'd) (see comments, pp. 221-227)

OTHER OPPORTUNISTIC INFECTIONS IN HIV		
Infection	Preferred Therapy	Alternate Therapy
CMV retinitis *Initial therapy*	Initiate systemic CMV therapy pending ophthalmology consult Ganciclovir 5 mg/kg (IV) q12h x 2-3 weeks **or** Valganciclovir 900 mg (PO) q12h x 3 weeks **or** Foscarnet 60 mg/kg (IV) q8h or 90 mg/kg (IV) q12h x 2-3 weeks	Initiate systemic CMV therapy pending ophthalmology consult Cidofovir 5 mg/kg (IV) once weekly x 2, then every 2 weeks. Give probenecid 2 gm (PO) 3 hours before and 1 gm (PO) 2 and 8 hours after cidofovir to preserve renal function
Maintenance therapy	Intraocular ganciclovir release device (Vitrasert) **plus either** Valganciclovir 900 mg (PO) q24h indefinitely[†] **or** Ganciclovir 1 gm (PO) q8h indefinitely[†]	No Vitrasert Valganciclovir 900 mg (PO) q24h indefinitely[†] **or** Ganciclovir 5 mg/kg (IV) q24h indefinitely[†] **or** Foscarnet 90 mg/kg (IV) q24h indefinitely[†]
Candida vaginitis *Initial infection*	Intravaginal miconazole suppository 200 mg q24h x 3 days or miconazole cream (2%) x 7 days **or** Fluconazole 150 mg (PO) x 1 dose (higher dose/longer course sometimes required)	Clotrimazole cream (1%) x 7 days or clotrimazole tablets 100 mg (PO) q24h x 7 days (or 100 mg q12h x 3 days, or 500 mg x 1 dose)
Frequent relapses	Fluconazole 100 mg (PO) q24h or 200 mg (PO) once weekly indefinitely.* Higher dose sometimes required	Not applicable

*   Consider discontinuation of therapy if CD₄ > 200 for ≥ 6 months in response to antiretroviral therapy

†   Consider discontinuation of therapy if CD₄ > 100-150 for ≥ 6 months in response to antiretroviral therapy,
     in consultation with ophthalmologist

Pneumocystis carinii Pneumonia (PCP)

Clinical Presentation: Fever, cough, dyspnea; often indolent presentation. Physical exam is usually normal. Chest x-ray is variable, but commonly shows a diffuse interstitial pattern. Elevated LDH and exercise desaturation are highly suggestive of PCP

Diagnostic Considerations: Diagnosis by immunofluorescent stain of induced sputum or bronchoscopy specimen. Check ABG if O₂ saturation is abnormal or respiratory rate is increased

Pitfalls: Slight worsening of symptoms is common after starting therapy, especially if not treated with steroids. Do not overlook superimposed bacterial pneumonia or other secondary infections while on pentamidine. Patients receiving second-line agents for PCP prophylaxis—in particular aerosolized pentamidine—may present with atypical radiographic findings, including apical infiltrates, multiple small-walled cysts, pleural effusions, pneumothorax, or single/multiple nodules

Therapeutic Considerations: Outpatient therapy is possible for mild disease, but only when close follow-up is assured. Adverse reactions to TMP-SMX (rash, fever, GI symptoms, hepatitis, hyperkalemia, leukopenia, hemolytic anemia) occur in 25-50% of patients, many of whom will need a second-line regimen to complete therapy (e.g., trimethoprim-dapsone or atovaquone). Unless an adverse reaction to TMP-SMX is particularly severe (e.g., Stevens-Johnson syndrome or other life-threatening problem), TMP-SMX may be considered for PCP prophylaxis, since prophylaxis requires a much lower dose (only 10-15% of treatment dose). Patients being treated for severe PCP who do not improve after one week may be switched to pentamidine, although there are no prospective data to confirm this approach. In general, patients receiving antiretroviral therapy when PCP develops should have their treatment continued, since intermittent antiretroviral therapy can lead to drug resistance. For newly-diagnosed or antiretroviral-naive HIV patients, treatment of PCP may be completed before starting antiretroviral therapy. Steroids should be tapered (p. 216), not discontinued abruptly. Adjunctive steroids increase the risk of thrush/herpes simplex infection, but probably not CMV, TB, or disseminated fungal infection
Prognosis: Usually responds to treatment. Adverse prognostic factors include ↑ A-a gradient, hypoxemia, ↑ LDH

Bacterial Pneumonia (see p. 47)

Pulmonary Tuberculosis (TB) (Mycobacterium tuberculosis)
Clinical Presentation: May present atypically. HIV patients with high (> 500) CD_4 cell counts are more likely to have a typical pulmonary presentation, but patients with advanced HIV disease may have a diffuse interstitial pattern, hilar adenopathy, or a normal chest x-ray. Tuberculin skin testing (TST) is reliable if positive, but unreliable if negative
Diagnostic Considerations: In many urban areas, TB is one of the most common HIV-related respiratory illnesses. In other areas, HIV-related TB occurs infrequently except in immigrants or patients arriving from highly TB endemic areas. Maintain a high Index of suspicion for TB in HIV patients with unexplained fevers/pulmonary infiltrates
Pitfalls: Extrapulmonary and pulmonary TB often coexist, especially in advanced HIV disease
Therapeutic Considerations: Duration of therapy should be extended if therapeutic response at end of 8-week induction is delayed (failure of sputum culture to convert to negative, lack of clinical response)
Prognosis: Usually responds to treatment. Relapse rates are related to the degree of immunosuppression and local risk of re-exposure to TB

Invasive Pulmonary Aspergillosis
Clinical Presentation: Pleuritic chest pain, hemoptysis, cough in a patient with advanced HIV disease
Diagnostic Considerations: Diagnosis by bronchoscopy with biopsy/culture. Open lung biopsy is sometimes required. Radiographic appearance includes cavitation, nodules, sometimes focal consolidation. Dissemination to CNS may occur, and manifests as focal neurological deficits
Pitfalls: Positive sputum culture for Aspergillus in advanced HIV disease should heighten awareness of possible infection
Therapeutic Considerations: Decrease/discontinue corticosteroids, if possible. Consider granulocyte-colony stimulating factor (G-CSF) if neutropenic
Prognosis: Poor unless immune deficits can be corrected

Toxoplasma Encephalitis (Toxoplasma gondii)
Clinical Presentation: Wide spectrum of neurologic symptoms, including sensorimotor deficits, seizures, confusion, ataxia. Fever/headache are common
Diagnostic Considerations: Diagnosis by characteristic radiographic appearance and response to empiric therapy in a Toxoplasma seropositive patient
Pitfalls: Use folinic acid 10 mg (PO) daily with pyrimethamine-containing regimens, not folate. Radiographic improvement may lag behind clinical response

Therapeutic Considerations: Alternate agents include atovaquone, azithromycin, clarithromycin, minocycline (all with pyrimethamine if possible). Decadron 4 mg (PO or IV) q6h is useful for edema/mass effect

Prognosis: Usually responds to treatment if able to tolerate drugs. Clinical response is evident by 1 week in 70%, by 2 weeks in 90%. Radiographic improvement is usually apparent by 2 weeks. Neurologic recovery is variable

Cryptococcal Meningitis (Cryptococcus neoformans)

Clinical Presentation: Often indolent onset of fever, headache, subtle cognitive deficits. Occasional meningeal signs and focal neurologic findings, though non-specific presentation is most common

Diagnostic Considerations: Diagnosis by CSF cryptococcal antigen; India ink stain is less sensitive. Diagnosis is essentially excluded with a negative serum cryptococcal antigen (sensitivity of test in AIDS patients approaches 100%). If serum cryptococcal antigen is positive, CSF antigen may be negative in disseminated disease without spread to CNS/meninges. Brain imaging is often normal, but CSF analysis is usually abnormal with a markedly elevated opening pressure

Pitfalls: Be sure to obtain a CSF opening pressure, since reduction of increased intracranial pressure is mandatory for successful treatment. Remove sufficient CSF during the initial lumbar puncture (LP) to reduce closing pressure to < 200 mm H_2O or 50% of opening pressure. Increased intracranial pressure requires repeat daily LPs (until CSF pressure stabilizes), placement of a lumbar drain, or ventriculo-peritoneal shunting. Adjunctive corticosteroids are not recommended

Therapeutic Considerations: Optimal total dose/duration of amphotericin B prior to fluconazole switch is unknown (2-3 weeks is reasonable if patient is doing well). Treatment with 5-FC is optional; however, since 5-FC is associated with more rapid sterilization of CSF, it is reasonable to start 5 FC and then discontinue it for toxicity (neutropenia, nausea). Fluconazole is preferred over itraconazole for life-long maintenance therapy

Prognosis: Variable. Mortality up to 40%. Adverse prognostic factors include increased intracranial pressure, abnormal mental status

CMV Encephalitis/Polyradiculitis

Clinical Presentation: Encephalitis presents as fever, mental status changes, and headache evolving over 1-2 weeks. True meningismus is rare. CMV encephalitis occurs in advanced HIV disease (CD_4 < 50/mm^3), often in patients with prior CMV retinitis. Polyradiculitis presents as rapidly evolving weakness/sensory disturbances in the lower extremities, often with bladder/bowel incontinence. Anesthesia in "saddle distribution" with reduced sphincter tone may be present

Diagnostic Considerations: CSF may show lymphocytic or neutrophilic pleocytosis; glucose is often decreased. For CMV encephalitis, characteristic findings on brain MRI include confluent periventricular abnormalities with variable degrees of enhancement. Diagnosis is confirmed by CSF CMV PCR (preferred), CMV culture, or brain biopsy

Pitfalls: For CMV encephalitis, a wide spectrum of radiographic findings are possible, including mass lesions (rare). Obtain ophthalmologic evaluation to exclude active retinitis. For polyradiculitis, obtain sagittal MRI of the spinal cord to exclude mass lesions, and CSF cytology to exclude lymphomatous involvement (can cause similar symptoms)

Therapeutic Considerations: Ganciclovir plus foscarnet may be beneficial as initial therapy for severe cases. Consider discontinuation of valganciclovir maintenance therapy if CD_4 increases to > 100-150/mm^3 x 6 months or longer in response to antiretroviral therapy

Prognosis: Unless immune reconstitution occurs, response to therapy is usually transient, followed by progression of symptoms

Progressive Multifocal Leukoencephalopathy (PML)

Clinical Presentation: Hemiparesis, ataxia, aphasia, other focal neurologic defects, which may progress over weeks to months. Usually alert without headache or seizures on presentation

Diagnostic Considerations: Demyelinating disease caused by reactivation of latent papovavirus (JC strain most common). Diagnosis by clinical presentation and MRI showing patchy demyelination of white matter ± cerebellum/brainstem. JC virus PCR of CSF is useful for non-invasive diagnosis. Biopsy may be needed to distinguish PML from other opportunistic infections or CNS lymphoma. Affects ~ 5% of AIDS patients

Pitfalls: Primary HIV-related encephalopathy has a similar appearance on MRI

Therapeutic Considerations: Most effective therapy is antiretroviral therapy with immune reconstitution. May attempt cidofovir (experience is limited)

Prognosis: Rapid progression to death over weeks to months is common. Best chance for survival is immune reconstitution in response to antiretroviral therapy

Oral Thrush (Candida)

Clinical Presentation: Dysphagia/odynophagia. More common/severe in advanced HIV disease

Diagnostic Considerations: Pseudomembranous (most common), erythematous, and hyperplastic (leukoplakia) forms. Pseudomembranes (white plaques on inflamed base) on buccal muscosa/tongue/gingiva/palate scrape off easily, hyperplastic lesions do not. Diagnosis by clinical appearance ± KOH/gram stain of scraping showing yeast/pseudomycelia. Other oral lesions in AIDS patients include herpes simplex, aphthous ulcers, Kaposi's sarcoma, oral hairy leukoplakia

Pitfalls: Patients may be asymptomatic

Therapeutic Considerations: Fluconazole is superior to topical therapy in preventing relapses of thrush and treating Candida esophagitis. Continuous treatment with fluconazole may lead to fluconazole-resistance, which is best treated initially with itraconazole suspension and, if no response, with IV amphotericin. Chronic suppressive therapy is usually only considered for severely immunosuppressed patients

Prognosis: Improvement in symptoms are often seen within 24-48 hours

Candida Esophagitis

Clinical Presentation: Dysphagia/odynophagia, almost always in the setting of oropharyngeal thrush. Fever is uncommon

Diagnostic Considerations: Most common cause of esophagitis in HIV disease. For persistent symptoms despite therapy, endoscopy with biopsy/culture is recommended to confirm diagnosis and assess azole-resistance. Other causes of esophagitis include CMV, herpes simplex, aphthous ulcers

Pitfalls: May extend into stomach and perforate. Kaposi's sarcoma, non-Hodgkin's lymphoma, zidovudine, dideoxycytidine, and other infections may cause esophageal symptoms

Therapeutic Considerations: Systemic therapy is preferred over topical therapy. Failure to improve on empiric therapy mandates endoscopy to look for other causes, especially herpesviruses/aphthous ulcers. Consider maintenance therapy with fluconazole for frequent relapses, although the risk of fluconazole resistance is increased

Prognosis: Relapse rate related to degree of immunosuppression

CMV Esophagitis/Colitis

Clinical Presentation: Localizing symptoms, including odynophagia, abdominal pain, diarrhea, sometimes bloody stools

Diagnostic Considerations: Diagnosis by finding CMV inclusions on biopsy. CMV can affect the entire GI tract, resulting in oral/esophageal ulcers, gastritis, and colitis (most common). CMV colitis varies greatly in severity, but typically causes fever, abdominal cramping, and sometimes bloody stools

Pitfalls: CMV colitis may cause colonic perforation and should be considered in any AIDS patient presenting with an acute abdomen, especially if radiography demonstrates free intraperitoneal air

Therapeutic Considerations: Consider chronic suppressive therapy for recurrent disease. Screen for CMV retinitis

Prognosis: Relapse rate is greatly reduced with immune reconstitution due to antiretroviral therapy

Salmonella Enteritis (see p. 63)

Cryptosporidia Enteritis
Clinical Presentation: High-volume watery diarrhea with weight loss and electrolyte disturbances, especially in advanced HIV disease
Diagnostic Considerations: Spore-forming protozoa. Diagnosis by AFB smear of stool demonstrating characteristic oocyte. Malabsorption may occur
Pitfalls: No fecal leukocytes
Therapeutic Considerations: Anecdotal reports of antimicrobial success. Immune reconstitution in response to antiretroviral therapy is the most effective therapy, and may induce prolonged remissions. Anti-diarrheal agents (Lomotil, Pepto-Bismol) are useful to control symptoms. Hyperalimentation may be required for severe cases
Prognosis: Related to degree of immunosuppression/response to antiretroviral therapy

Microsporidia Enteritis
Clinical Presentation: Intermittent chronic diarrhea without fever/fecal leukocytes
Diagnostic Considerations: Spore-forming protozoa (S. intestinalis, E. bieneusi). Diagnosis by modified trichrome or fluorescent antibody stain of stool. Microsporidia can rarely disseminate to sinuses/cornea. Severe malabsorption may occur
Pitfalls: Cannot be detected by routine microscopic examination of stool due to small size
Therapeutic Considerations: Albendazole is less effective for E. bieneusi than S. intestinalis, but speciation is usually not possible
Prognosis: Related to degree of immunosuppression/response to antiretroviral therapy

Isospora Enteritis
Clinical Presentation: Severe chronic diarrhea without fever/fecal leukocytes
Diagnostic Considerations: Spore-forming protozoa (Isospora belli). Oocyst on AFB smear of stool larger that Cryptosporidium (20-30 microns vs. 4-6 microns). More common in HIV patients from the Tropics (e.g., Haiti). Less common than Cryptosporidium or Microsporidia. Malabsorption may occur
Pitfalls: Multiple relapses are possible
Therapeutic Considerations: Chronic suppressive therapy may be required
Prognosis: Related to degree of immunosuppression/response to antiretroviral therapy

Antibiotic-Associated Diarrhea/Colitis (Clostridium difficile) (see p. 64)

Disseminated Mycobacterium avium-intracellulare (MAI)
Clinical Presentation: Typically presents as a febrile wasting illness in advanced HIV disease ($CD_4 <$ 50/mm^3). Focal invasive disease is possible, especially in patients with advanced immunosuppression after starting antiretroviral therapy. Focal disease likely reflects restoration of pathogen-specific immune response to subclinical infection ("immune reconstitution" syndrome), and typically manifests as lymphadenitis (mesenteric, cervical, thoracic) or rarely disease in the spine mimicking Pott's disease. Immune reconstitution syndrome usually occurs within weeks to months after starting antiretroviral therapy for the first time, but may occur a year or more later
Diagnostic Considerations: Diagnosis by isolation of organism from a normally sterile body site (blood, lymph node, bone marrow, liver biopsy). Lysis centrifugation (DuPont isolators) is the preferred blood culture method. Anemia/↑ alkaline phosphatase are occasionally seen
Pitfalls: Isolator blood cultures may be negative, especially in immune reconstitution syndrome
Therapeutic Considerations: Some studies suggest benefit for addition of rifabutin 300 mg (PO) q24h, others do not. Rifabutin is contraindicated in patients receiving delavirdine or hard-gel saquinavir. For concurrent use with nelfinavir, indinavir, or amprenavir, decrease rifabutin to 150 mg (PO) q24h. For concurrent use with ritonavir, decrease rifabutin to 150 mg (PO) 2-3x/week. For concurrent use

with efavirenz, increase rifabutin to 450-600 mg (PO) q24h. The dose of PIs or NNRTIs may need to be increased by 20-25%. Monitor carefully for rifabutin drug toxicity (arthralgias, uveitis, leukopenia). Treat immune reconstitution syndrome the same as for disseminated MAI; corticosteroids may be necessary to control fevers. Optimal long-term management is unknown
Prognosis: Depends on immune reconstitution in response to antiretroviral therapy. Adverse prognostic factors include high-grade bacteremia or severe wasting

Extrapulmonary Tuberculosis
Clinical Presentation: Multiple presentations possible (e.g., lymphadenitis, osteomyelitis, meningitis, hepatitis). Dissemination is more common in patients with low CD_4 counts (< $100/mm^3$)
Diagnostic Considerations: Diagnosis by isolator blood cultures or tissue biopsy
Pitfalls: Patients with disseminated disease frequently have pulmonary disease, which has implications for infection control
Therapeutic Considerations: Response to therapy may be slower than in normal hosts
Prognosis: Usually responsive to therapy

Non-meningeal Cryptococcus (see index for site-specific disease)

Disseminated Histoplasmosis
Clinical Presentation: Two general forms: Mild disease with fever/lymph node enlargement (e.g., cervical adenitis), or severe disease with fever, wasting ± diarrhea/meningitis/GI ulcerations
Diagnostic Considerations: Diagnosis by urine/serum histoplasmosis antigen, sometimes by culture of bone marrow/liver or isolator blood cultures. May occur in patients months to years after having lived/moved from an endemic area
Pitfalls: Relapse is common after discontinuation of therapy
Therapeutic Considerations: Initial therapy depends on severity of illness on presentation. Extremely sick patients should be started on amphotericin B. Mildly ill patients can be started on itraconazole. All patients require chronic suppressive therapy, with possible discontinuation for immune reconstitution with CD_4 counts > $100/mm^3$ for at least 6 months
Prognosis: Usually responds to treatment, except in fulminant cases

Herpes Simplex (genital/oral)
Clinical Presentation: Painful, grouped vesicles on an erythematous base that rupture, crust, and heal within 2 weeks. Lesions may be chronic, severe, ulcerative with advanced immunosuppression
Diagnostic Considerations: Diagnosis by Herpes culture of swab from lesion base/roof of blister
Pitfalls: Acyclovir prophylaxis is not required in patients receiving ganciclovir or foscarnet
Therapeutic Considerations: In refractory cases, consider acyclovir resistance and treat with foscarnet. Topical trifluridine ophthalmic solution (Viroptic 1%) may be considered for direct application to small, localized areas of refractory disease; clean with hydrogen peroxide, then debride lightly with gauze, apply trifluridine, and cover with bacitracin/polymyxin ointment and nonadsorbent gauze
Prognosis: Responds well to treatment except in severely immunocompromised patients, in whom acyclovir resistance may develop

Herpes Zoster (Varicella-Zoster Virus, VZV)
Clinical Presentation: Primary varicella (chickenpox) presents as clear vesicles on an erythematous base that heal with crusting and sometimes scarring. Zoster usually presents as painful tense vesicles on an erythematous base in a dermatomal distribution. In AIDS, primary varicella is more severe/prolonged, and zoster is more likely to involve multiple dermatomes/disseminate
Diagnostic Considerations: Diagnosis is clinical. Immunofluorescence can be used to distinguish herpes zoster from herpes simplex
Pitfalls: Extend duration of therapy for slowly responsive lesions
Therapeutic Considerations: IV therapy is generally indicated for severe disease/cranial nerve zoster

Prognosis: Usually responds slowly to treatment

CMV Retinitis
Clinical Presentation: Blurred vision, scotomata, field cuts common. Often bilateral, even when initial symptoms are unilateral
Diagnostic Considerations: Diagnosis by characteristic hemorrhagic ("tomato soup and milk") retinitis on funduscopic exam. Consult ophthalmology in suspected cases
Pitfalls: May develop immune reconstitution vitreitis
Therapeutic Considerations: Oral ganciclovir should not be used as sole initial therapy. Maintenance therapy with oral ganciclovir is nearly as effective as IV ganciclovir, but should be avoided with lesions near the optic nerve or fovea; consult an ophthalmologist. Life-long maintenance therapy for CMV retinitis is required for CD_4 counts < 100, but may be discontinued if CD_4 counts increase to > 100-150 for 6 or more months in response to antiretroviral therapy (in consultation with ophthalmologist)
Prognosis: Good initial response to therapy. High relapse rate

Candida Vaginitis
Clinical Presentation: White, cheesy, vaginal discharge or vulvar rash ± itching/pain
Diagnostic Considerations: Local infection. Not a manifestation of disseminated disease
Pitfalls: Women with advanced AIDS receiving fluconazole may develop fluconazole-resistant Candida
Therapeutic Considerations: For recurrence, consider maintenance treatment with daily or weekly fluconazole
Prognosis: Good response to therapy. Relapses common

FEVER OF UNKNOWN ORIGIN (FUO)

A. Differential Diagnosis. Fever without localizing symptoms or signs is common in HIV disease. Infectious causes of fever in patients with CD_4 cell counts > 500/mm^3 are similar to immunocompetent hosts. With CD_4 cell counts of 200-500/mm^3, the most common causes of fever include respiratory bacterial infections (especially S pneumoniae, H. influenzae), TB, and complications of IV drug use. Patients with advanced HIV disease can have any cause of fever listed in Table 9, including typical opportunistic infections and non-infectious causes, such as neoplasm (especially non-Hodgkin's lymphoma) or drug fever. Common causes of drug fever include sulfonamides, dapsone, beta-lactams, phenytoin, carbamazepine, thalidomide, and pentamidine. NNRTIs such as nevirapine, delavirdine, and efavirenz can also cause fevers ± rash. Abacavir hypersensitivity reactions occur in ~ 3%, and are usually associated with fever and multisystem complaints (GI disturbances, rash, respiratory symptoms), rechallenge is contraindicated (can be fatal).

B. Key Historical Features. Level of immunosuppression; travel/residence history; medication history (new agents, prophylaxis); need for central venous access; intravenous drug use; prior opportunistic infections.

C. Diagnostic Approach. Begin with non-invasive tests and become more invasive if fevers persist, weight loss is evident, or the illness appears to be progressing. Physical examination/labs should focus on possible clues suggesting a diagnosis, including skin rashes (disseminated fungal infections; Cryptococcus may cause a molluscum-like rash), oral ulcerations (histoplasmosis, CMV), new or regional lymphadenopathy (lymphoma, immune reconstitution MAI), retinal lesions (CMV), hepatosplenomegaly (histoplasmosis, MAI, disseminated Pneumocystis carinii), new cytopenias (bone marrow infiltrative process), ↑ LDH (lymphoma, Pneumocystis carinii), ↑ alkaline phosphatase (liver infiltrative process), hilar adenopathy on chest x-ray (histoplasmosis, TB, lymphoma). Abdominal CT scan often shows mesenteric adenopathy in MAI disease, and chest CT may show faint infiltrates of early PCP not evident on plain films. Routine blood cultures are useful for detecting endocarditis, Salmonella bacteremia, or line infections, and isolator blood cultures are useful for detecting disseminated MAI, other mycobacterium, or histoplasmosis. Serum cryptococcal antigen, urine histoplasmosis antigen, and CMV antigenemia studies may be appropriate if further testing is needed. Yields from liver/bone marrow biopsy range from 20-80%. In general, ↑ alkaline phosphatase increases the likelihood of a diagnostic liver biopsy.

Table 9. Causes of Pulmonary, CNS, Diarrheal Disease and FUO in HIV Disease

	Very Common	Somewhat Common	Rare
Respiratory disease	PCP S. pneumoniae H. influenzae M. tuberculosis[†]	Enteric gram (−) rods H. capsulatum C. neoformans CMV Aspergillus sp. Pulmonary lymphoma Heart failure Kaposi's sarcoma	N. asteroides Legionella spp. MAI T. gondii Cryptosporidia R. equii Primary pulmonary hypertension
CNS disease	C. neoformans T. gondii* Drug reactions Psychiatric illness HIV PML* CNS lymphoma*	M. tuberculosis[†] CMV Bacterial brain abscess*	N. asteroides* H. capsulatum C. immitis Aspergillus sp.* L. monocytogenes VZV, HSV* T. pallidum Acanthamoeba sp.* T. cruzi
Diarrheal disease	CMV C. difficile Salmonella MAI Giardia Protease inhibitors	Shigella Campylobacter Microsporidia Cryptosporidia Isospora Cyclospora	Amebiasis S. stercoralis GI lymphoma Kaposi's sarcoma Enteroaggretative E. coli
FUO	MAI M. tuberculosis[†] CMV Drug fever Sinusitis Central line infection Early PCP, HIV	C. neoformans H. capsulatum Endocarditis Lymphoma	Extrapulmonary PCP B. henselae C. immitis M. kansasii P. marneffei Leishmania sp. T. gondii

† Incidence highly dependent on local rates of TB
* Generally characterized by focal lesions on MRI/CT

POST-EXPOSURE PROPHYLAXIS (PEP)

The CDC estimates > 600,000 significant exposures to blood-borne pathogens occur yearly. Of 56 confirmed cases of HIV acquisition in healthcare workers, more than 90% involved percutaneous exposure, with the remaining cases due to mucous membrane/skin exposure. Estimates of HIV seroconversion rates after percutaneous and mucous membrane exposure to HIV-infected blood are 0.3% and 0.09%, respectively; lower rates of transmission occur after nonintact skin exposure. (By comparison, the risks of seroconversion after percutaneous exposure to Hepatitis B and Hepatitis C viruses are 30% and 3%, respectively.) Risk factors for increased risk of HIV transmission after percutaneous exposure include deep injury (OR 16.1), visible blood on device (OR 5.2), source patient is terminally ill (OR 6.4), or needle was in source patient's artery/vein (OR 5.1); AZT prophylaxis reduces the risk of transmission (OR 0.2). All guidelines suggest PEP should be administered as soon as possible after exposure, but there is no absolute window (e.g., within 1-2 weeks) after which PEP should be withheld following serious exposure. Because clear-cut efficacy data for patient selection and PEP regimens are lacking, most experts rely on CDC guidelines, which emphasize the type of exposure and potential infectivity of the source patient (Tables 10, 11). There are no formal guidelines for non-occupational PEP, but it is reasonable to consider PEP for serious exposures (e.g., rape victims, shared needle use). The latest U.S. Public Health Service (USPHS) guidelines for the management of occupational exposure to HIV and postexposure prophylaxis are summarized below, and are detailed in Morbidity Mortality Weekly Review 50(RR11):1-52, June 29, 2001, or at www.cdc.gov/mmwr/preview/mmwrhtml/rr5011a1.htm. Other occupational exposure resources include the National Clinicians' Postexposure Prophylaxis Hotline (www.ucsf.edu/hivcntr), Needlestick! (www.needlestick.mednet.ucla,edu), and HIV Antiretroviral Pregnancy Registry (www.glaxowellcome.com/preg[underscore]reg/antiretroviral). Occupationally acquired HIV infections and PEP failures can be reported to the CDC at (800) 893-0485.

Recommendations from the updated 2001 USPHS guidelines include:
- Initiate PEP as soon as possible after exposure (preferably within hours), and continue PEP for 4 weeks if tolerated (Tables 10, 11)
- Seek expert consultation if viral resistance is suspected
- Offer pregnancy testing to all women of childbearing age not known to be pregnant
- Advise exposed persons to seek medical evaluation for any acute illness during follow-up
- Perform HIV-antibody testing and HIV viral load testing for any illness compatible with an acute retroviral syndrome (e.g., pharyngitis, fever, rash, myalgia, fatigue, malaise, lymphadenopathy)
- Perform HIV-antibody testing for at least 6 months postexposure (at baseline, 6 weeks, 3 months, and 6 months)
- Advise exposed persons to use precautions to prevent secondary transmission during follow-up, especially during the first 6-12 weeks, when most HIV-infected patients will seroconvert. Precautions include sexual abstinence or use of condoms, refrain from

donating blood, plasma, organs, tissue or semen, and discontinuation of breast-feeding after high-risk exposures
• Evaluate exposed persons taking PEP within 72 hours after exposure, and monitor for drug toxicity for at least 2 weeks. Approximately 50% will experience nausea, malaise, headache, or anorexia, and about one-third will discontinue PEP due to drug toxicity. Lab monitoring should include (at a minimum) a CBC, serum creatinine, liver function tests, serum glucose (if receiving a protease inhibitor to detect hyperglycemia), and monitoring for crystalluria, hematuria, hemolytic anemia, and hepatitis (if indinavir is prescribed). Serious adverse events should be reported to the FDA's MedWatch Program

Table 10. Recommendations for HIV Postexposure Prophylaxis (see Table 11 for basic and expanded PEP regimens)

Exposure Type	Infection Status of Source Patient				
	HIV (+) Class 1*	HIV (+) Class 2*	HIV status unknown[†]	Unknown source[††]	HIV (–)
Percutaneous injuries *Less severe*[+]	Recommend basic 2-drug PEP	Recommend expanded 3-drug PEP	Generally no PEP warranted; consider basic 2-drug PEP[†††] for source with HIV risk factors**	Generally no PEP warranted; consider basic 2-drug PEP[†††] if exposure to HIV-infected persons is likely	No PEP warranted
More severe[+]	Recommend expanded 3-drug PEP	Recommend expanded 3-drug PEP			
Mucous membrane/nonintact skin exposure *Small volume*[++]	Consider basic 2-drug PEP	Recommend basic 2-drug PEP			
Large volume[++]	Recommend expanded 3-drug PEP	Recommend expanded 3-drug PEP			

HIV (+) = HIV-positive, HIV (–) = HIV-negative, PEP = postexposure prophylaxis
*   Class 1: Asymptomatic HIV infection or known low viral load (e.g., < 1500 RNA copies/mL)
     Class 2: Symptomatic HIV infection, AIDS, acute seroconversion, or known high viral load. If drug resistance is a concern, obtain expert consultation; do not delay PEP pending consultation
**   Source with HIV risk factors: If PEP is administered and the source patient is later determined to be HIV-negative, PEP should be discontinued
†   HIV status unknown: for example, source patient is deceased with no samples available for HIV testing
††   Unknown source: for example, a needle from a sharps disposal container (percutaneous injury), or a splash from inappropriately disposed blood (mucous membrane/nonintact skin exposure)
††† PEP is optional; discuss with patient and individualize decision
+   Less severe: for example, a solid needle and superficial injury. More severe: for example, a large-bore hollow needle, deep puncture, visible blood on device, or needle used in patient's artery/vein
++   Small volume: a few drops. Large volume: major blood splash
From: Updated U.S. Public Health Service Guidelines for the Management of Occupational Exposures to HBV, HCV, and HIV and Recommendations for Postexposure Prophylaxis, MMWR, 50 (RR11) June 29, 2001 (www.cdc.gov/mmwr/preview/mmwrhtml/rr5011a1.htm)

**Table 11. Basic and Expanded HIV Postexposure Prophylaxis Regimens
(see Table 10 for patient selection guidelines)**

Regimen	Dosage	Comments
Basic regimen *Preferred*	Combivir (zidovudine 300 mg + lamivudine 150 mg) 1 tablet (PO) q12h x 4 weeks	Most experience; serious toxicity rare; side effects common but usually manageable with antimotility/antiemetic agents; probably safe during pregnancy; source patient virus may be resistant
Alternate	Lamivudine 150 mg (PO) q12h + stavudine 40 mg (PO) q12h* x 4 weeks	Well-tolerated; good adherence; serious toxicity rare; source patient virus may be resistant
	Didanosine 400 mg (PO) q24h** on empty stomach + stavudine 40 mg (PO) q12h* x 4 weeks	Likely to be effective against HIV strains from source patients taking zidovudine and lamivudine; serious toxicity may occur (e.g., neuropathy, pancreatitis, hepatitis); careful monitoring required; side effects common (anticipate diarrhea and low adherence)
Expanded regimen *(basic regimen plus one of the following drugs)*	Indinavir 800 mg (PO) q8h on empty stomach x 4 weeks	Potent HIV inhibitor; serious toxicity may occur (e.g., nephrolithiasis); 8 glasses of fluid required per day; hyperbilirubinemia is common; avoid during late pregnancy; cannot be co-administered with didanosine in chewable/dispersible buffered tablet formulation (doses must be separated by at least 1 hour); many drug interactions possible
	Nelfinavir 750 mg (PO) q8h or 1250 mg (PO) q12h with food x 4 weeks	Potent HIV inhibitor; may accelerate clearance of certain drugs, including oral contraceptives; many drug interactions possible
	Efavirenz 600 mg (PO) q24h at bedtime x 4 weeks	Once daily dosing may improve adherence; may cause severe rash with rare progression to Stevens-Johnson syndrome; CNS side effects common (e.g., dizziness, somnolence, insomnia, abnormal dreaming); severe psychiatric symptoms possible; avoid during pregnancy; many drug interactions possible
	Abacavir 300 mg (PO) q12h x 4 weeks	Potent HIV inhibitor; well-tolerated; severe hypersensitivity reactions may occur; available as combination tablet (Trizivir = abacavir 300 mg + lamivudine 150 mg + zidovudine 300 mg)
For PEP only with expert consultation	Ritonavir, saquinavir, amprenavir, delavirdine, lopinavir + ritonavir	Poor tolerability; drug toxicity common; many drug interactions

*   If < 60 kg, give 30 mg (PO) q12h
** If < 60 kg, give 125 mg (PO) q12h
Adapted from: U.S. Public Health Service Guidelines. MMWR 50(RR11):47-52, June 29, 2001,
www.cdc..gov/mmwr/preview/mmwrhtml/rr5011a4.htm

References and Readings: See pp. 344-346

Chapter 6

Antibiotic Prophylaxis and Immunizations*

Burke A. Cunha, M.D.

* For prophylaxis of opportunistic infections in HIV/AIDS, see Chapter 5, pp. 212-215

ANTIBIOTIC PROPHYLAXIS

Antibiotic prophylaxis is designed to prevent infection for a defined period of time. Prophylaxis is most likely to be effective when given for a short duration against a single pathogen with a known sensitivity pattern, and least likely to be effective when given for a long duration against multiple organisms with varying/unpredictable sensitivity patterns (Table 1). It is a common misconception that antibiotics used for prophylaxis should not be used for therapy and vice versa. The only difference between prophylaxis and therapy is the inoculum size and the duration of antibiotic administration: In prophylaxis, there is no infection, so the inoculum is minimal/none and antibiotics are administered only for the duration of exposure/surgical procedure. With therapy, the inoculum is large (infection already exists), and antibiotics are continued until the infection is eradicated.

Table 1. Factors Affecting the Efficacy of Surgical Antibiotic Prophylaxis

Number of Organisms	Susceptibility Pattern	Duration of Protection	Efficacy of Prophylaxis
Single organism	Predictable	Short	Excellent
Multiple organisms	Predictable	Short	Excellent
Single organism	Unpredictable	Short	Good
Single organism	Predictable	Long	Good
Multiple organisms	Unpredictable	Long	Poor/none

SURGICAL PROPHYLAXIS

Antibiotic prophylaxis is designed to achieve maximum antibiotic serum/tissue concentrations at the time of initial surgical incision, and is maintained throughout the "vulnerable period" of the procedure (i.e., time between skin incision and skin closure) to protect against transient bacteremias (Table 2). If prophylaxis is given too early, antibiotic levels will be suboptimal/nonexistent when protection is needed. Appropriate pre-operative prophylaxis is mandatory, since antibiotics given after skin closure are unlikely to be effective. When no infection exists prior to surgery (clean/clean contaminated surgery), single-dose prophylaxis is preferred. When infection is present/likely prior to surgery ("dirty" surgery, e.g., perforated colon, TURP in the presence of positive urine cultures, repair of open fracture), antibiotics are given for > 1 day and represent early therapy, not true prophylaxis. Parenteral cephalosporins are commonly used for surgical prophylaxis, and ordinarily given as a bolus injection/rapid IV infusion 15-30 minutes prior to the procedure. Prophylaxis with vancomycin or gentamicin is given by slow IV infusion over 1 hour, starting ~ 1 hour prior to the procedure.

Table 2. Surgical Prophylaxis

Procedure	Usual Organisms	Preferred Prophylaxis	Alternate Prophylaxis	Comments
CNS shunt (VP/VA) placement, craniotomy, open CNS trauma	S. epidermidis S. aureus	<u>MRSA/MRSE unlikely</u> Cefotaxime 2 gm (IV) x 1 dose **or** Ceftizoxime 2 gm (IV) x 1 dose <u>MRSA/MRSE likely</u> Linezolid 600 mg (IV) x 1 dose	<u>MRSA/MRSE unlikely</u> Minocycline 200 mg (IV) x 1 dose <u>MRSA/MRSE likely</u> Linezolid 600 mg (PO) x 1 dose **or** Vancomycin 1 gm (IV) x 1 dose	Administer immediately prior to procedure. Vancomycin protects against wound infections, but may not prevent CNS infections. Give vancomycin slowly IV over 1 hour prior to procedure
Thoracic (non-cardiac) surgery	S. aureus (MSSA)	Cefazolin 1 gm (IV) x 1 dose	Cefotaxime 2 gm (IV) x 1 dose **or** Ceftizoxime 2 gm (IV) x 1 dose	Administer immediately prior to procedure
Cardiac valve replacement surgery	S. epidermidis (MSSE/MRSE) S. aureus (MSSA/MRSA) Enterobacter	Vancomycin 1 gm (IV) x 1 dose **plus** Gentamicin 240 mg (IV) x 1 dose	Linezolid 600 mg (IV) x 1 dose **plus** Gentamicin 240 mg (IV) x 1 dose	Administer vancomycin and gentamicin slowly IV over 1 hour prior to procedure
Coronary artery bypass graft (CABG) surgery	S. aureus (MSSA)	Cefazolin 2 gm (IV) x 1 dose	Cefotaxime 2 gm (IV) x 1 dose **or** Ceftizoxime 2 gm (IV) x 1 dose	Administer immediately prior to procedure. Repeat dose intraoperatively for procedures lasting > 3 hours
Biliary tract surgery	E. coli Klebsiella Enterococci	Ampicillin 1 gm (IV) x 1 dose **plus** Cefazolin 1 gm (IV) x 1 dose	Levofloxacin 500 mg (IV) x 1 dose	Administer immediately prior to procedure (anaerobic coverage unnecessary)
Hepatic surgery	E. coli Klebsiella Enterococci B. fragilis	Ampicillin/sulbactam 3 gm (IV) x 1 dose **or** Piperacillin/tazobactam 4.5 gm (IV) x 1 dose	Meropenem 1 gm (IV) x 1 dose **or** Moxifloxacin 400 mg (IV) x 1 dose	Administer immediately prior to procedure

Table 2. Surgical Prophylaxis (cont'd)

Procedure	Usual Organisms	Preferred Prophylaxis	Alternate Prophylaxis	Comments
Stomach, upper small bowel surgery	S. aureus Group A streptococci	Cefazolin 1 gm (IV) x 1 dose	Cefotaxime 2 gm (IV) x 1 dose **or** Ceftizoxime 2 gm (IV) x 1 dose	Administer immediately prior to procedure (anaerobic coverage unnecessary)
Distal small bowel, colon surgery	E. coli Klebsiella B. fragilis Enterococci	Ampicillin/ sulbactam 3 gm (IV) x 1 dose **or** Piperacillin/ tazobactam 4.5 gm (IV) x 1 dose **or** Meropenem 1 gm (IV) x 1 dose	Metronidazole 1 gm (IV) x 1 dose **plus either** Levofloxacin 500 mg (IV) x 1 dose **or** Gentamicin 240 mg (IV) x 1 dose	Administer immediately prior to procedure. Give gentamicin slowly IV over 1 hour
Pelvic (OB/GYN) surgery	Aerobic gram-negative bacilli Anaerobic streptococci B. fragilis	Ceftizoxime 2 gm (IV) x 1 dose	Cefotetan 2 gm (IV) x 1 dose **or** Cefoxitin 2 gm (IV) x 1 dose	Administer immediately prior to procedure
Orthopedic prosthetic implant surgery (total hip/knee replacement)	S. epidermidis S. aureus	<u>MRSA/MRSE unlikely</u> Cefazolin 2 gm (IV) x 1 dose <u>MRSA/MRSE likely</u> Vancomycin 1 gm (IV) x 1 dose	<u>MRSA/MRSE unlikely</u> Cefotaxime 2 gm (IV) x 1 dose **or** Ceftizoxime 2 gm (IV) x 1 dose <u>MRSA/MRSE likely</u> Linezolid 600 mg (IV) x 1 dose	Administer immediately prior to procedure. Post-operative doses are ineffective and unnecessary
Arthroscopy	S. aureus Enteric gram-negative bacilli	Cefazolin 1 gm (IV) x 1 dose	Cefotaxime 2 gm (IV) x 1 dose **or** Ceftizoxime 2 gm (IV) x 1 dose	Pre-procedure prophylaxis is usually unnecessary in clean surgical procedures
Orthopedic surgery (open fracture)	S. aureus Aerobic gram negative bacilli	Cefotaxime 2 gm (IV) q6h x 3-7 days **or** Ceftizoxime 2 gm (IV) q8h x 3-7 days	Clindamycin 600 mg (IV) q8h x 3-7 days **plus** Gentamicin 240 mg (IV) q24h x 3-7 days	Represents early therapy, not true prophylaxis. Duration of post-op antibiotics depends on severity of infection

Table 2. Surgical Prophylaxis (cont'd)

Procedure	Usual Organisms	Preferred Prophylaxis	Alternate Prophylaxis	Comments
Urological implant surgery	S. aureus Enteric gram negative bacilli	Ceftizoxime 2 gm (IV) x 1 dose	Cefotaxime 2 gm (IV) x 1 dose	Administer immediately prior to procedure
TURP, cystoscopy	P. aeruginosa P. cepacia P. maltophilia E. faecalis Enteric gram negative bacilli	Piperacillin 4 gm (IV) x 1 dose	Ciprofloxacin 400 mg (IV) x 1 dose	Prophylaxis given to TURP patients with positive pre-op urine cultures. Represents early therapy, not true prophylaxis. No prophylaxis required for TURP if pre-op urine culture is negative
	E. faecium (VRE)	Linezolid 600 mg (IV) x 1 dose	Quinupristin/ dalfopristin 7.5 mg/kg (IV) x 1 dose	

MSSA/MRSA = methicillin-sensitive/resistant S. aureus; MSSE/MRSE = methicillin-sensitive/resistant S. epidermidis.

POST-EXPOSURE MEDICAL PROPHYLAXIS (Table 3)

Some infectious diseases can be prevented by post-exposure prophylaxis (PEP). To be maximally effective, PEP should be administered within 24 hours of the exposure, since the effectiveness of prophylaxis > 24 hours after exposure decreases rapidly in most cases. PEP is usually reserved for persons with close face-to-face/intimate contact with an infected individual. Casual contact usually does not warrant PEP.

Table 3. Post-Exposure Medical Prophylaxis

Exposure	Usual Organisms	Preferred Prophylaxis	Alternate Prophylaxis	Comments
Meningitis	N. meningitidis	Levofloxacin 500 mg (PO) x 1 dose **or** Ciprofloxacin 500 mg (PO) x 1 dose	Minocycline 100 mg (PO) q12h x 2 days **or** Rifampin 600 mg (PO) q12h x 2 days	Must be administered within 24 hours of close face-to-face exposure to be effective. Otherwise, observe and treat if infection develops
	H. influenzae	Rifampin 600 mg (PO) q24h x 3 days	Levofloxacin 500 mg (PO) q24h x 3 days	Must be administered within 24 hours of close face-to-face exposure to be effective. H. influenzae requires 3 days of prophylaxis

Table 3. Post-Exposure Medical Prophylaxis (cont'd)

Exposure	Usual Organisms	Preferred Prophylaxis	Alternate Prophylaxis	Comments
Viral influenza	Influenza virus (type A)	Rimantadine 200 mg (PO) q24h x 4-6 weeks	Amantadine 100 mg (PO) q12h x 4-6 weeks	Give to non-immunized contacts. Begin at onset and continue for duration of outbreak
Pertussis	B. pertussis	Erythromycin 500 mg (PO) q6h x 2 weeks	TMP-SMX 1 SS tablet (PO) q12h x 2 weeks **or** Levofloxacin 500 mg (PO) q24h x 2 weeks	Administer as soon as possible after exposure. Effectiveness is greatly reduced after 24 hours
Diphtheria	C. diphtheriae	Erythromycin 500 mg (PO) q6h x 1 week **or** Benzathine penicillin 1.2 mu (IM) x 1 dose	Azithromycin 500 mg (PO) q24h x 3 days	Administer as soon as possible after exposure. Effectiveness is greatly reduced after 24 hours
TB	M. tuberculosis	INH 300 mg (PO) q24h x 6-12 months	Rifampin 600 mg (PO) q24h x 6-12 months	For INH, monitor SGOT/SGPT weekly x 4, then monthly x 3. Mild elevations are common and resolve spontaneously. INH should be stopped for SGOT/SGPT levels ≥ 5 x normal
Gonorrhea	N. gonorrhoeae	Ceftriaxone 125 mg (IM) x 1 dose	Spectinomycin 2 gm (IM) x 1 dose **or** Any oral quinolone x 1 dose	Administer as soon as possible after sexual exposure (≤ 72 hours). Ceftriaxone also treats incubating syphilis
Syphilis	T. pallidum	Benzathine penicillin 2.4 mu (IM) x 1 dose	Doxycycline 100 mg (PO) q12h x 1 week	Administer as soon as possible after sexual exposure. Obtain HIV serology
Chancroid	H. ducreyi	Ceftriaxone 250 mg (IM) x 1 dose	Azithromycin 1 gm (PO) x 1 dose **or** Any oral quinolone x 3 days	Administer as soon as possible after sexual exposure. Obtain HIV and syphilis serologies

Table 3. Post-Exposure Medical Prophylaxis (cont'd)

Exposure	Usual Organisms	Preferred Prophylaxis	Alternate Prophylaxis	Comments
Non-gonococcal urethritis (NGU)	C. trachomatis U. urealyticum M. genitalium	Azithromycin 1 gm (PO) x 1 dose **or** Doxycycline 100 mg (PO) q12h x 1 week	Any oral quinolone x 1 week	Administer as soon as possible after sexual exposure. Also test for gonorrhea/Ureaplasma
Varicella (chicken-pox)	VZV	Varicella vaccine 0.5 mL (SC) x 1 dose. Repeat in 4 weeks	Varicella-zoster immune globulin (VZIG) 625 mcg (IM) x 1 dose	Administer as soon as possible after exposure (< 72 hours). Varicella vaccine is a live attenuated vaccine and should not be given to immunocompromised patients
Hepatitis B (HBV)	Hepatitis B virus	<u>Unvaccinated</u> Hepatitis B immune globulin (HBIG) 0.06 mL/kg (IM) x 1 dose **plus** HBV vaccine (40 mcg HBsAg/mL) deep deltoid (IM) at 0, 1, 6 months (can use 10-mcg dose in healthy adults < 40 years)	<u>Previously vaccinated</u> *Known responder* (anti-HBsAg antibody levels ≥ 10 IU/mL): No treatment *Known non-responder* (anti-HBsAg antibody levels < 10 IU/mL): Treat as if unvaccinated *Antibody status unknown*: Obtain HBsAg antibody levels to determine immunity status. If testing is not possible or results are not available within 24 hours of exposure, give HBIG plus 1 dose of HBV vaccine (booster)	
Hepatitis A (HAV)	Hepatitis A virus	HAV vaccine 1 mL (IM) x 1 dose	Immune serum globulin (IG) 0.02 mL/kg (IM) x 1 dose	HAV vaccine is effective post-exposure. Give at onset/once notified of outbreak
Rocky Mountain spotted fever	R. rickettsia	Doxycycline 100 mg (PO) q12h x 1 week	Any oral quinolone x 1 week	Administer prophylaxis after removal of Dermacentor tick
Lyme disease	B. burgdorferi	Doxycycline 200 mg (PO) x 1 dose **or** Amoxicillin* 1 gm (PO) q8h x 3 days	Any oral 1st gen. cephalosporin* x 3 days **or** Azithromycin* 500 mg (PO) q24h x 3 days	If tick is in place ≥ 72 hours or is grossly engorged, prophylaxis may be given after tick is removed. Otherwise, prophylaxis is usually not recommended
		* Although experience is limited, single-dose prophylaxis with these agents is probably also effective		

Table 3. Post-Exposure Medical Prophylaxis (cont'd)

Exposure	Usual Organisms	Preferred Prophylaxis	Alternate Prophylaxis	Comments
Zoonotic diseases (plague, anthrax)	B. anthracis Y. pestis	Doxycycline 100 mg (PO) q12h for duration of exposure	Any oral quinolone for duration of exposure	Provides protection against most bacterial systemic infections by zoonotic pathogens if continued for the duration of exposure/outbreak
Rabies	Rabies virus	<u>No Previous Immunization</u> HRIG 20 IU/kg* **plus either** PCEC 1 mL (IM) in deltoid **or** RVA 1 mL (IM) in deltoid **or** HDCV 1 mL (IM) in deltoid PCEC, RVA, HDCV given on days 0, 3, 7, 14, and 28 post-exposure	<u>Previous Immunization</u> PCEC 1 mL (IM) in deltoid on days 0 and 3 **or** RVA 1 mL (IM) in deltoid on days 0 and 3 **or** HDCV 1 mL (IM) in deltoid on days 0 and 3	Following unprovoked or suspicious dog or cat bite, immediately begin prophylaxis if animal develops rabies during a 10-day observation period. If dog or cat is suspected of being rabid, begin vaccination sequence immediately. Raccoon, skunk, bat, fox and most wild carnivore bites should be regarded as rabid, and bite victims should be vaccinated against rabies immediately (contact local health department regarding rabies potential of animals in your area). All potential rabies wounds should immediately be thoroughly cleaned with soap and water. Do not inject rabies vaccine IV (may cause hypotension/shock). Serum sickness may occur with HDCV

HDCV = human diploid cell vaccine, HRIG = human rabies immune globulin, PCEC = purified chick embryo cells, RVA = rabies vaccine absorbed

* All or as much of the full dose should be injected into the tissues surrounding the bite wound, and the remaining vaccine should be injected IM into the deltoid. Do not give HRIG at the same site or through the same syringe with PCEC, RVA, or HDCV

CHRONIC MEDICAL PROPHYLAXIS/SUPPRESSION (Table 4)

Some infectious diseases are prone to recurrence/relapse and may benefit from intermittent or chronic suppressive therapy. The goal of suppressive therapy is to minimize the frequency/severity of recurrent infectious episodes.

Table 4. Chronic Medical Prophylaxis/Suppression

Disorder	Usual Organisms	Preferred Prophylaxis	Alternate Prophylaxis	Comments
Asplenia	S. pneumonia H. influenzae N. meningitidis	Levofloxacin 500 mg (PO) q24h indefinitely	Amoxicillin 1 gm (PO) q24h indefinitely	Chemoprophylaxis is uniformly effective, but needs to be given long-term. Pneumococcal, H. influenzae, and meningococcal vaccines should be given if possible, but are not always protective
UTIs (recurrent)	Gram-negative bacilli Enterococci	Nitrofurantoin 100 mg (PO) q24h x 6 months	Amoxicillin 500 mg (PO) q24h x 6 months **or** TMP-SMX 1 SS tablet (PO) q24h x 6 months	Prophylaxis is indicated for frequent (≥ 3 per year) UTIs caused by reinfection; usually taken at bedtime. Recurrent UTIs of the "relapse" variety (same organism/serotype for each UTI) should be investigated for stones, abscesses, or structural abnormalities
Asymptomatic bacteriuria in pregnancy	Gram-negative bacilli	Nitrofurantoin 100 mg (PO) q24h x 1 week	Amoxicillin 1 gm (PO) q24h x 1 week	Treat to prevent symptomatic infections
Recurrent genital herpes *(treatment of episodic recurrences)*	H. simplex (HSV-2)	Acyclovir 400 mg (PO) q8h x 5 days	Famciclovir 125 mg (PO) q12h x 5 days **or** Valacyclovir 1 gm (PO) q12h x 5 days	Begin therapy as soon as lesions appear

Table 4. Chronic Medical Prophylaxis/Suppression (cont'd)

Disorder	Usual Organisms	Preferred Prophylaxis	Alternate Prophylaxis	Comments
Recurrent genital herpes *(chronic suppressive therapy)*	H. simplex (HSV-1)	Acyclovir 400 mg (PO) q12h x 1 year	Famciclovir 250 mg (PO) q12h x 1 year **or** Valacyclovir 500 mg (PO) q12h x 1 year	Suppressive therapy is indicated for frequent recurrences (≥ 3/year)
Acute exacerbation of chronic bronchitis (AECB)	S. pneumoniae H. influenzae M. catarrhalis	Levofloxacin 500 mg (PO) q24h x 1-2 weeks **or** Gatifloxacin 400 mg (PO) q24h x 1-2 weeks	Doxycycline 100 mg (PO) q12h x 1-2 weeks **or** Cefprozil 500 mg (PO) q12h x 1-2 weeks	Two commonly used approaches: Treat each episode x 1-2 weeks, or treat x 3 months during the winter
Acute rheumatic fever (ARF)	Group A streptococci	Benzathine penicillin 1.2 mu (IM) monthly until age 30	Amoxicillin 500 mg (PO) q24h until age 30 **or** Azithromycin 500 mg (PO) q72h until age 30	Group A streptococcal pharyngitis and acute rheumatic fever are uncommon after age 30
Neonatal Group B streptococcal (GBS) infection (primary prevention)	Group B streptococci	Ampicillin 2 gm (IV) q4h at onset of labor until delivery	Clindamycin 600 mg (IV) q8h at onset of labor until delivery **or** Vancomycin 1 gm (IV) q12h at onset of labor until delivery	Indicated for previous infant with GBS infection, maternal GBS colonization/infection during pregnancy, or vaginal/rectal culture of GBS after week 35 of gestation. Also indicated for delivery ≤ week 37 of gestation without labor/ruptured membranes, for ruptured membranes ≥ 12 hours, or for intrapartum temperature ≥ 100.4°F
Febrile neutropenia (PMNs ≤ 1000/mm^3)	P. aeruginosa Aerobic gram-negative bacilli	See p. 115		

ENDOCARDITIS PROPHYLAXIS (Tables 5-7)

Endocarditis prophylaxis is designed to prevent native/prosthetic cardiac valve infections by preventing procedure-related bacteremias due to cardiac pathogens. For procedures above-the-waist, usual pathogens are viridans streptococci from the mouth. For procedures below-the-waist, usual pathogens are enterococci. Since procedure-related bacteremias are usually asymptomatic and last less than 15 minutes, single-dose oral regimens prior to the procedure provide effective prophylaxis. Parenteral SBE prophylaxis is preferred for patients with previous endocarditis, shunts, or prosthetic heart valves. Regimens vary among the experts, and no regimen is fully protective. Since erythromycin-based regimens have had the highest failure rate in the past, macrolides have not been included in the recommendations.

Table 5. Indications for Infective Endocarditis (IE) Prophylaxis*

Subset	Prophylaxis Recommended (Column A)	Prophylaxis Not Recommended (Column B)
Cardiac conditions	• Ostium primum ASD • Prosthetic heart valves, including bioprosthetic and homograft valves • Previous infective endocarditis • Most congenital cardiac malformations • Rheumatic valve disease • Hypertrophic cardiomyopathy • MVP with valvular regurgitation	• Isolated ostium secundum ASD • Surgical repair without residue beyond 6 months of ostium secundum ASD or PDA • Previous coronary artery bypass surgery • MVP without valvular regurgitation • Physiologic, functional, or innocent murmurs • Previous Kawasaki's cardiac disease or rheumatic fever without valve disease
Procedures	• Dental procedures known to induce gingival/mucosal bleeding, including dental cleaning • Tonsillectomy or adenoidectomy • Surgical operations involving intestinal or respiratory mucosa • Rigid bronchoscopy • Sclerotherapy for esophageal varices • Esophageal dilation • Gallbladder surgery • Cystoscopy or urethral dilation • Urethral catheterization or urinary tract surgery if UTI is present • Prostate surgery • I & D of infected tissue • Vaginal hysterectomy • Vaginal delivery, D & C, IUD insertion/removal, or therapeutic abortion in the presence of infection	• Dental procedures not likely to induce gingival bleeding • Tympanostomy tube insertion • Flexible bronchoscopy ± biopsy • Endotracheal intubation • Endoscopy ± gastrointestinal biopsy • Cesarean section • D & C, IUD insertion/removal, or therapeutic abortion in the absence of infection • Cardiac pacemaker/defibrillator insertion • Coronary stent implantation • Percutaneous transluminal coronary angioplasty (PTCA) • Cardiac catheterization

ASD = atrial septal defect, D & C = dilatation and curettage, I & D = incision and drain, IUD = intrauterine device, MVP = mitral valve prolapse, PDA = patent ductus arteriosus, UTI = urinary tract infection

* Prophylaxis is indicated for patients with cardiac conditions in Column A undergoing procedures in Column A. Prophylaxis is not recommended for patients or procedures in Column B. See Tables 6 and 7 for prophylaxis regimens for above-the-waist and below-the-waist procedures, respectively

Table 6.   Endocarditis Prophylaxis for Above-the-Waist (Dental, Oral, Esophageal, Respiratory Tract) Procedures*

Prophylaxis**	Reaction to Penicillin	Antibiotic Regimen
Oral prophylaxis	None	Amoxicillin 2 gm (PO) 1 hour pre-procedure[†]
	Non-anaphylactoid	Cephalexin 1 gm (PO) 1 hour pre-procedure
	Anaphylactoid	Clindamycin 300 mg (PO) 1 hour pre-procedure[††]
IV prophylaxis	None	Ampicillin 2 gm (IV) 30 minutes pre-procedure
	Non-anaphylactoid	Cefazolin 1 gm (IV) 15 minutes pre-procedure
	Anaphylactoid	Clindamycin 600 mg (IV) 30 minutes pre-procedure

*   Endocarditis prophylaxis is directed against Streptococcus viridans, the usual SBE pathogen above the waist. Macrolide regimens are less effective than other regimens; clarithromycin/azithromycin regimens (500 mg PO 1 hour pre-procedure) are of unproven efficacy
** Oral prophylaxis is preferred to IV prophylaxis, except in patients with previous endocarditis, shunts, or prosthetic heart valves
†   Some recommend a 3 gm dose of amoxicillin, which is excessive given the sensitivity of viridans streptococci to amoxicillin
††   Some recommend a 600 mg dose of clindamycin, but a 300 mg dose gives adequate blood levels and is better tolerated (less diarrhea)

Table 7.   Endocarditis Prophylaxis for Below-the-Waist (Genitourinary, Gastrointestinal) Procedures*

Prophylaxis**	Reaction to Penicillin	Antibiotic Regimen
Oral prophylaxis	None	Amoxicillin 2 gm (PO) 1 hour pre-procedure
	Non-anaphylactoid, anaphylactoid	Linezolid 600 mg (PO) 1 hour pre-procedure
IV prophylaxis	None	Ampicillin 2 gm (IV) 30 minutes pre-procedure **plus** Gentamicin 80 mg (IM) or (IV) over 1 hour 60 minutes pre-procedure
	Non-anaphylactoid, anaphylactoid	Vancomycin 1 gm (IV) over 1 hour 60 minutes pre-procedure **plus** Gentamicin 80 mg (IM) or (IV) over 1 hour 60 minutes pre-procedure

*   Endocarditis prophylaxis is directed against Enterococcus faecalis, the usual SBE pathogen below the waist
** Oral prophylaxis is preferred to IV prophylaxis, except in patients with previous endocarditis, shunts, or prosthetic heart valves

TRAVEL PROPHYLAXIS (Tables 8, 9)

Travelers may acquire infectious diseases from ingestion of fecally-contaminated water/food, exchange of infected body secretions, inhalation of aerosolized droplets, direct inoculation via insect bites, or from close contact with infected birds/animals. Recommendations to prevent infection in travelers consist of general travel precautions (Table 8), and specific travel prophylaxis regimens (Table 9).

Table 8. General Infectious Disease Travel Precautions

Exposure	Risk	Precautions
Unsafe water (fecally-contaminated)	Diarrhea/dysentery, viral hepatitis (HAV)	• Avoid ingestion of unbottled/unpotable water. Be sure bottled water has an unbroken seal and has not been opened/refilled with tap water • Avoid ice cubes made from water of uncertain of origin/handling, and drinking from unclean glasses • Drink only pasteurized bottled drinks. Be sure bottles/cans are opened by you or in your presence • Avoid drinking unpasteurized/warm milk; beer, wine, and pure alcoholic beverages are safe • Eat only canned fruit or fresh fruit peeled by you or in your presence with clean utensils • Avoid eating soft cheeses • Avoid eating raw tomatoes/uncooked vegetables that may have been exposed to contaminated water • Avoid using hotel water for tooth brushing/rinsing unless certain of purity. Many hotels use common lines for bath/sink water that is unsuitable for drinking • Avoid wading/swimming/bathing in lakes or rivers
Food-borne (fecally-contaminated)	Diarrhea/dysentery	• Eat only seafood/poultry/meats that are freshly cooked and served hot. Avoid eating at roadside stands or small local restaurants with questionable sanitary practices • "Boil it, peel it, or forget it"
Body fluid secretions	Viral hepatitis (HBV, HCV, etc.), STDs, HIV/other retroviruses	• Do not share utensils/glasses/straws or engage in "risky behaviors" involving body secretion exchange • Avoid blood transfusion (use blood expanders instead) • Treat dental problems before travel
Animal bite	Animal bite-associated infections	• Do not pet/play with stray dogs/cats. Rabies and other infections are common in wild animals
Flying insects	Malaria, arthropod-borne infections	• Avoid flying/biting insects by wearing dark protective clothing (long sleeves/pants) and using insect repellent on clothes/exposed skin, especially during evening hours • Minimize dawn-to-dusk outdoor exposure • Use screens/mosquito nets when possible • Do not use perfume, after shave, or scented deodorants/toiletries that will attract flying insects

Table 9. Travel Prophylaxis Regimens

Exposure	Usual Pathogens	Prophylaxis Regimens	Comments
Traveler's diarrhea	E. coli Salmonella Shigella Non-cholera vibrios V. cholerae Aeromonas Plesiomonas Rotavirus Norwalk virus Giardia lamblia Campylobacter Yersinia Cryptosporidium Cyclospora Enteroviruses Amebiasis	Doxycycline 100 mg (PO) q24h for duration of exposure **or** Any quinolone (PO) for duration of exposure **or** TMP-SMX 1 SS tablet (PO) q24h for duration of exposure	Observe without prophylaxis and treat mild diarrhea symptomatically with loperimide (2 mg). Persons with medical conditions adversely affected by diarrhea may begin prophylaxis after arrival in country and continue for 1 day after returning home. Should severe diarrhea/dysentery occur, continue/switch to a quinolone, maximize oral hydration, and see a physician if possible. Anti-spasmodics may be used for symptomatic relief of mild, watery diarrhea, but should be avoided in severe diarrhea/dysentery (may make infection worse). Bismuth subsalicylate is less effective than antibiotic prophylaxis. Traveler's diarrhea usually presents as acute watery diarrhea with low-grade fever after ingestion of fecally-contaminated water. Most cases are due to enterotoxigenic E. coli. TMP-SMX is active against most bacterial pathogens and Cyclospora, but not against E. histolytica or enteroviral pathogens (e.g., Rotavirus, Norwalk agent). Doxycycline is active against most bacterial pathogens and E. histolytica, but misses Campylobacter, Cryptosporidium, Cyclospora, Giardia, and enteroviral pathogens. Levofloxacin and ciprofloxacin are active against most pathogens except Giardia, Cryptosporidium, Cyclospora, E. histolytica, and enteroviral pathogens. All antibiotics are inactive against viral/parasitic pathogens causing diarrhea
Meningococcal meningitis	N. meningitidis	<u>Pre-travel prophylaxis</u> Meningococcal vaccine 0.5 mL (SC) ≥ 1 month prior to travel to outbreak area <u>Post-exposure prophylaxis</u> See p. 236	Acquired via close face-to-face contact (airborne aerosol/droplet exposure). Vaccine is highly protective against N. meningitidis serotypes A, C, Y, and W-135, but misses B serotype

Table 9. Travel Prophylaxis Regimens (cont'd)

Exposure	Usual Pathogens	Prophylaxis Regimens	Comments
Hepatitis A (HAV)	Hepatitis A virus	HAV vaccine 1 mL (IM) ≥ 2 weeks prior to travel, then follow with a one-time booster ≥ 6 months later	HAV vaccine is better than immune globulin for prophylaxis. Take care to avoid direct/indirect ingestion of fecally-contaminated water. HAV vaccine is recommended for travel to all developing countries. Protective antibody titers develop after 2 weeks
Typhoid fever	S. typhi	ViCPS vaccine 0.5 mL (IM). Booster every 2 yrs for repeat travelers **or** Oral Ty21a vaccine 1 capsule (PO) q48h x 4 doses. Booster every 5 years for repeat travelers	Do not co-administer with antibiotics. Contraindicated in compromised hosts and children ≤ 6 years old. Take oral capsules with cold water. Degree of protective immunity is limited with vaccine. Some prefer chemoprophylaxis for Traveler's diarrhea (p. 245)
Yellow fever	Yellow fever virus	Yellow fever vaccine 0.5 mL (SC). Booster every 10 years for repeat travelers	Vaccine is often required for travel to or from Tropical South America or Tropical Central Africa. Administer 1 month apart from other live vaccines. Contraindicated in children < 4 months old; caution in children ≤ 1 year old. Reactions may occur in persons with egg allergies. Immunity is life-long, but booster every 10 years is needed for vaccination certification by some countries
Japanese encephalitis (JE)	Japanese encephalitis virus	JE vaccine 1 mL (SC) on days 0, 7, and 14 or 30. Booster schedule not established	Recommended for travelers planning prolonged (> 3 week) visits during the rainy season to rural, endemic areas of Asia (e.g., Eastern Russia, Indian subcontinent, China, Southeast Asia, Thailand, Korea, Laos, Cambodia, Vietnam, Malaysia, Philippines). Administer ≥ 2 weeks before exposure. Children < 3 years may be given 0.5 mL (SC) on same schedule as adults
Rabies	Rabies virus	HDCV, PCEC, or RVA 1 mL (IM) on days 0, 7, and 21 or 28. Booster: HDCV, PCEC, or RVA 1 mL (IM) **or** HDCV 1 mL (ID) on days 0, 7, and 21 or 28. Booster: HDCV 1 mL (ID)	Avoid contact with wild dogs/animals during travel. Dose of rabies vaccine for adults and children are the same. Booster given on days 0 and 3 after rabies exposure/bite

Table 9. Travel Prophylaxis Regimens (cont'd)

Exposure	Usual Pathogens	Prophylaxis Regimens	Comments
Malaria	P. vivax P. ovale P. malariae P. falciparum (chloroquine sensitive)	Chloroquine phosphate 500 mg (300 mg base) (PO) weekly **or** Mefloquine 250 mg (228 mg base) (PO) weekly **or** Malarone (atovaquone 250 mg + proguanil 100 mg) 1 tablet (PO) q24h	Acquired from female Anopheles mosquito bites. Avoid mosquito exposure using long-sleeved shirts/long pants at dawn/dusk when mosquitoes feed. Screens/mosquito nets are the best natural protection. DEET/pyrethrin sprays on clothing is helpful. Begin anti-malarial prophylaxis 1 week before travel to malarious areas (most of Africa, Latin America, Indian subcontinent, Southeast Asia), and continue for 4 weeks after returning home. Chemoprophylaxis reduces but does not eliminate the risk of malaria. Malarone prophylaxis may be given 1 day before travel, daily during malaria exposure, and for 1 week after returning home. Malarone is effective against sensitive/resistant P. falciparum strains, but not hepatic stages of P. vivax/P. ovale. Chloroquine-resistant P. falciparum is seen in sub-Saharan Africa, South America (except Chile, Argentina), Indian subcontinent, and Southern Asia (Burma, Thailand, Cambodia). Only areas without chloroquine-resistant P. falciparum are Middle East (except Saudi Arabia), Central America (west of Panama Canal), Haiti, and Dominican Republic. Fansidar resistance is common in chloroquine-resistant areas of Asia, Latin American, Africa. Mefloquine (but not doxycycline) resistance is seen in Thailand. Doxycycline is contraindicated in pregnancy, but chloroquine and proguanil are safe, and mefloquine is probably safe late in pregnancy. If pregnant, try to delay travel to malarial areas until after delivery
	P. falciparum (chloroquine resistant)	Doxycycline 100 mg (PO) q24h **or** Mefloquine 250 mg (228 mg base) (PO) weekly **or** Malarone (atovaquone 250 mg + proguanil 100 mg) 1 tablet (PO) q24h	

HDCV = human diploid cell vaccine, PCEC = purified chick embryo cell vaccine, RVA = rabies vaccine absorbed, RIG = rabies immune globulin

TETANUS PROPHYLAXIS (Table 10)

Current information suggests that immunity lasts for decades/life-time after tetanus immunization. A tetanus booster should not be routinely given for minor wounds, but is recommended for wounds with high tetanus potential (e.g., massive crush wounds, soil-contaminated wounds, or deep puncture wounds).

Table 10. Tetanus Prophylaxis in Routine Wound Management

History of Adsorbed Tetanus Toxoid	Wound Type	Recommendations
Unknown or < 3 doses	Clean, minor wounds	Td‡
	Tetanus-prone wounds†	Td‡ plus TIG
≥ 3 doses	Clean, minor wounds	No prophylaxis needed
	Tetanus-prone wounds†	Td‡ if > 10 years since last dose*

DT = diphtheria and tetanus toxoids adsorbed (pediatrics), DTP = diphtheria and tetanus toxoids and pertussis vaccine adsorbed, Td = tetanus and diphtheria toxoids adsorbed (adult), TIG = tetanus immune globulin
†   For example, massive crush wounds; wounds contaminated with dirt, soil, feces, or saliva; deep puncture wounds; or significant burn wounds or frostbite
‡   For children < 7 years, DTP (DT if pertussis is contraindicated) is preferred to tetanus toxoid alone. For children ≥ 7 years old and adults, Td is preferred to tetanus toxoid alone
*   More frequent booster doses are unnecessary and can increase side effects. Protection lasts > 20 yrs
Adapted from: Centers for Disease Control and Prevention. MMWR Rep 40 (RR-10):1-28. 1991

IMMUNIZATIONS (Table 11)

Immunizations are designed to reduce infections in large populations, and may prevent/decrease the severity of infection in non-immunized individuals. Compromised hosts with altered immune systems may not develop protective antibody titers to antigenic components of various vaccines. Immunizations are not fully protective, but are recommended (depending on the vaccine) for most normal hosts, since some protection is better than none. Post-exposure prophylaxis and travel prophylaxis are described on pp. 236-239 and 244-247, respectively.

Table 11. Adult Immunizations

Vaccine	Indications	Dosage	Comments
Bacille Calmette Guérin (BCG)	Possibly beneficial for adults at high-risk of multiple-drug resistant tuberculosis	Primary: 1 dose (intradermal). Booster not recommended	Live attenuated vaccine. PPD remains positive for years/life. Contraindicated in immuno-compromised hosts. Side effects include injection site infection or disseminated infection (rare)

Table 11. Adult Immunizations (cont'd)

Vaccine	Indications	Dosage	Comments
Hemophilus influenzae (type B)	Patients with splenic dysfunction	Primary: 0.5 mL dose (IM). Booster not recommended	Capsular polysaccharide conjugated to diphtheria toxoid. Safety in pregnancy unknown. Mild local reaction in 10%
Hepatitis A (HAV)	Adults at increased risk for HAV	Primary: 1 mL dose (IM). One-time booster ≥ 6 months later	Inactivated whole virus. Pregnancy risk not fully evaluated. Mild soreness at injection site. Occasional headache/malaise
Hepatitis B (HBV)	Household/sexual contact with carrier, IV drug use, multiple sex partners (heterosexual), homosexual male activity, blood product recipients, hemodialysis, occupational exposure to blood, residents/staff of institutions for developmentally disabled, prison inmates, residence ≥ 6 months in areas of high endemicity, others at high risk	Primary (3 dose series): Recombivax 10 mcg (1 mL) or Engerix-B 20 mcg (1 mL) IM in deltoid at 0, 1, and 6 months. Alternate schedule for Engerix-B: 4 dose series at 0, 1, 2, and 12 months. Booster not routinely recommended	Recombinant vaccine comprised of hepatitis B surface antigen. For compromised hosts (including dialysis patients), use specially packaged Recombivax 40-mcg doses (1 mL vial containing 40 mcg/mL). HBsAb titers should be obtained 6 months after 3-dose primary series. Those with non-protective titers (≤ 10 mIU/mL) should receive 1 dose monthly (with subsequent HbsAb testing) up to a maximum of 3 doses. Safety to fetus unknown; pregnancy not a contraindication in high-risk females. Mild local reaction in 10-20%. Occasional fever, headache, fatigue, nausea
Influenza	Healthy persons ≥ 50 years, healthcare personnel, adults with high-risk conditions (e.g., heart disease, lung disease, diabetes, renal dysfunction, hemoglobinopathies, immunosuppression)	Annual vaccine. Single 0.5 mL dose (IM) between October and November (before flu season) is optimal, but can be given anytime during flu season	Trivalent inactivated whole and split virus. Contraindications include anaphylaxis to eggs or sensitivity to thimerosal. Mild local reaction in up to 30%. Occasional malaise/myalgia beginning 6-12 hours after vaccination. Neurologic and allergic reactions are rare. For pregnancy, administer in 2nd or 3rd trimester during flu season
Lyme disease	Chronically, heavily exposed individuals	Primary: 0.5 mL (IM) in deltoid at 0, 1, and 12 months. Need for booster unknown	Bacterial capsular antigen. Efficacy ~ 80%, but short duration of antibody response and potential immune mimicry have limited use of vaccine

Table 11. Adult Immunizations (cont'd)

Vaccine	Indications	Dosage	Comments
Measles	Adults born after 1956 without live-virus immunization or measles diagnosed by a physician or immunologic test. Also indicated for revaccination of persons given killed measles vaccine between 1963-67	Primary: 0.5 mL dose (SC). A second dose (≥ 1 month later) is recommended for certain adults at increased risk of exposure (e.g., healthcare workers, travelers to developing countries)	Live virus vaccine (usually given in MMR). Contraindicated in compromised hosts, pregnancy, history of anaphylaxis to eggs or neomycin. Ineffective if given 3-11 months after blood products. Side effects include low-grade fever 5-21 days after vaccination (5-15%), transient rash (5%), and local reaction in 4-55% of persons previously immunized with killed vaccine (1963-67)
Mumps	Non-immune adults	Primary: 0.5 mL dose (SC)	Live attenuated vaccine (usually given in MMR). Contraindicated in pregnancy, immuno-compromised hosts, history of anaphylaxis to eggs or neomycin. Side effects include mild allergic reactions (uncommon), parotitis (rare)
Rubella	Non-immune adults, particularly women of childbearing age	Primary: 0.5 mL dose (SC)	Live virus (RA 27/3 strain) vaccine (usually given in MMR). Contraindicated in immuno-compromised hosts, pregnancy, history of anaphylactic reaction to neomycin. Joint pains and transient arthralgias in up to 40%, beginning 3-25 days after vaccination and lasting 1-11 days; frank arthritis in < 2%
Tetanus-diphtheria	Adults	Primary: Two 0.5 mL doses (IM), 1-2 months apart; third dose 6-12 months after second dose. No booster (unless develop a tetanus-prone wound, p. 248)	Adsorbed toxoid vaccine. Contraindicated if hypersensitivity/neurological reaction or severe local reaction to previous doses. Side effects include local reactions, occasional fever, systemic symptoms, Arthus-like reaction in persons with multiple previous boosters, and systemic allergy (rare)

Table 11. Adult Immunizations (cont'd)

Vaccine	Indications	Dosage	Comments
Varicella (VZV) chickenpox	Non-immune adolescents and adults, especially healthcare workers and others likely to be exposed	Primary: Two 0.5 mL doses (SC), 4-8 weeks apart. Vaccine must be stored frozen and used within 30 minutes after thawing and reconstitution. No booster	Live attenuated vaccine. Contraindications include pregnancy, active untreated TB, immunocompromised host, malignancy of bone marrow or lymphatic system, anaphylactic reaction to gelatin/neomycin, or blood product recipient within previous 6 months (may prevent development of protective antibody). Mild febrile illness in 10%. Injection site symptoms in 25-30% (local rash in 3%). Mild diffuse rash in 5%

Avery RK. Immunizations in Adult Immunocompromised Patients: Which to Use and Which to Avoid. Cleve Clin J Med 68:337-348,2001. Reid KC, Grizzard TA, Poland GA. Adult Immunizations: Recommendations for Practice. Mayo Clin Proc 74:377-384,1999.

Table 12. Immunizations in Pregnancy

Recommendations	Vaccines
Should be considered if otherwise indicated	Hepatitis B, influenza, tetanus/diphtheria, meningococcal, rabies
Contraindicated in pregnancy	Measles*, mumps*, rubella*, varicella*, BCG*, vaccinia*
Inadequate information for recommendation	Hepatitis A, pneumococcal, polio (oral polio virus*, injectable polio virus), cholera, Japanese encephalitis, plague, yellow fever*, typhoid (parenteral, Ty21a*)

* Live attenuated vaccine
From: CDC: ACIP Guidelines for Vaccinating Pregnant Women, October 1998.

Chapter 7
Antimicrobial Drug Summaries
Burke A. Cunha, M.D.

This section contains prescribing information pertinent to the clinical use of 130 antimicrobial agents, as compiled from a variety of sources (pp. 343-344). The information provided is not exhaustive, and the reader is referred to other drug information references and the manufacturer's product literature for further information. Clinical use of the information provided and any consequences that may arise from its use are the responsibilities of the prescribing physician. The authors, editors, and publisher do not warrant or guarantee the information contained in this section, and do not assume and expressly disclaim any liability for errors or omissions or any consequences that may occur from such. The use of any drug should be preceded by careful review of the package insert, which provides indications and dosing approved by the U.S. Food and Drug Administration.

Drugs are listed alphabetically by generic name; trade names follow in parentheses. To search by trade name, consult the index (pp. 347-360). Each drug summary contains the following information:

Usual dose. Represents the usual dose to treat most susceptible infections in adult patients with normal hepatic and renal function. Dosing for special situations is listed under the comments section, and may also be found in Chapters 2, 4, and 5. Loading doses for doxycycline, fluconazole, itraconazole, voriconazole, caspofungin, ganciclovir, and valganciclovir are described in either the usual dose or comments section. Meningeal doses of antimicrobials used for CNS infection are described at the end of the comments section.

Peak serum level. Refers to the peak serum concentration (mcg/ml) after the usual dose is administered. Peak serum level is useful in calculating the "kill ratios," the ratio of peak serum level to minimum inhibitory concentration (MIC) of the organism. The higher the "kill ratio," the more effective the antimicrobial is likely to be against a particular organism.

Bioavailability. Refers to the percentage of the dose reaching the systemic circulation from the site of administration (PO or IM). For PO antibiotics, bioavailability refers to the percentage of dose adsorbed from the GI tract. For IV antibiotics, "not applicable" appears next to bioavailability, since the entire dose reaches the systemic circulation. Antibiotics with high bioavailability (> 90%) are ideal for IV to PO switch therapy. Antibiotics with low bioavailability are effective if their "kill ratios" are favorable.

Excreted unchanged. Refers to the percentage of drug excreted unchanged, and provides an indirect measure of drug concentration in the urine/feces. Antibiotics excreted unchanged in the urine in low percentage are unlikely to be useful for urinary tract infections.

Serum half-life (normal/ESRD). The serum half-life ($T_{1/2}$) is the time (in hours) in which serum concentration falls by 50%. Serum half-life is useful in determining dosing interval. If the half-life of drugs eliminated by the kidneys is prolonged in end-stage renal disease (ESRD), then the total daily dose is reduced in proportion to the degree of renal dysfunction. If the half-life in ESRD is similar to the normal half-life, then the total daily dose does not change.

Plasma protein binding. Expressed as the percentage of drug reversibly bound to serum albumin. It is the unbound (free) portion of a drug that equilibrates with tissues and imparts antimicrobial activity. Plasma protein binding is not typically a factor in antimicrobial effectiveness unless binding exceeds 95%, and then only if the "kill ratio" is relatively low. Decreases in serum albumin (nephrotic syndrome, liver disease) or competition for protein binding from other drugs or endogenously produced substances (uremia, hyperbilirubinemia) will increase the percentage of free drug available for antimicrobial activity, and may require a decrease in dosage. Increases in serum binding proteins (trauma, surgery, critical illness) will decrease the percentage of free drug available for antimicrobial activity, and may require an increase in dosage.

Volume of distribution (V_d). Represents the apparent volume into which the drug is distributed, and is calculated as the amount of drug in the body divided by the serum concentration (in liters/kilogram). V_d is related to total body water distribution (V_d $H_2O = 0.7$ L/kg). Hydrophilic (water soluble) drugs are restricted to extracellular fluid and have a $V_d \leq 0.7$ L/kg. In contrast, hydrophobic (highly lipid soluble) drugs penetrate most fluids/tissues of the body and have a large V_d. Drugs that are concentrated in certain tissues (e.g., liver) can have a V_d greatly exceeding total body water. V_d is affected by organ profusion, membrane diffusion/permeability, lipid solubility, protein binding, and state of equilibrium between body compartments. For hydrophilic drugs, increases in V_d may occur with burns, heart failure, dialysis, sepsis, cirrhosis, or mechanical ventilation; decreases in V_d may occur with trauma, hemorrhage, pancreatitis (early), or GI fluid losses. Increases in V_d may require an increase in total daily drug dose for antimicrobial effectiveness; decreases in V_d may require a decrease in drug dose. In addition to drug distribution, V_d reflects binding avidity to cholesterol membranes and concentration within organ tissues (e.g., liver).

Mode of elimination. Refers to the primary route of inactivation/excretion of the antibiotic, which impacts dosing adjustments in renal/hepatic failure.

Dosage adjustments. Each grid provides dosing adjustments based on renal and hepatic function, and indicates the supplemental dose required immediately after hemodialysis (post–HD), peritoneal dialysis (post–PD), or continuous veno–venous hemofiltration (post–CVVH). Following the supplemental dose, antimicrobial dosing should resume as indicated for a CrCl < 10 mL/min. "No change" indicates no change from the usual dose. "Avoid" indicates the drug should be avoided in the setting described. "None" indicates no supplemental dose is required. "No information" indicates there are insufficient data from which to make a dosing recommendation. Dosing recommendations are based on data, experience, or pharmacokinetic parameters. Post–CVVH dosing recommendations represent general guidelines, since antibiotic removal is dependent on area/type of filter, ultrafiltration rates, and sieving coefficients; replacement dosing should be individualized and guided by serum levels, if possible. Creatinine clearance (CrCl) is used to gauge the degree of renal insufficiency, and can be estimated by the following calculation: CrCl (mL/min) = [(140 − age) x weight (kg)] / [72 x serum creatinine (mg/dL)]. The calculated value is multiplied by 0.85 for females. It is important to recognize that due to age-dependent decline in renal function, elderly patients with "normal" serum creatinines may have low CrCls requiring dosage adjustments. (For example, a 70-year-old, 50-kg female with a serum creatinine of 1.2 mg/dL has an estimated CrCl of 34 mL/min.) "Antiretroviral Dosage Adjustment" grids indicate recommended dosage adjustments when protease inhibitors (PIs) and non-nucleoside reverse transcriptase inhibitor (NNRTIs) are combined or used in conjunction with rifampin or rifabutin. These grids were compiled from "Guidelines for the Use of Antiretroviral Agents in HIV-Infected Adults and Adolescents," Panel on Clinical Practices for Treatment of HIV Infection, Department of Health and Human Services, April 23, 2001 (www.hivatis.org)

Drug interactions. Refers to common/important drug interactions, as compiled from various sources. If a specific drug interaction is well-documented (e.g, antibiotic X with lovastatin), than other drugs from the same drug class (e.g., atorvastatin) may also be listed, based on theoretical considerations. Drug interactions may occur as a consequence of altered absorption (e.g., metal ion chelation of tetracycline), altered distribution (e.g., sulfonamide displacement of barbiturates from serum albumin), altered metabolism (e.g., rifampin–induced hepatic P-450 metabolism of theophylline/warfarin; chloramphenicol inhibition of phenytoin metabolism), or altered excretion (e.g., probenecid competition with penicillin for active transport in the kidney).

Adverse side effects. Common/important side effects are indicated.

Resistance potential. Described as low, moderate, or high. "Low" resistance potential indicates the drug has not been associated with widespread resistance problems, even with extensive use. Episodic reports of clonal resistance outbreaks may occur, but not as a widespread phenomenon related to antibiotic use. "High" resistance potential indicates that resistance may occur even if the antibiotic is used on a limited basis. The usual organisms associated with moderate/high resistance potential antibiotics are indicated in parentheses.

Allergic potential. Described as low or high. Refers to the likelihood of a hypersensitivity reaction to a particular antimicrobial.

Safety in pregnancy. Designated by the U.S. Food and Drug Administration's (USFDA) use-in-pregnancy letter code (Table 1).

Table 1. USFDA Use-in-Pregnancy Letter Code

Category	Interpretation
A	**Controlled studies show no risk.** Adequate, well-controlled studies in pregnant women have not shown a risk to the fetus in any trimester of pregnancy
B	**No evidence of risk in humans.** Adequate, well-controlled studies in pregnant women have not shown increased risk of fetal abnormalities despite adverse findings in animals, or, in the absence of adequate human studies, animal studies show no fetal risk. The chance of fetal harm is remote, but remains a possibility
C	**Risk cannot be ruled out.** Adequate, well-controlled human studies are lacking, and animal studies have shown a risk to the fetus or are lacking. There is a chance of fetal harm if the drug is administered during pregnancy, but potential benefit from use of the drug may outweigh potential risk
D	**Positive evidence of risk.** Studies in humans or investigational or post-marketing data have demonstrated fetal risk. Nevertheless, potential benefit from use of the drug may outweigh potential risk. For example, the drug may be acceptable if needed in a life-threatening situation or serious disease for which safer drugs cannot be used or are ineffective
X	**Contraindicated in pregnancy.** Studies in animals or humans or investigational or post-marketing reports have demonstrated positive evidence of fetal abnormalities or risk which clearly outweigh any possible benefit to the patient

Comments. Includes various useful information for each antimicrobial agent.

Cerebrospinal fluid penetration. Indicated as a percentage relative to peak serum concentration. If an antimicrobial is used for CNS infections, then its meningeal dose is indicated directly above CSF penetration. No meningeal dose is given if CSF penetration is inadequate for treatment of meningitis due to susceptible organisms.

Biliary tract penetration. Indicated as a percentage relative to peak serum concentrations. Percentages > 100% reflect concentration within the biliary system. This information is useful for the treatment of biliary tract infections.

Selected references. These references are classic, important, or recent. General reference texts relating to antimicrobial therapy are listed on pp. 343-344.

Abacavir (Ziagen)

Drug Class: Antiretroviral NRTI (nucleoside reverse transcriptase inhibitor)
Usual Dose: 300 mg (PO) q12h
Pharmacokinetic Parameters:
Peak serum level: 3 mcg/mL
Bioavailability: 83%
Excreted unchanged: 1.2%
Serum half-life (normal/ESRD): 1.5 hrs/no data
Plasma protein binding: 30%
Volume of distribution (V_d): 0.86 L/kg
Primary Mode of Elimination: Hepatic
Dosage Adjustments:

CrCl ~ 40–60 mL/min	No change
CrCl ~ 10–40 mL/min	No change
CrCl < 10 mL/min	No change
Post–HD dose	None
Post–PD dose	None
Post–CVVH dose	None
Moderate hepatic insufficiency	No information
Severe hepatic insufficiency	No information

Drug Interactions: Amprenavir (↑ amprenavir levels); zidovudine (no interaction)
Adverse Effects: Drug fever/rash, abdominal pain/diarrhea, nausea, vomiting, anorexia, insomnia, weakness, headache, ↑ SGOT/SGPT, hyperglycemia, hypertriglyceridemia, lactic acidosis with hepatic steatosis (rare, but potentially life-threatening toxicity with use of NRTIs). Abacavir may cause severe hypersensitivity reactions during the first 4 weeks of therapy, which may be fatal. Avoid co-administration with other drugs with high hypersensitivity potential (e.g., TMP-SMX). Alcohol may ↑ abacavir serum levels ~ 40% and may ↑ toxicity
HIV Resistance Potential: Low (triple therapy); high (mono/double drug therapy)
Allergic Potential: High
Safety in Pregnancy: C

Comments: May be taken with or without foods. Discontinue abacavir and do not restart in patients with signs/symptoms of hypersensitiviy reaction (which may include fever, rash, fatigue, nausea, vomitiing, diarrhea, abdominal pain, anorexia, respiratory symptoms). Report cases of hypersensitivity syndrome to Abacavir Hypersensitivity Registry at 1-800-270-0425. Effective antiretroviral therapy consists of at least 3 antiretrovirals (same/different classes)
Cerebrospinal Fluid Penetration: 30%

REFERENCES:
Katalama C, Clotet B, Plettenberg A, et al. The role of abacavir (AVC, 1592) in antiretroviral therapy-experiences patients: results from randomized, double-blind, trial. CNA3002 European Study Team. AIDS 14:781-9, 2000.
Keating MR. Antiviral agents. Mayo Clin Proc 67:160-78, 1992.
McDowell JA, Lou Y, Symonds WS, et al. Multiple-dose pharmacokinetics and pharmacodynamics of abacavir alone and in combination with zidovudine in human immunodeficiency virus-infected adults. Antimicrob Agents Chemother 44:2061-7, 2000.
Panel on Clinical Practices for Treatment of HIV Infection. Guidelines for the Use of Antiretroviral Agents in HIV-Infected Adults and Adolescents. Department of Health and Human Services. April 23, 2001. www.hivatis.org

Abacavir + lamivudine + zidovudine (Trizivir)

Drug Class: Antiretroviral NRTI combination
Usual Dose: Trizivir tablet = abacavir 300 mg + lamivudine 150 mg + zidovudine 300 mg. Usual dose = 1 tablet (PO) q12h
Pharmacokinetic Parameters:
Peak serum level: 3/1.5/1.2 mcg/mL
Bioavailability: 83/82/65%
Excreted unchanged: 1.2/90/16%
Serum half-life (normal/ESRD): [1.5/6/1] / [no data/20/1.4] hrs
Plasma protein binding: 30/36/20%
Volume of distribution (V_d): 0.86/1.3/1.6 L/kg
Primary Mode of Elimination: Hepatic/renal

---

* Resume dosing for CrCl < 10 mL/min after supplemental dose. "Usual dose" assumes normal renal and hepatic function. CrCl = creatinine clearance; CVVH = continuous veno-venous hemofiltration; HD = hemodialysis; PD = peritoneal dialysis. See pp. 252-255 for definitions/explanations, p. 1 for abbreviations

Dosage Adjustments:

CrCl ~ 40–60 mL/min	1 tablet (PO) q24h
CrCl ~ 10–40 mL/min	Avoid
CrCl < 10 mL/min	Avoid
Post–HD dose	Avoid
Post–PD dose	Avoid
Post–CVVH dose	Avoid
Moderate hepatic insufficiency	No information
Severe hepatic insufficiency	No information

Drug Interactions: Acetaminophen (↑ Trizivir toxicity, neutropenia); acyclovir (↑ lethargy, fatigue); amprenavir, atovaquone (↑ zidovudine levels); clarithromycin (↓ zidovudine levels); cidofovir (↑ zidovudine levels, flu-like symptoms); dapsone, doxorubicin (neutropenia); TMP-SMX (↑ lamivudine and zidovudine levels)
Adverse Effects: Vomiting, diarrhea, anorexia, nausea, fatigue, insomnia, hyperglycemia, hypertriglyceridemia, peripheral neuropathy, anemia, leukopenia, myopathy, steatosis, pancreatitis. Abacavir may cause severe/fatal rash/hypersensitivity hepatitis; do not co-administer with other drugs with high allergic/hypersensitivity potential (eg, TMP-SMX)
HIV Resistance Potential: Low (triple therapy); high (mono/double drug therapy)
Allergic Potential: High
Safety in Pregnancy: C
Comments: Avoid in patients requiring dosage adjustments of NRTIs; avoid in patients ≤ 40 kg. May be taken with or without food. HBV hepatitis may relapse if lamivudine is discontinued

REFERENCES:
Havlir DV, Lange JM. New antiretrovirals and new combinations. AIDS 12(Suppl A):S165-74, 1998.
McDowell JA, Lou Y, Symonds WS, et al. Multiple-dose pharmacokinetics and pharmacodynamics of abacavir alone and in combination with zidovudine in human immunodeficiency virus-infected adults. Antimicrob Agents Chemother 44:2061-7, 2000.

Three new drugs for HIV infection. Med Lett Drugs Ther 40:114-6, 1998.
Weverling GJ, Lange JM, Jurriaans S, et al. Alternative multidrug regimen provides improved suppression of HIV-1 replication over triple therapy. AIDS 12:117-22, 1998.

Acyclovir (Zovirax)

Drug Class: Antiviral
Usual Dose: <u>HSV</u>: 5 mg/kg (IV) q8h until able to take PO, then 400 mg (PO) 5x/day.
<u>VZV</u>: 10 mg/kg (IV) q8h until able to take PO, then 800 mg (PO) 5x/day
Pharmacokinetic Parameters:
Peak serum level: 7.7 mcg/mL
Bioavailability: 30%
Excreted unchanged: 70%
Serum half-life (normal/ESRD): 3/20 hrs
Plasma protein binding: 30%
Volume of distribution (V_d): 0.7 L/kg
Primary Mode of Elimination: Renal
Dosage Adjustments:

CrCl ~ 40–60 mL/min	5 mg/kg (IV/PO) q12h
CrCl ~ 10–30 mL/min	5 mg/kg (IV/PO) q24h
CrCl < 10 mL/min	2.5 mg/kg (IV/PO) q24h
Post–HD dose*	5 mg/kg (IV/PO)
Post–PD dose*	2.5 mg/kg (IV/PO)
Post–CVVH dose*	5 mg/kg (IV/PO)
Moderate hepatic insufficiency	No change
Severe hepatic insufficiency	No change

Drug Interactions: Cimetidine, probenecid (↑ acyclovir levels); nephrotoxic drugs (↑ nephrotoxicity); zidovudine (lethargy)
Adverse Effects: Seizures/tremors (dose related), crystalluria. Base dose on ideal body weight in the elderly to minimize adverse effects
Resistance Potential: Low
Allergic Potential: Low
Safety in Pregnancy: C
Comments: Na^+ content = 4 mEq/g. CSF levels

---

* Resume dosing for CrCl < 10 mL/min after supplemental dose. "Usual dose" assumes normal renal and hepatic function. CrCl = creatinine clearance; CVVH = continuous veno-venous hemofiltration; HD = hemodialysis; PD = peritoneal dialysis. See pp. 252-255 for definitions/explanations, p. 1 for abbreviations

may be increased with probenecid.
Meningeal dose = VZV/HSV encephalitis dose
Cerebrospinal Fluid Penetration: 50%

REFERENCES:
Keating MR. Antiviral Agents. Mayo Clin Proc 67:160-78, 1992.
Geers TA, Isada CM. Update on antiviral therapy for genital herpes infection. Cleve Clinic J Med 67:567-73, 2000.
Owens RC, Ambrose PG. Acyclovir. Antibiotics for Clinicians 1:85-93, 1997
Whitley RJ, Gnann JW Jr. Acyclovir: a decade later. N Engl J Med 327:782-3, 1992.

Amantadine (Symmetrel)

Drug Class: Antiviral
Usual Dose: 200 mg (PO) q24h
Pharmacokinetic Parameters:
Peak serum level: 0.6 mcg/mL
Bioavailability: 90%
Excreted unchanged: 90%
Serum half-life (normal/ESRD): 12/500 hrs
Plasma protein binding: 60%
Volume of distribution (V_d): 6.6 L/kg
Primary Mode of Elimination: Renal
Dosage Adjustments:

CrCl ~ 40–60 mL/min	100 mg (PO) q24h
CrCl ~ 10–30 mL/min	100 mg (PO) q48h
CrCl < 10 mL/min	200 mg (PO) qweek
Post–HD dose	None
Post–PD dose	None
Post–CVVH dose	None
Moderate hepatic insufficiency	No change
Severe hepatic insufficiency	No change

Drug Interactions: Alcohol (↑ CNS effects); benztropine, trihexyphenidyl (↑ interacting drug effect: dry mouth, ataxia); CNS stimulants (additive stimulation); digoxin (↑ digoxin levels); trimethoprim (↑ amantadine and trimethoprim levels); scopolamine (↑ scopolamine effect:

blurred vision, slurred speech, toxic psychosis)
Adverse Effects: Confusion/delusions, dysarthria, ataxia, anticholinergic effects (blurry vision, dry mouth, orthostatic hypotension, urinary retention, constipation), livedo reticularis, may ↑ QT_c interval
Resistance Potential: Low
Allergic Potential: Low
Safety in Pregnancy: C
Comments: May precipitate heart failure. Avoid co-administration with anticholinergics, MAO inhibitors, or antihistamines
Cerebrospinal Fluid Penetration:
Non-inflamed meninges = 15%
Inflamed meninges = 20%

REFERENCES:
Douglas RG, Jr. Prophylaxis and treatment of influenza. N Engl J Med 322:443-50, 1990.
Gubareva LV, Kaiser L, Hayden FG. Influenza virus neuraminidase inhibitors. Lancet 355:827-5,2000.
Keyers LA, Karl M, Nafziger AN, et al. Comparison of central nervous system adverse effects of amantadine and rimantadine used as sequential prophylaxis of influenza A in elderly nursing home patients. Arch Intern Med 160:1485-8, 2000.
Somani S, Degelau J, Cooper SL, et al. Comparison of pharmacokinetic and safety profiles of amantadine 50- and 100-mg daily doses in elderly nursing home residents. Pharmacotherapy 11:460-6, 1991.

Amikacin (Amikin)

Drug Class: Aminoglycoside
Usual Dose: 15 mg/kg or 1 gm (IV) q24h (preferred to q12h dosing)
Pharmacokinetic Parameters:
Peak serum level: 20-30 mcg/mL (q12h dosing); 65-75 mcg/mL (q24h dosing)
Bioavailability: < 5%
Excreted unchanged: 95%
Serum half-life (normal/ESRD): 2/50 hrs
Plasma protein binding: < 5%
Volume of distribution (V_d): 0.25 L/kg
Primary Mode of Elimination: Renal
Dosage Adjustments:

CrCl ~ 40–60 mL/min	7.5 mg/kg (IV) q24h or 500 mg (IV) q24h

---

* Resume dosing for CrCl < 10 mL/min after supplemental dose. "Usual dose" assumes normal renal and hepatic function. CrCl = creatinine clearance; CVVH = continuous veno-venous hemofiltration; HD = hemodialysis; PD = peritoneal dialysis. See pp. 252-255 for definitions/explanations, p. 1 for abbreviations

CrCl ~ 10–30 mL/min	7.5 mg/kg (IV) q48h or 500 mg (IV) q48h
CrCl < 10 mL/min	3.75 mg/kg (IV) q48h or 250 mg (IV) q48h
Post–HD dose*	7.5 mg/kg (IV) or 500 mg (IV)
Post–PD dose*	3.75 mg/kg (IV) or 250 mg (IV)
Post–CVVH dose*	7.5 mg/kg (IV) or 500 mg (IV)
Moderate hepatic insufficiency	No change
Severe hepatic insufficiency	No change

Drug Interactions: Amphotericin B, cephalothin, cyclosporine, enflurane, methoxyflurane, NSAIDs, polymyxin B, radiographic contrast, vancomycin (↑ nephrotoxicity); cis-platinum (↑ nephrotoxicity, ↑ ototoxicity); loop diuretics (↑ ototoxicity); neuromuscular blocking agents (↑ apnea, prolonged paralysis); non-polarizing muscle relaxants (↑ apnea)

Adverse Effects: Neuromuscular blockade with rapid infusion/absorption. Nephrotoxicity only with prolonged/extremely high serum trough levels; may cause reversible non–oliguric renal failure (ATN). Ototoxicity associated with prolonged/extremely high peak serum levels (usually irreversible): Cochlear toxicity (1/3 of ototoxicity) manifests as decreased high frequency hearing, but deafness is unusual. Vestibular toxicity (2/3 of ototoxicity) develops before ototoxicity, and typically manifests as tinnitus

Resistance Potential: Low
Allergic Potential: Low
Safety in Pregnancy: C
Comments: Dose for synergy = 7.5 mg/kg (IV) q24h or 500 mg (IV) q24h. Single daily dosing greatly reduces nephrotoxic/ototoxic potential. Incompatible with solutions containing β–lactams, erythromycin, chloramphenicol, furosemide, sodium bicarbonate. IV infusion should be given slowly over 1 hour. May be given IM. Avoid intraperitoneal infusion due to risk of neuromuscular blockade. Avoid intratracheal/aerosolized intrapulmonary instillation, which may predispose to antibiotic resistance. V_d increases with edema/ascites, trauma, burns, cystic fibrosis; may require ↑ dose. V_d decreases with dehydration, obesity; may require ↓ dose. Renal cast counts are the best indicator of aminoglycoside nephrotoxicity, not serum creatinine. Dialysis removes ~ 50% of amikacin from serum. Na^+ content = 1.3 mEq/g

Therapeutic Serum Concentrations:
Peak (q24h/q12h dosing): 65-75/20-30 mcg/mL
Trough (q24h/q12h dosing): 0/4-8 mcg/mL
Intrathecal (IT) dose = 10–20 mg (IT) q24h
Cerebrospinal Fluid Penetration:
Non-inflamed meninges = 15%
Inflamed meninges = 20%
Bile Penetration: 30%

REFERENCES:
Cunha BA. Aminoglycosides: Current role in antimicrobial therapy. Pharmacotherapy 8: 334-50,1988.
Edson RS, Terrel CL. The Aminoglycosides. Mayo Clin Proc 74:519-28, 1999.
Lortholoary O, Tod M, Cohen Y, et al. Aminoglycosides. Med Clin North Am 79:761-87, 1995.
Nicolau DP, Freeman CD, Belliveau PP, et al. Experience with a once-daily aminoglycoside program administered to 2184 adult patients. Antimicrob Chemother 39:650-59, 1995.
Van der Auwera P. Pharmacokinetic evaluation of single dose amikacin. J Antimicrob Chemother 27:63-71,1991.

Amoxicillin (Amoxil, A-cillin, Polymox, Trimox, Wymox)

Drug Class: Aminopenicillin
Usual Dose: 1 gm (PO) q8h
Pharmacokinetic Parameters:
Peak serum level: 20 mcg/mL
Bioavailability: 90%
Excreted unchanged: 80%
Serum half-life (normal/ESRD): 1.2/16 hrs
Plasma protein binding: 17%
Volume of distribution (V_d): 0.26 L/kg
Primary Mode of Elimination: Renal

* Resume dosing for CrCl < 10 mL/min after supplemental dose. "Usual dose" assumes normal renal and hepatic function. CrCl = creatinine clearance; CVVH = continuous veno-venous hemofiltration; HD = hemodialysis; PD = peritoneal dialysis. See pp. 252-255 for definitions/explanations, p. 1 for abbreviations

Dosage Adjustments:

CrCl ~ 40–60 mL/min	500 mg (PO) q8h
CrCl ~ 10–30 mL/min	500 mg (PO) q12h
CrCl < 10 mL/min	500 mg (PO) q24h
Post–HD dose*	500 mg
Post–PD dose	None
Post–CVVH dose*	1 gm
Moderate hepatic insufficiency	No change
Severe hepatic insufficiency	No change

Drug Interactions: Allopurinol (↑ frequency of rash)
Adverse Effects: Drug fever/rash, ↑ SGOT/SGPT
Resistance Potential: Low
Allergic Potential: High
Safety in Pregnancy: B
Comments: No irritative diarrhea with 1 gm (PO) q8h dose due to nearly complete proximal GI absorption. Na$^+$ content = 2.7 mEq/g
Cerebrospinal Fluid Penetration:
Non-inflamed meninges = 1%
Inflamed meninges = 8%
Bile Penetration: 3000%

REFERENCES:
Cunha BA. The aminopenicillins. Urology 40:186-190,1992.
Cupo J. Amoxicillin. Antibiotics for Clinicians 1:21-28,1997.
Donowitz GR, Mandell GL. Beta-lactam antibiotics. N Engl J Med 318:419-26 and 318:490-500, 1993.
Wright AJ, Wilkowske CJ. The penicillins. Mayo Clin Proc 66:1047-63, 1991.

Amoxicillin/Clavulanic Acid (Augmentin)

Drug Class: Aminopenicillin/β-lactamase inhibitor combination
Usual Dose: 875/125 mg (PO) q12h
Pharmacokinetic Parameters:

Peak serum level: 15/2 mcg/mL
Bioavailability: 90/60%
Excreted unchanged: 80/40%
Serum half-life (normal/ESRD): [1.2/16]/[1/2] hrs
Plasma protein binding: 60/30%
Volume of distribution (V_d): 0.26/0.3 L/kg
Primary Mode of Elimination: Renal
Dosage Adjustments:

CrCl ~ 40–60 mL/min	500/125 mg (PO) q12h
CrCl ~ 10–30 mL/min	500/125 mg (PO) q24h
CrCl < 10 mL/min	250/125 mg (PO) q24h
Post–HD dose*	250/125 mg (PO)
Post–PD dose	None
Post–CVVH dose*	875/125 mg (PO)
Moderate hepatic insufficiency	No change
Severe hepatic insufficiency	No change

Drug Interactions: Allopurinol (↑ frequency of rash)
Adverse Effects: Drug fever/rash, diarrhea, ↑ SGOT/SGPT. Rash potential same as ampicillin
Resistance Potential: Low
Allergic Potential: High
Safety in Pregnancy: B
Comments: GI side effects much less with current formulation containing less clavulanate
Cerebrospinal Fluid Penetration:
Non-inflamed meninges = 1%
Inflamed meninges = 1%
Bile Penetration: 3000%

REFERENCES:
Cunha BA. Amoxicillin/clavulanic acid in respiratory infections: microbiologic and pharmacokinetic considerations. Clinical Therapeutics 14:418-25, 1992.
Donowitz GR, Mandell GL. Beta-lactam antibiotics. N Engl J Med 318:419-26 and 318:490-500, 1993.
Wright AJ, Wilkowske CJ. The penicillins. Mayo Clin Proc 66:1047-63, 1991.

---

* Resume dosing for CrCl < 10 mL/min after supplemental dose. "Usual dose" assumes normal renal and hepatic function. CrCl = creatinine clearance; CVVH = continuous veno-venous hemofiltration; HD = hemodialysis; PD = peritoneal dialysis. See pp. 252-255 for definitions/explanations, p. 1 for abbreviations

Amphotericin B (Fungizone)

Drug Class: Antifungal
Usual Dose: 1–1.5 mg/kg (IV) q24h
Pharmacokinetic Parameters:
Peak serum level: 1-2 mcg/mL
Bioavailability: Not applicable
Excreted unchanged: 5%
Serum half-life (normal/ESRD): 15/48 hrs
Plasma protein binding: 90%
Volume of distribution (V_d): 4 L/kg
Primary Mode of Elimination: Metabolized
Dosage Adjustments:

CrCl ~ 40–60 mL/min	No change
CrCl ~ 10–30 mL/min	No change
CrCl < 10 mL/min	No change
Post–HD dose	None
Post–PD dose	None
Post–CVVH dose	None
Moderate hepatic insufficiency	No change
Severe hepatic insufficiency	No change

Drug Interactions: Adrenocorticoids (hypokalemia); aminoglycosides, cyclosporine, polymyxin B (↑ nephrotoxicity); digoxin (↑ digitalis toxicity due to hypokalemia); flucytosine (↑ flucytosine effect); neuromuscular blocking agents (↑ neuromuscular blockade due to hypokalemia)
Adverse Effects: Fevers/chills, flushing thrombophlebitis, bradycardia, seizures, hypotension, distal renal tubular acidosis ($\downarrow K^+/\downarrow Mg^{++}$), anemia. If renal insufficiency is secondary to amphotericin, either ↓ daily dose by 50%, give dose every other day, or switch to an amphotericin lipid formulation
Resistance Potential: Low
Allergic Potential: Low
Safety in Pregnancy: B
Comments: Reconstitute in sterile water, not in dextrose, saline, or bacteriostatic water. Do not co-administer in same IV with other drugs. Give by slow IV infusion over 2 hours initially. Test dose unnecessary. Amphotericin B with granulocyte colony stimulating factor (GCSF) may result in ARDS. Amphotericin B with pentamidine may cause acute tubular necrosis in HIV/AIDS patients. Fevers/chills may be reduced by meperidine, aspirin, NSAIDs, hydrocortisone or acetaminophen, if given 30-60 minutes before infusion. For bladder irrigation, use 50 mg/mL until cultures are negative.
Meningeal dose = usual dose plus 0.5 mg 3-5x/week (IT) via Ommaya reservoir
Cerebrospinal Fluid Penetration: < 10%

REFERENCES:
Cruz JM, Peacock JE Jr., Loomer L, et al. Rapid intravenous infusion of Amphotericin B: A pilot study. Am J Med 93:123-30, 1992.
Gallis HA, Drew RH, Pickard WW. Amphotericin B: 30 years of clinical experience. Rev Infect Dis 12:308-29, 1990.
Lyman CA, Walsh TJ. Systemically administered antifungal agents: A review of their clinical pharmacology and therapeutic applications. Drugs 44:9-35, 1992.
Menzies D, Goel K, Cunha BA. Amphotericin B. Antibiotics for Clinicians 2:73-6, 1998.

Amphotericin B Lipid Complex (Abelcet) ABLC

Drug Class: Antifungal
Usual Dose: 5 mg/kg (IV) q24h
Pharmacokinetic Parameters:
Peak serum level: 1-2 mcg/mL
Bioavailability: Not applicable
Excreted unchanged: 5%
Serum half-life (normal/ESRD): 24/27 hrs
Plasma protein binding: 90%
Volume of distribution (V_d): 131 L/kg
Primary Mode of Elimination: Metabolized
Dosage Adjustments:

CrCl ~ 40–60 mL/min	No change
CrCl ~ 10–30 mL/min	No change
CrCl < 10 mL/min	No change
Post–HD dose	None

---

* Resume dosing for CrCl < 10 mL/min after supplemental dose. "Usual dose" assumes normal renal and hepatic function. CrCl = creatinine clearance; CVVH = continuous veno-venous hemofiltration; HD = hemodialysis; PD = peritoneal dialysis. See pp. 252-255 for definitions/explanations, p. 1 for abbreviations

Post–PD dose	None
Post–CVVH dose	None
Moderate hepatic insufficiency	No change
Severe hepatic insufficiency	No change

Drug Interactions: Adrenocorticoids (hypokalemia); aminoglycosides, cyclosporine, polymyxin B (↑ nephrotoxicity); digoxin (↑ digitalis toxicity due to hypokalemia); flucytosine (↑ flucytosine effect); neuromuscular blocking agents (↑ neuromuscular blockade due to hypokalemia)
Adverse Effects: Fevers/chills, flushing thrombophlebitis, bradycardia, seizures, hypotension, distal renal tubular acidosis ($\downarrow K^+/\downarrow Mg^{++}$), anemia. Fewer/less severe side effects and less nephrotoxicity than amphotericin B
Resistance Potential: Low
Allergic Potential: Low
Safety in Pregnancy: B
Comments: Useful in patients unable to tolerate amphotericin B or in patients with amphotericin B nephrotoxicity
Cerebrospinal Fluid Penetration: < 10%

REFERENCES:
Hiemenz JW, Walsh TJ. Lipid formulations of Amphotericin B: Recent progress and future directions. Clin Infect Dis 2:133-44, 1996.
Kauffman CA, Carver PL. Antifungal agents in the 1990s: Current status and future developments. Drugs 53:539-49, 1997.
Slain D. Lipid-based Amphotericin B for the treatment of fungal infections. Pharmacotherapy 19:306-23, 1999.

Amphotericin B Liposomal (AmBisome) L-AmB

Drug Class: Antifungal
Usual Dose: 3-5 mg/kg (IV) q24h
Pharmacokinetic Parameters:
Peak serum level: 7-57 mcg/mL
Bioavailability: Not applicable
Excreted unchanged: 5%
Serum half-life (normal/ESRD): 174 hrs/no data

Plasma protein binding: 90%
Volume of distribution (V_d): 0.44 L/kg
Primary Mode of Elimination: Metabolized
Dosage Adjustments:

CrCl ~ 40–60 mL/min	No change
CrCl ~ 10–30 mL/min	No change
CrCl < 10 mL/min	No change
Post–HD dose	None
Post–PD dose	None
Post–CVVH dose	None
Moderate hepatic insufficiency	No change
Severe hepatic insufficiency	No change

Drug Interactions: Adrenocorticoids (hypokalemia); aminoglycosides, cyclosporine, polymyxin B (↑ nephrotoxicity); digoxin (↑ digitalis toxicity due to hypokalemia); flucytosine (↑ flucytosine effect); neuromuscular blocking agents (↑ neuromuscular blockade due to hypokalemia)
Adverse Effects: Fevers/chills, flushing, thrombophlebitis, bradycardia, seizures, hypotension, distal renal tubular acidosis ($\downarrow K^+/\downarrow Mg^{++}$), anemia
Resistance Potential: Low
Allergic Potential: Low
Safety in Pregnancy: B
Comments: Less nephrotoxicity than amphotericin B and other amphotericin lipid preparations. For empiric therapy of fungemia, 3 mg/kg/day may be used; for suspected/known Aspergillus infection, use 5 mg/kg/day
Cerebrospinal Fluid Penetration: < 10%

REFERENCES:
De Marie S. Clinical use of liposomal and lipid-complexed amphotericin-B. J Antimicrob Chemother 33:907-16, 1994.
Hiemenz JW, Walsh TJ. Lipid formulations of amphotericin B: Recent progress and future directions. Clin Infect Dis 2:133-44, 1996.
Slain D. Lipid-based amphotericin B for the treatment of fungal infections. Pharmacotherapy 19:306-23, 1999.

* Resume dosing for CrCl < 10 mL/min after supplemental dose. "Usual dose" assumes normal renal and hepatic function. CrCl = creatinine clearance; CVVH = continuous veno-venous hemofiltration; HD = hemodialysis; PD = peritoneal dialysis. See pp. 252-255 for definitions/explanations, p. 1 for abbreviations

Amphotericin B Cholesteryl Sulfate Complex (Amphotec), ABCD (amphotericin B colloidal dispersion)

Drug Class: Antifungal
Usual Dose: 5 mg/kg (IV) q24h
Pharmacokinetic Parameters:
Peak serum level: 1-2 mcg/mL
Bioavailability: Not applicable
Excreted unchanged: 5%
Serum half-life (normal/ESRD): 28/29 hrs
Plasma protein binding: 90%
Volume of distribution (V_d): 4 L/kg
Primary Mode of Elimination: Metabolized
Dosage Adjustments:

CrCl ~ 40–60 mL/min	No change
CrCl ~ 10–30 mL/min	No change
CrCl < 10 mL/min	No change
Post–HD dose	None
Post–PD dose	None
Post–CVVH dose	None
Moderate hepatic insufficiency	No change
Severe hepatic insufficiency	No change

Drug Interactions: Adrenocorticoids (hypokalemia); aminoglycosides, cyclosporine, polymyxin B (↑ nephrotoxicity); digoxin (↑ digitalis toxicity due to hypokalemia); flucytosine (↑ flucytosine effect); neuromuscular blocking agents (↑ neuromuscular blockade due to hypokalemia)
Adverse Effects: Fevers/chills, flushing, thrombophlebitis, bradycardia, seizures, hypotension, distal renal tubular acidosis (↓ K⁺/↓ Mg⁺⁺), anemia. Fewer/less severe side effects/less nephrotoxicity vs. amphotericin B
Resistance Potential: Low
Allergic Potential: Low

Safety in Pregnancy: B
Comments: Reconstitute in sterile water, not dextrose, saline or bacteriostatic water. Do not co-administer with in same IV line with other drugs. Give by slow IV infusion over 2 hours. Test dose unnecessary
Cerebrospinal Fluid Penetration: < 10%

REFERENCES:
De Marie S. Clinical use of liposomal and lipid-complexed amphotericin B. J Antimicrob Chemother 33:907-16, 1994.
Kline S, Larsen TA, Fieber L, et al. Limited toxicity of prolonged therapy with high doses of amphotericin B lipid complex. Clin Infect Dis 21:1154-8, 1995.
Rapp RP, Gubbins PO, Evans ME. Amphotericin B lipid complex. Ann Pharmacother 31:1174-86, 1997.

Ampicillin (various)

Drug Class: Aminopenicillin
Usual Dose: 2 gm (IV) q4h, 500 mg (PO) q6h
Pharmacokinetic Parameters:
Peak serum level: 48 (IV) / 5 (PO) mcg/mL
Bioavailability: 40%
Excreted unchanged: 90%
Serum half-life (normal/ESRD): 0.8/10 hrs
Plasma protein binding: 20%
Volume of distribution (V_d): 0.25 L/kg
Primary Mode of Elimination: Renal
Dosage Adjustments:

CrCl ~ 40–60 mL/min	1 gm (IV) q4h; 250 mg (PO) q6h
CrCl ~ 10–30 mL/min	1 gm (IV) q8h; 250 mg (PO) q8h
CrCl < 10 mL/min	1 gm (IV) q12h; 250 mg (PO) q12h
Post–HD dose*	1 gm (IV) 500 mg (PO)
Post–PD dose	None
Post–CVVH dose*	2 gm (IV); 500 mg (PO)
Moderate hepatic insufficiency	No change

---
* Resume dosing for CrCl < 10 mL/min after supplemental dose. "Usual dose" assumes normal renal and hepatic function. CrCl = creatinine clearance; CVVH = continuous veno-venous hemofiltration; HD = hemodialysis; PD = peritoneal dialysis. See pp. 252-255 for definitions/explanations, p. 1 for abbreviations

Severe hepatic insufficiency	No change

Drug Interactions: Allopurinol (↑ frequency of rash); warfarin (↑ INR)
Adverse Effects: Drug fever/rash, nausea, GI upset, irritative diarrhea, h SGOT/SGPT, ↑ incidence of rash vs. penicillin in patients with EBV, HIV, lymphocytic leukemias, or allopurinol, C. difficile diarrhea/colitis
Resistance Potential: High (E. coli, H. influenzae, S. aureus)
Allergic Potential: High
Safety in Pregnancy: B
Comments: Incompatible in solutions containing amphotericin B, heparin, corticosteroids, erythromycin, aminoglycosides, or metronidazole. Na⁺ content = 2.9 mEq/g.
Meningeal dose = 2 gm (IV) q4h
Cerebrospinal Fluid Penetration:
Non-inflamed meninges = 1%
Inflamed meninges = 10%
Bile Penetration: 3000%

REFERENCES:
Donowitz GR, Mandell GL. Beta-lactam antibiotics. N Engl J Med 318:419-26 and 318:490-500, 1993.
Wright AJ. The penicillins. Mayo Clin Proc 74:290-307, 1999.
Wright AJ, Wilkowske CJ. The penicillins. Mayo Clin Proc 66:1047-63, 1991.

Ampicillin/sulbactam (Unasyn)

Drug Class: Aminopenicillin/β-lactamase inhibitor combination
Usual Dose: 3 gm (IV) q6h
Pharmacokinetic Parameters:
Peak serum level: 60/120 mcg/mL
Bioavailability: Not applicable
Excreted unchanged: 90/75%
Serum half-life (normal/ESRD): [0.8/10]/[1/10] hrs
Plasma protein binding: 28/38%
Volume of distribution (V_d): 0.25/0.38 L/kg
Primary Mode of Elimination: Renal/hepatic
Dosage Adjustments:

CrCl ~ 40–60 mL/min	1.5 gm (IV) q6h
CrCl ~ 10–30 mL/min	1.5 gm (IV) q8h
CrCl < 10 mL/min	1.5 gm (IV) q12h
Post–HD dose*	1.5 gm (IV)
Post–PD dose	None
Post–CVVH dose*	3 gm (IV)
Moderate hepatic insufficiency	No change
Severe hepatic insufficiency	No change

Drug Interactions: Probenecid (↑ ampicillin/sulbactam levels)
Adverse Effects: Drug fever/rash, ↑ SGOT/SGPT, C. difficile diarrhea/colitis
Resistance Potential: Low
Allergic Potential: High
Safety in Pregnancy: B
Comments: Pseudoresistance with E. coli/Klebsiella (resistant in-vitro, not in-vivo). Na⁺ content = 4.2 mEq/g
Cerebrospinal Fluid Penetration: < 10%

REFERENCES:
Itokazu GS, Danziger LH. Ampicillin-sulbactam and ticarcillin-clavulanic acid: A comparison of their in vitro activity and review of their clinical efficacy. Pharmacotherapy 11:382-414, 1991.
Sensakovic JW, Smith LG. Beta-lactamase inhibitor combinations. Med Clin North Am 79:695-704, 1995.
Wright AJ. The penicillins. Mayo Clin Proc 73:290-307,1999.

Amprenavir (Agenerase)

Drug Class: Antiretroviral protease inhibitor
Usual Dose: > 50 kg: 1200 mg (PO) q12h (capsules) or 1400 mg (PO) q12h (solution); < 50 kg: 20 mg/kg (PO) q12h (capsules) or 1.5 ml/kg (PO) q12h (15 mg/mL solution)
Pharmacokinetic Parameters:
Peak serum level: 5.4 mcg/mL
Bioavailability: 63%
Excreted unchanged: 1%
Serum half-life (normal/ESRD): 7-10/7-10 hrs
Plasma protein binding: 90%

---

* Resume dosing for CrCl < 10 mL/min after supplemental dose. "Usual dose" assumes normal renal and hepatic function. CrCl = creatinine clearance; CVVH = continuous veno-venous hemofiltration; HD = hemodialysis; PD = peritoneal dialysis. See pp. 252-255 for definitions/explanations, p. 1 for abbreviations

Volume of distribution (V$_d$): 6.1 L/kg
Primary Mode of Elimination: Hepatic
Dosage Adjustments:

CrCl ~ 40–60 mL/min	No change
CrCl ~ 10–30 mL/min	No change
CrCl < 10 mL/min	No change
Post–HD dose	None
Post–PD dose	None
Post–CVVH dose	None
Moderate hepatic insufficiency	450 mg (PO) q12h
Severe hepatic insufficiency	300 mg (PO) q12h

Antiretroviral Dosage Adjustments:

Delavirdine	No information
Efavirenz	Amprenavir 1200 mg q8h as single PI, or 1200 mg q12h + ritonavir 200 mg q12h
Indinavir	No changes
Lopinavir/ritonavir	Amprenavir 600-750 mg q12h
Nelfinavir	No information
Nevirapine	No information
Ritonavir	Limited data for amprenavir 600-1200 mg q12h + ritonavir 100-200 mg q12h
Saquinavir	No information
Rifampin	Avoid combination
Rifabutin	Rifabutin 150 mg q24h or 300 mg 2-3x/week

Drug Interactions: Antiretrovirals, rifabutin, rifampin (see dose adjustment grid, above);

astemizole, terfenadine, bepridil, cisapride, ergotamine, statins, benzodiazepines, St. John's wort (avoid if possible); carbamazepine, phenobarbital, phenytoin (may ↑ amprenavir levels, monitor anticonvulsant levels)
Adverse Effects: Drug fever/rash, E. multiforme/Stevens-Johnson syndrome, GI upset, headache, depression, taste perversion, perioral paresthesias, hyperglycemia (including worsening diabetes, new-onset diabetes, DKA), ↑ cholesterol/triglycerides (evaluate risk for coronary disease/pancreatitis), fat redistribution, ↑ SGOT/SGPT, possible increased bleeding in hemophilia
HIV Resistance Potential: Low (triple therapy); high (mono/double drug therapy)
Allergic Potential: High
Safety in Pregnancy: C
Comments: Can be taken with or without food, but avoid high fat meals (may ↓ absorption). High vitamin E content. Capsules and solution are not interchangeable on a mg per mg basis. Decrease dosage in moderate or severe liver disease; use with caution. Oral solution contains propylene glycol: avoid in pregnancy, hepatic/renal failure, patients taking disulfiram or metronidazole, or children < 4 years old. Effective antiretroviral therapy consists of three antiretrovirals (same/different classes)

REFERENCES:
Adkins JC, Faulds D. Amprenavir. Drugs 55:837-42,1998.
Go J, Cunha BA. Amprenavir. Antibiotics for Clinicians 4:49-55, 2000.
Kaul DR, Cinti SK, Carver PL, et al. HIV protease inhibitors: Advances in therapy and adverse reactions, including metabolic complications. Pharmacotherapy 19:281-98, 1999.
Panel on Clinical Practices for Treatment of HIV Infection. Guidelines for the use of antiretroviral agents in HIV-infected adults and adolescents. Department of Health and Human Services. April 23, 2001. www.hivatis.org

Atovaquone (Mepron)

Drug Class: Antiprotozoal
Usual Dose: 750 mg (PO) q12h (with food)
Pharmacokinetic Parameters:
Peak serum level: 38 mcg/mL

---

* Resume dosing for CrCl < 10 mL/min after supplemental dose. "Usual dose" assumes normal renal and hepatic function. CrCl = creatinine clearance; CVVH = continuous veno venous hemofiltration; HD = hemodialysis; PD = peritoneal dialysis. See pp. 252-255 for definitions/explanations, p. 1 for abbreviations

Bioavailability: 30% (3-fold ↑ with high fat meal)
Excreted unchanged: 1%
Serum half-life (normal/ESRD): 2.9/2.9 days
Plasma protein binding: 99.9%
Volume of distribution (V_d): 3.5 L/kg
Primary Mode of Elimination: Metabolized
Dosage Adjustments:

CrCl ~ 40–60 mL/min	No change
CrCl ~ 10–30 mL/min	No change
CrCl < 10 mL/min	No change
Post–HD dose	None
Post–PD dose	None
Post–CVVH dose	None
Moderate hepatic insufficiency	No information
Severe hepatic insufficiency	No information

Drug Interactions: Metoclopramide, rifabutin, rifampin, ritonavir, tetracycline (↓ atovaquone effect); zidovudine (↑ zidovudine levels)
Adverse Effects: Rifampin decreases atovaquone levels by 50%. Headache, fever, cough, neurovascular, diarrhea, anemia, leukopenia, ↑ SGOT/SGPT
Resistance Potential: Low
Allergic Potential: Low
Safety in Pregnancy: B
Comments: Active against T. gondii, P. carinii, Plasmodia, and Babesia

REFERENCES:
Artymowicz RJ, James VE. Atovaquone: A new anti-pneumocystis agent. Clin Pharmacol 12:563-70, 1993.
Bonoan JT, Johnson DH, Schoch PE, Cunha BA. Life threatening babesiosis treated by exchange transfusion with azithromycin and atovaquone. Heart & Lung 27:42-8, 1998.
Chan C, Montaner J, LeFebvre BA, et al. Atovaquone suspension compared with aerosolized pentamidine for prevention of Pneumocystis carinii pneumonia in human immunodeficiency virus infected subsets intolerant of trimethoprim or sulfamethoxazole. J Infect Dis 180:369-376, 1999.
Haile LG, Flaherty JF. Atovaquone: A review. Ann Pharmacother 27:1488-94, 1993.

Atovaquone + proguanil (Malarone)

Drug Class: Antimalarial
Usual Dose: Malarone tablet = 250 mg atovaquone + 100 mg proguanil. Usual dose = 1 tablet (PO) q24h (see comments)
Pharmacokinetic Parameters:
Peak serum level: 38 mcg/mL
Bioavailability: 23/90%
Excreted unchanged: 94/50%
Serum half-life (normal/ESRD): [2.9/2.9]/[21/no data] hrs
Plasma protein binding: 99/75%
Volume of distribution (V_d): 3.5/42 L/kg
Primary Mode of Elimination: Metabolized
Dosage Adjustments:

CrCl ~ 40–60 mL/min	No change
CrCl ~ 10–30 mL/min	No change
CrCl < 10 mL/min	No change
Post–HD dose	No information
Post–PD dose	No information
Post–CVVH dose	No information
Moderate hepatic insufficiency	No information
Severe hepatic insufficiency	No information

Drug Interactions: Chloroquine (↑ incidence of mouth ulcers); metoclopramide, rifabutin, rifampin, tetracycline (↓ atovaquone + proguanil effect); ritonavir (↑ or ↓ atovaquone + proguanil effect); typhoid vaccine (↓ typhoid vaccine effect)
Adverse Effects: Headache, dizziness, nausea, vomiting, diarrhea, abdominal pain, anorexia, myalgias, fever
Resistance Potential: Low
Allergic Potential: Low
Safety in Pregnancy: C
Comments: Effective against chloroquine sensitive/resistant strains of P. falciparum, but not P. ovale, P. vivax, or P. malariae.

---

* Resume dosing for CrCl < 10 mL/min after supplemental dose. "Usual dose" assumes normal renal and hepatic function. CrCl = creatinine clearance; CVVH = continuous veno-venous hemofiltration; HD = hemodialysis; PD = peritoneal dialysis. See pp. 252-255 for definitions/explanations, p. 1 for abbreviations

Malaria prophylaxis: 1 tablet (PO) q24h for 2 days before entering endemic area, daily during exposure, and daily x 1 week post-exposure
Therapy: 4 tablets (PO) as single dose x 3 days

REFERENCES:

Atovaquone/proguanil (Malarone) for malaria. Med Lett Drugs Ther 42:109-11, 2000.

Looareesuwan S, Chulay JD, Canfield CJ. Malarone (atovaquone and proguanil hydrochloride): a review of its clinical development for treating malaria. Malarone clinical trials study group. Am J Trop Med Hyg 60:533-41, 1999.

Nosten F. Prophylactic effect of malarone against malaria: all good news? Lancet 356:1864-5, 2000.

Azithromycin (Zithromax)

Drug Class: Macrolide (Azolide)
Usual Dose: 500 mg (IV/PO) x 1 dose, then 250 mg (IV/PO) q24h
Pharmacokinetic Parameters:
Peak serum level: 3.6 (IV)/0.3 (PO) mcg/mL
Bioavailability: 35%
Excreted unchanged: 10%
Serum half-life (normal/ESRD): 68/68 hrs
Plasma protein binding: 50%
Volume of distribution (V_d): 18 L/kg
Primary Mode of Elimination: Hepatic
Dosage Adjustments:

CrCl ~ 40–60 mL/min	No change
CrCl ~ 10–30 mL/min	No change
CrCl < 10 ml/min	No change
Post–HD dose	None
Post–PD dose	None
Post–CVVH dose	None
Moderate hepatic insufficiency	No change
Severe hepatic insufficiency	250 mg (IV/PO) q24h

Drug Interactions: Carbamazepine, cisapride, clozapine, corticosteroids, midazolam, triazolam, valproic acid (not studied/not reported); cyclosporine (↑ cyclosporine levels with toxicity); digoxin (↑ digoxin levels); pimozide (may ↑ QT interval, torsade de pointes)
Adverse Effects: Nausea, GI upset, diarrhea
Resistance Potential: Low
Allergic Potential: Low
Safety in Pregnancy: B
Comments: May ↑ QT_c interval. Bioavailability is decreased by food. For C. trachomatis urethritis, use 1 gm (PO) x 1 dose. For N. gonorrhoea urethritis, use 2 gm (PO) x 1 dose. For MAI prophylaxis, use 1200 mg (PO) weekly. For MAI therapy, use 600 mg (PO) q24h
Cerebrospinal Fluid Penetration: < 10%
Bile/serum ratio: > 3000%

REFERENCES:

Alvarez-Elcoro S, Enzler MJ. The macrolides: Erythromycin, clarithromycin and azithromycin. Mayo Clin Proc 74:613-34, 1999.

Cunha BA. Macrolides, doxycycline, and fluoroquinolones in the treatment of Legionnaires' Disease. Antibiotics for Clinicians 2:117-8, 1998.

Paradisi F, Corti G. Azithromycin. Antibiotics for Clinicians 3:1-8, 1999

Schlossberg D. Azithromycin and clarithromycin. Med Clin N Amer 79:803-816, 1995.

Zuckerman JM, Kaye KM. The newer macrolides, azithromycin and clarithromycin. Infect Dis Clin N Am 9:731-45, 1995.

Aztreonam (Azactam)

Drug Class: Monobactam
Usual Dose: 2 g (IV) q8h
Pharmacokinetic Parameters:
Peak serum level: 222 mcg/mL
Bioavailability: Not applicable
Excreted unchanged: 75%
Serum half-life (normal/ESRD): 1.7/7 hrs
Plasma protein binding: 56%
Volume of distribution (V_d): 0.2 L/kg
Primary Mode of Elimination: Renal
Dosage Adjustments:

CrCl ~ 40–60 mL/min	1 gm (IV) q8h
CrCl ~ 10–30 mL/min	1 gm (IV) q12h
CrCl < 10 mL/min	1gm (IV) q24h
Post–HD dose*	1 gm (IV)

Post–PD dose*	500 mg (IV)
Post–CVVH dose*	2 gm (IV)
Moderate hepatic insufficiency	No change
Severe hepatic insufficiency	No change

Drug Interactions: None
Adverse Effects: None
Resistance Potential: Low
Allergic Potential: Low
Safety in Pregnancy: B
Comments: Incompatible in solutions containing vancomycin or metronidazole. No cross allergenicity with penicillins, β-lactams; safe to use in penicillin allergic patients. Meningeal dose = 2 gm (IV) q6h
Cerebrospinal Fluid Penetration:
Non-inflamed meninges = 1%
Inflamed meninges = 40%
Bile Penetration: 300%

REFERENCES:
Brogden RN, Heal RC. Aztreonam: A review of its antibacterial activity, pharmacokinetic properties, and therapeutic use. Drugs 31:96-130, 1986.
Cunha BA. Cross allergenicity of penicillin with carbapenems and monobactams. J Crit Illness 13:344, 1998.
Cunha BA. Aztreonam: A review. Urology 41:249-58, 1993.
Hellinger WC, Brewer NS. Carbapenems and monobactams: Imipenem, meropenem, and aztreonam. Mayo Clin Proc 74:420-34, 1999.
Johnson, Cunha BA. Aztreonam. Med Clin North Am 79:733-43, 1995.

Bacampicillin (Spectrobid)

Drug Class: Aminopenicillin
Usual Dose: 800 mg (PO) q12h
Pharmacokinetic Parameters:
Peak serum level: 14 mcg/mL
Bioavailability: 96%
Excreted unchanged: 90%
Serum half-life (normal/ESRD): 1.1/11 hrs
Plasma protein binding: 20%
Volume of distribution (V_d): 0.25 L/kg
Primary Mode of Elimination: Renal

Dosage Adjustments:

CrCl ~ 40–60 mL/min	400 mg (PO) q12h
CrCl ~ 10–30 mL/min	400 mg (PO) q12h
CrCl < 10 mL/min	400 mg (PO) q24h
Post–HD dose*	400 mg (PO)
Post–PD dose	None
Post–CVVH dose*	800 mg (PO)
Moderate hepatic insufficiency	No change
Severe hepatic insufficiency	No change

Drug Interactions: None
Adverse Effects: Drug fever/rash, ↑ SGOT/SGPT. Rash potential same as ampicillin
Resistance Potential: Low
Allergic Potential: High
Safety in Pregnancy: B
Comments: No irritative diarrhea due to nearly complete upper GI absorption
Cerebrospinal Fluid Penetration: < 10%

REFERENCES:
Cunha BA. The aminopenicillins. Urology 40:186-190, 1992.
Cupo J. Amoxicillin. Antibiotics for Clinicians 21-28, 1997.
Donowitz GR, Mandell GL. Beta-lactam antibiotics. N Engl J Med 318:419-26 and 318:490-500, 1993.
Wright AJ, Wilkowske CJ. The penicillins. Mayo Clin Proc 66:1047-63, 1991.

Capreomycin (Capastat)

Drug Class: Anti-TB drug
Usual Dose: 1 gm (IM) q24h
Pharmacokinetic Parameters:
Peak serum level: 30 mcg/mL
Bioavailability: Not applicable
Excreted unchanged: 90%
Serum half-life (normal/ESRD): 5/75 hrs
Plasma protein binding: No data
Volume of distribution (V_d): No data
Primary Mode of Elimination: Renal

---

* Resume dosing for CrCl < 10 mL/min after supplemental dose. "Usual dose" assumes normal renal and hepatic function. CrCl = creatinine clearance; CVVH = continuous veno-venous hemofiltration; HD = hemodialysis; PD = peritoneal dialysis. See pp. 252-255 for definitions/explanations, p. 1 for abbreviations

Dosage Adjustment:

CrCl ~ 40–60 mL/min	500 mg (IM) q24h
CrCl ~ 10–30 mL/min	500 mg (IM) q48h
CrCl < 10 mL/min	500 mg (IM) q72h
Post–HD dose	No information
Post–PD dose	No information
Post–CVVH dose	No information
Moderate hepatic insufficiency	No change
Severe hepatic insufficiency	No change

Drug Interactions: None
Adverse Effects: Eosinophilia, leukopenia, drug fever/rash, ototoxicity (vestibular), nephrotoxicity (glomerular/tubular)
Resistance Potential: Low
Allergic Potential: Moderate
Safety in Pregnancy: C
Comments: Pain/phlebitis at IM injection site. Additive toxicity with aminoglycosides/viomycin
Cerebrospinal Fluid Penetration: < 10%

REFERENCES:
Davidson PT, Le HQ. Drug treatment of tuberculosis - 1992. Drugs 43:651-73, 1992.
Drugs for tuberculosis. Med Lett Drugs Ther 35:99-101, 1993.
Iseman MD. Treatment of multidrug resistant tuberculosis. N Engl J Med 329:784-91, 1993.

Carbenicillin (Geocillin)

Drug Class: Oral anti-pseudomonal penicillin
Usual Dose: 382 mg (PO) q6h (for UTIs only)
Pharmacokinetic Parameters:
Peak serum level: 6.5 mcg/mL
Bioavailability: 35%
Excreted unchanged: 90%
Serum half-life (normal/ESRD): 1/14 hrs
Plasma protein binding: 50%
Volume of distribution (V_d): No data
Primary Mode of Elimination: Renal

Dosage Adjustments:

CrCl ~ 40–60 mL/min	382 mg (PO) q12h
CrCl ~ 10–30 mL/min	382 mg (PO) q24h
CrCl < 10 mL/min	382 mg (PO) q48h
Post–HD dose*	382 mg (PO)
Post–PD dose	None
Post–CVVH dose*	382 mg (PO)
Moderate hepatic insufficiency	No change
Severe hepatic insufficiency	No change

Drug Interactions: Aminoglycosides (inactivation of carbenicillin in renal failure); warfarin (↑ INR); oral contraceptives (↓ oral contraceptive effect); cefoxitin (↓ carbenicillin effect)
Adverse Effects: Drug fever/rash, E. multiforme/Stevens–Johnson syndrome, diarrhea, anaphylactic reactions (hypotension, laryngospasm, bronchospasm), hives, serum sickness, seizures, ↓ Ca^{++}, ↓ Mg^{++}
Resistance Potential: High (P. aeruginosa)
Allergic Potential: High
Safety in Pregnancy: B
Comments: Serum concentrations inadequate for systemic infections. Indanyl carbenicillin (oral carbenicillin) useful only for UTIs. Na^+ content = 4.7 mEq/g
Cerebrospinal Fluid Penetration: < 10%

REFERENCES:
Donowitz GR, Mandell GL. Beta-lactam antibiotics. N Engl J Med 318:419-26 and 318:490-500, 1993.
Ortega AM, Cunha BA. Acute prostatitis. Contemporary Urology 18:73-80, 1997.
Wright AJ. The penicillins. Mayo Clin Proc 74:290-307, 1999.

Caspofungin (Cancidas)

Drug Class: Echinocandin antifungal
Usual Dose: 70 mg (IV) x 1 dose, then 50 mg (IV) q24h
Pharmacokinetic Parameters:

---

* Resume dosing for CrCl < 10 mL/min after supplemental dose. "Usual dose" assumes normal renal and hepatic function. CrCl = creatinine clearance, CVVH = continuous veno-venous hemofiltration; HD = hemodialysis; PD = peritoneal dialysis. See pp. 252-255 for definitions/explanations, p. 1 for abbreviations

Peak serum level:
70 mg: 12.1 14.83 mcg/mL (multiple dose)
50 mg: 7.6 8.7 mcg/mL (multiple doses)
Bioavailability: Not applicable
Excreted unchanged: 1.4%
Serum half-life (normal/ESRD): 10/10 hrs
Plasma protein binding: 97%
Volume of distribution (V_d): No data
Primary Mode of Elimination: Hepatic
Dosage Adjustments:

CrCl ~ 40–60 mL/min	No change
CrCl ~ 10–30 mL/min	No change
CrCl < 10 mL/min	No change
Post–HD dose	None
Post–PD dose	None
Post–CVVH dose	None
Moderate hepatic insufficiency	35 mg (IV) q24h (maintenance dose)
Severe hepatic insufficiency	No information

Drug Interactions: Carbamazepine, rifampin, dexamethasone, efavirenz, nelfinavir, nevirapine, phenytoin (↓ caspofungin levels; ↑ caspofungin maintenance dose to 70 mg/day); cyclosporine (↑ caspofungin levels, ↑ SGOT/SGPT); tacrolimus (↓ tacrolimus levels, ↑ SGOT/SGPT)
Adverse Effects: Drug fever/rash
Resistance Potential: Low
Allergic Potential: Low
Safety in Pregnancy: C
Comments: Administer by slow IV infusion over 1 hour; do not give IV bolus. Do not mix/co-infuse with glucose solution. If co-administered with drugs that ↓ caspofungin levels or for highly-resistant organisms, then 70 mg (IV) q24h dosing may be used
Cerebrospinal Fluid Penetration: No data

REFERENCES:
Abruzzo GK, Gill CJ, Flattery AM, et al. Efficacy of the echinocandin caspofungin against disseminated aspergillosis and candidiasis in cyclophosphamide-induced immunosuppressed mice. Antimicrob Agents Chemother 44:2310- 8, 2000.

Andriole VT. Current and future antifungal therapy: New targets for antifungal agents. J Antimicrob Chemother 44:151-62, 1999.
Barchiesi F, Schimizzi AM, Fothergill AW, et al. In vitro activity of the new echinocandin antifungal against common and uncommon clinical isolates of Candida species. Eur J Clin Microbiol Infect Dis 18:302-4, 1999.
Lomaestro BM. Caspofungin. Hospital Formulary 36:527-36, 2001.

Cefaclor (Ceclor)

Drug Class: 2nd generation oral cephalosporin
Usual Dose: 500 mg (PO) q8h
Pharmacokinetic Parameters:
Peak serum level: 9.3 mcg/mL
Bioavailability: 93%
Excreted unchanged: 80%
Serum half-life (normal/ESRD): 0.8/3 hrs
Plasma protein binding: 25%
Volume of distribution (V_d): 0.30 L/kg
Primary Mode of Elimination: Renal
Dosage Adjustments:

CrCl ~ 40–60 mL/min	250 mg (PO) q8h
CrCl ~ 10–30 mL/min	250 mg (PO) q12h
CrCl < 10 mL/min	250 mg (PO) q12h
Post–HD dose*	500 mg (PO)
Post–PD dose*	250 mg (PO)
Post–CVVH dose*	500 mg (PO)
Moderate hepatic insufficiency	No change
Severe hepatic insufficiency	No change

Drug Interactions: None
Adverse Effects: Drug fever/rash
Resistance Potential: Low
Allergic Potential: High
Safety in Pregnancy: B
Comments: Limited penetration into respiratory secretions
Cerebrospinal Fluid Penetration: < 10%.
Bile Penetration: 60%

REFERENCES:
Cazzola M, Di Perna F, Boveri B. Interrelationship

---

* Resume dosing for CrCl < 10 mL/min after supplemental dose. "Usual dose" assumes normal renal and hepatic function. CrCl = creatinine clearance; CVVH = continuous veno-venous hemofiltration; HD = hemodialysis; PD = peritoneal dialysis. See pp. 252-255 for definitions/explanations, p. 1 for abbreviations

between the pharmacokinetics and pharmacodynamics of cefaclor advanced formulation in patients with acute exacerbation of chronic bronchitis. J Chemother 12:216-22, 2000.

Mazzei T, Novelli A, Esposito S, et al. New insight into the clinical pharmacokinetics of cefaclor: Tissue penetration. J Chemother 12:53-62, 2000.

Meyers BR. Cefaclor revisited. Clin Ther 22:154-66, 2000.

REFERENCES:
Cunha BA. Antibiotics selection for the treatment of sinusitis, otitis media, and pharyngitis. Infect Dis Pract 7:S324-S326, 1998.

Donowitz GR, Mandell GL. Beta-lactam antibiotics. N Engl J Med 318:419-26 and 318:490-500, 1993.

Gustaferro CA, Steckelberg JM. Cephalosporins: Antimicrobic agents and related compounds. Mayo Clin Proc 66:1064-73, 1991.

Smith GH. Oral cephalosporins in perspective. DICP 24:45-51, 1990.

Cefadroxil (Duricef, Ultracef)

Drug Class: 1st generation oral cephalosporin
Usual Dose: 500 mg (PO) q12h
Pharmacokinetic Parameters:
Peak serum level: 18 mcg/mL
Bioavailability: 99%
Excreted unchanged: 90%
Serum half-life (normal/ESRD): 1.5/22 hrs
Plasma protein binding: 20%
Volume of distribution (V_d): 0.31 L/kg
Primary Mode of Elimination: Renal
Dosage Adjustments:

CrCl ~ 40–60 mL/min	500 mg (PO) q24h
CrCl ~ 10–30 mL/min	500 mg (PO) q24h
CrCl < 10 mL/min	250 mg (PO) q24h
Post–HD dose*	500 mg (PO)
Post–PD dose*	250 mg (PO)
Post–CVVH dose*	500 mg (PO)
Moderate hepatic insufficiency	No change
Severe hepatic insufficiency	No change

Drug Interactions: None
Adverse Effects: Drug fever/rash
Resistance Potential: Low
Allergic Potential: High
Safety in Pregnancy: B
Comments: Penetrates oral/respiratory secretions well
Cerebrospinal Fluid Penetration: < 10%
Bile Penetration: 20%

Cefamandole (Mandol)

Drug Class: 2nd generation cephalosporin
Usual Dose: 2 gm (IV) q6h
Pharmacokinetic Parameters:
Peak serum level: 165 mcg/mL
Bioavailability: Not applicable
Excreted unchanged: 95%
Serum half-life (normal/ESRD): 1/11 hrs
Plasma protein binding: 76%
Volume of distribution (V_d): 0.29 L/kg
Primary Mode of Elimination: Renal
Dosage Adjustments:

CrCl ~ 40–60 mL/min	1 gm (IV) q6h
CrCl ~ 10–30 mL/min	1 gm (IV) q8h
CrCl < 10 mL/min	1 gm (IV) q12h
Post–HD dose*	1 gm (IV)
Post–PD dose	None
Post–CVVH dose*	2 gm (IV)
Moderate hepatic insufficiency	No change
Severe hepatic insufficiency	No change

Drug Interactions: Alcohol (disulfiram-like reaction); antiplatelet agents, heparin, thrombolytics, warfarin (↑ risk of bleeding)
Adverse Effects: Drug fever/rash, ↑ INR
Resistance Potential: High (H. influenzae, Enterobacter)
Allergic Potential: High
Safety in Pregnancy: B
Comments: Incompatible in solutions with

---

* Resume dosing for CrCl < 10 mL/min after supplemental dose. "Usual dose" assumes normal renal and hepatic function. CrCl = creatinine clearance; CVVH = continuous veno-venous hemofiltration; HD = hemodialysis; PD = peritoneal dialysis. See pp. 252-255 for definitions/explanations, p. 1 for abbreviations

Mg^{++} or Ca^{++}. Contains MTT side chain, but no increase in clinical bleeding. Na^+ content = 3.3 mEq/g

Cerebrospinal Fluid Penetration: < 10%
Bile Penetration: 300%

REFERENCES:
Cunha BA, Klimek JJ, Qunitiliani R. Cefamandole nafate in respiratory and urinary tract infections. Curr Ther Res 25:584-9, 1971.
Gentry LO, Zeluff BJ, Cooley DA. Antibiotic prophylaxis in open-heart surgery: A comparison of cefamandole, cefuroxime, and cefazolin. Ann Thorac Surg 46:167-71, 1988.
Peterson CD, Lake KD, Arom KV. Antibiotic prophylaxis in open-heart surgery patients: Comparison of cefamandole and cefuroxime. Drug Intell Clin Pharmacol 21:728-32, 1987.

Cefazolin (Ancef, Kefzol)

Drug Class: 1st generation cephalosporin
Usual Dose: 1 gm (IV) q8h
Pharmacokinetic Parameters:
Peak serum level: 200 mcg/mL
Bioavailability: Not applicable
Excreted unchanged: 96%
Serum half-life (normal/ESRD): 1.8/18 hrs
Plasma protein binding: 85%
Volume of distribution (V_d): 0.2 L/kg
Primary Mode of Elimination: Renal
Dosage Adjustments:

CrCl ~ 40–60 mL/min	500 mg (IV) q8h
CrCl ~ 10–30 mL/min	500 mg (IV) q12h
CrCl < 10 mL/min	500 mg (IV) q24h
Post–HD dose*	500 mg (IV)
Post–PD dose	None
Post–CVVH dose*	1 gm (IV)
Moderate hepatic insufficiency	No change
Severe hepatic insufficiency	No change

Drug Interactions: None
Adverse Effects: Drug fever/rash

Resistance Potential: Low
Allergic Potential: High
Safety in Pregnancy: B
Comments: Incompatible in solutions containing erythromycin, aminoglycosides, cimetidine, theophylline. Na^+ content = 2 mEq/g

Cerebrospinal Fluid Penetration: < 10%
Bile Penetrations: 300%

REFERENCES:
Gentry LO, Zeluff BJ, Cooley DA. Antibiotic prophylaxis in open-heart surgery: A comparison of cefamandole, cefuroxime, and cefazolin. Ann Thorac Surg 46:167-71, 1988.
Cunha BA, Gossling HR, Pasternak HS, et al. Penetration of cephalosporins into bone. Infection 12:80-4, 1984.
Marshall WF, Blair JE. The cephalosporins. Mayo Clin Proc 74:187-95, 1999.
Nightingale CH, Klimek JJ, Quintiliani R. Effect of protein binding on the penetration of nonmetabolized cephalosporins into atrial appendage and pericardial fluids in open-heart surgical patients. Antimicrob Agents Chemother 17:595-8, 1980.
Quintiliani R, Nightingale CH. Cefazolin. Ann Intern Med 89:650-6, 1978.

Cefdinir (Omnicef)

Drug Class: 3rd generation oral cephalosporin
Usual Dose: 600 mg (PO) q24h
Pharmacokinetic Parameters:
Peak serum level: 2.9 mcg/mL
Bioavailability: 16%
Excreted unchanged: 11.6%
Serum half-life (normal/ESRD): 1.7/3 hrs
Plasma protein binding: 70%
Volume of distribution (V_d): 0.35 L/kg
Primary Mode of Elimination: Renal
Dosage Adjustments:

CrCl ~ 40–60 mL/min	No change
CrCl ~ 10–30 mL/min	No change
CrCl < 10 mL/min	300 mg (PO) q24h
Post–HD dose*	300 mg (PO)
Post–PD dose	None
Post–CVVH dose*	600 mg (PO)

----

* Resume dosing for CrCl < 10 mL/min after supplemental dose. "Usual dose" assumes normal renal and hepatic function. CrCl = creatinine clearance; CVVH = continuous veno-venous hemofiltration; HD = hemodialysis; PD = peritoneal dialysis. See pp. 252-255 for definitions/explanations, p. 1 for abbreviations

Moderate hepatic insufficiency	No change
Severe hepatic insufficiency	No change

Drug Interactions: Probenecid (↑ cefdinir levels)
Adverse Effects: Drug fever/rash
Resistance Potential: No data
Allergic Potential: High
Safety in Pregnancy: B
Comments: Good activity against bacterial respiratory pathogens. Available as capsules or suspension. Treat community-acquired pneumonia with 300 mg (PO) q12h; for other respiratory pathogens, use 600 mg (PO) q24h
Cerebrospinal Fluid Penetration: No data

REFERENCES:

Cefdinir: A new oral cephalosporin. Med Lett Drugs Therap 40:85-7, 1998.

Fogarty CM, Bettis RB, Griffin TJ, et al. Comparison of a 5 day regimen of cefdinir with a 10 day regimen of cefprozil for treatment of acute exacerbations of chronic bronchitis. J Antimicrob Chemother 45:851-8,2000.

Nemeth MA, Gooche WM 3rd, Hedrick J, et al. Comparison of cefdinir and penicillin for the treatment of pediatric streptococcal pharyngitis. Clin Ther 21:1525-32, 1999.

Cefditoren (Spectracef)

Drug Class: 3rd generation oral cephalosporin
Usual Dose: 400 mg (PO) q12h
Pharmacokinetic Parameters:
Peak serum level: 4.1 mcg/mL
Bioavailability: No data
Excreted unchanged: 20%
Serum half-life (normal/ESRD): 1.5/5 hrs
Plasma protein binding: 88%
Volume of distribution (V_d): No data
Primary Mode of Elimination: Renal
Dosage Adjustments:

CrCl ~ 40–60 mL/min	No change
CrCl ~ 10–30 mL/min	200 mg (PO) q12h
CrCl < 10 mL/min	200 mg (PO) q24h

Post–HD dose	No information
Post–PD dose	No information
Post–CVVH dose	No information
Moderate hepatic insufficiency	No change
Severe hepatic insufficiency	No change

Drug Interactions: No data
Adverse Effects: Drug fever/rash
Resistance Potential: No data
Allergic Potential: Low
Safety in Pregnancy: B
Comments: Serum concentrations increased ~ 50% if taken without food
Cerebrospinal Fluid Penetration: No data

REFERENCES:

Chow J, Russel M, Bolk S. et al. Efficacy of cefditoren pivoxil vs. amoxicillin-clavulanic in acute maxillary sinusitis. Presented at the 40th Interscience Conference on Antimicrobial Agents and Chemotherapy; Abstract 835, Toronto, ON 2000.

Feimagham D, Robbins MJ, Ghosh G, et al. An in vitro characterization of cefditoren: A new oral cephalosporin. Drugs Exp Clin Res 20:127-47, 1994.

Kuti JL, Quintiliani R. Cefditoren pivoxil: A novel broad-spectrum oral cephalosporin. Formulary 3 6:265-75, 2001.

Cefepime (Maxipime)

Drug Class: 4th generation cephalosporin
Usual Dose: 2 gm (IV) q8h
Pharmacokinetic Parameters:
Peak serum level: 193 mcg/mL
Bioavailability: Not applicable
Excreted unchanged: 85%
Serum half-life (normal/ESRD): 2.2/18 hrs
Plasma protein binding: 18%
Volume of distribution (V_d): 0.29 L/kg
Primary Mode of Elimination: Renal
Dosage Adjustments:

CrCl ~ 40–60 mL/min	No change
CrCl ~ 10–30 mL/min	2 gm (IV) q12h

CrCl < 10 mL/min	1 gm (IV) q24h
Post–HD dose*	1 gm (IV)
Post–PD dose	None
Post–CVVH dose*	2 gm (IV)
Moderate hepatic insufficiency	No change
Severe hepatic insufficiency	No change

Drug Interactions: None
Adverse Effects: Drug fever/rash
Resistance Potential: Low
Allergic Potential: Moderate
Safety in Pregnancy: B
Comments: For proven serious systemic P. aeruginosa infections or febrile neutropenia, use 2 gm (IV) q8h. For other infections, 2 gm (IV) q12h may be used. Effective against most strains of ceftazidime–resistant P. aeruginosa and ESBLs. Meningeal dose = usual dose
Cerebrospinal Fluid Penetration:
Non-inflamed meninges = 1%
Inflamed meninges = 15%
Bile Penetration: 10%

REFERENCES:
Barrade B, Bryson HM. Cefepime: A review of its antibacterial activity, pharmacokinetic properties, and therapeutic use. Drugs 47:471-505, 1994.
Cunha BA, Gill MV. Cefepime. Med Clin North Am 79:721-32, 1995.
Okamoto MP, Nakahiro RK, Chin A, et al. Cefepime: A new fourth-generation cephalosporin. Am J Hosp Pharm 51:463-77, 1994.
Paradisi F, Corti G, Strohmeyer M. Cefepime. Antibiotics for Clinicians 3:41-50, 1999.

Volume of distribution (V_d): 0.1 L/kg
Primary Mode of Elimination: Renal
Dosage Adjustments:

CrCl ~ 40–60 mL/min	No change
CrCl ~ 10–30 mL/min	200 mg (PO) q12h
CrCl < 10 mL/min	200 mg (PO) q24h
Post–HD dose*	200 mg (PO)
Post–PD dose	None
Post–CVVH dose*	400 mg (PO)
Moderate hepatic insufficiency	No change
Severe hepatic insufficiency	No change

Drug Interactions: Carbamazepine (↑ carbamazepine levels)
Adverse Effects: Drug fever/rash, diarrhea
Resistance Potential: Low
Allergic Potential: High
Safety in Pregnancy: B
Comments: Little/no activity against S. aureus (MSSA)
Cerebrospinal Fluid Penetration: < 10%
Bile Penetration: 800%

REFERENCES:
Markham A, Brogden RN. Cefixime: A review of its therapeutic efficacy in lower respiratory tract infections. Drugs 49:1007-22, 1995.
Marshall WF, Blair JE. The cephalosporins . Mayo Clin Proc 74:187-95, 1999.
Quintiliani R. Cefixime in the treatment of patients with lower respiratory tract infections: Results of US clinical trials. Clinical Therapeutics 18:373-90, 1996.

Cefixime (Suprax)

Drug Class: 3rd generation oral cephalosporin
Usual Dose: 400 mg (PO) q12h
Pharmacokinetic Parameters:
Peak serum level: 3.7 mcg/mL
Bioavailability: 50%
Excreted unchanged: 35%
Serum half-life (normal/ESRD): 3.1/11 hrs
Plasma protein binding: 65%

Cefoperazone (Cefobid)

Drug Class: 3rd generation cephalosporin
Usual Dose: 2 gm (IV) q12h
Pharmacokinetic Parameters:
Peak serum level: 240 mcg/mL
Bioavailability: Not applicable
Excreted unchanged: 20%
Serum half-life (normal/ESRD): 2.4/2.4 hrs
Plasma protein binding: 90%

* Resume dosing for CrCl < 10 mL/min after supplemental dose. "Usual dose" assumes normal renal and hepatic function. CrCl = creatinine clearance; CVVH = continuous veno-venous hemofiltration; HD = hemodialysis; PD = peritoneal dialysis. See pp. 252-255 for definitions/explanations, p. 1 for abbreviations

Volume of distribution (V_d): 0.17 L/kg
Primary Mode of Elimination: Hepatic
Dosage Adjustments:

CrCl ~ 40–60 mL/min	No change
CrCl ~ 10–30 mL/min	No change
CrCl < 10 mL/min	No change
Post–HD dose	None
Post–PD dose	None
Post–CVVH dose	None
Moderate hepatic insufficiency	No change
Severe hepatic insufficiency	1 gm (IV) q12h

Drug Interactions: Alcohol (disulfiram-like reaction); antiplatelet agents, heparin, thrombolytics, warfarin (↑ risk of bleeding)
Adverse Effects: Drug fever/rash. ↑ INR due to MTT side chain, but no increase in clinical bleeding. Prophylactic vitamin K unnecessary
Resistance Potential: Low
Allergic Potential: Low
Safety in Pregnancy: B
Comments: One of the few antibiotics to penetrate into an obstructed biliary tract. May be administered IM. Concentration dependent serum half life. Na$^+$ content = 1.5 mEq/g. Meningeal dose = 2 gm (IV) q8h
Cerebrospinal Fluid Penetration:
Non-inflamed meninges = 1%
Inflamed meninges = 10%
Bile Penetration: 1200%

REFERENCES:
Cunha BA: 3rd generation cephalosporins: A review. Clin Ther 14:616-52, 1992.
Klein NC, Cunha BA. Third-generation cephalosporins. Med Clin North Am 79:705-19, 1995.
Marshall WF, Blair JE. The cephalosporins. Mayo Clin Proc 74:187-95, 1999.

Cefotaxime (Claforan)

Drug Class: 3rd generation cephalosporin
Usual Dose: 2 gm (IV) q6h

Pharmacokinetic Parameters:
Peak serum level: 214 mcg/mL
Bioavailability: Not applicable
Excreted unchanged: 60%
Serum half-life (normal/ESRD): 1/15 hrs
Plasma protein binding: 37%
Volume of distribution (V_d): 0.25 L/kg
Primary Mode of Elimination: Renal
Dosage Adjustments:

CrCl ~ 40–60 mL/min	1 gm (IV) q6h
CrCl ~ 10–30 mL/min	1 gm (IV) q8h
CrCl < 10 mL/min	1 gm (IV) q12h
Post–HD dose*	1 gm (IV)
Post–PD dose	None
Post–CVVH dose*	2 gm (IV)
Moderate hepatic insufficiency	No change
Severe hepatic insufficiency	No change

Drug Interactions: None
Adverse Effects: Drug fever/rash
Resistance Potential: Low
Allergic Potential: Moderate
Safety in Pregnancy: B
Comments: Incompatible in solutions containing sodium bicarbonate, metronidazole, or aminoglycosides. Desacetyl metabolite ($t_{1/2}$ = 1.5 hrs) synergistic with cefotaxime against S. aureus/B. fragilis. Na$^+$ content = 2.2 mEq/g. Meningeal dose = 3 gm (IV) q6h
Cerebrospinal Fluid Penetration:
Non-inflamed meninges = 1%
Inflamed meninges = 10%
Bile Penetration: 75%

REFERENCES:
Brogden RN, Spencer CM. Cefotaxime: A reappraisal of its antibacterial activity and pharmacokinetic properties and a review of its therapeutic efficacy when administered twice daily for the treatment of mild to moderate infections. Drugs 53:483-510, 1987.
Klein NC, Cunha BA. Third-generation cephalosporins. Med Clin North Am 79:705-19, 1995.

Marshall WF, Blair JE. The cephalosporins. Mayo Clin Proc 74:187-95, 1999.

Patel KB, Nicolau DP, Nightingale CH, et al. Comparative serum bactericidal activities of ceftizoxime and cefotaxime against intermediately penicillin-resistant Streptococcus pneumoniae. Antimicrob Agents Chemother 40:2805-8, 1996.

Cefotetan (Cefotan)

Drug Class: 2nd generation cephalosporin (Cephamycin)
Usual Dose: 2 gm (IV) q12h
Pharmacokinetic Parameters:
Peak serum level: 237 mcg/mL
Bioavailability: Not applicable
Excreted unchanged: 75%
Serum half-life (normal/ESRD): 4/20 hrs
Plasma protein binding: 85%
Volume of distribution (V_d): 0.17 L/kg
Primary Mode of Elimination: Renal
Dosage Adjustments:

CrCl ~ 40–60 mL/min	1 gm (IV) q12h
CrCl ~ 10–30 mL/min	1 gm (IV) q24h
CrCl < 10 mL/min	1 gm (IV) q48h
Post–HD dose*	1 gm (IV)
Post–PD dose	None
Post–CVVH dose*	2 gm (IV)
Moderate hepatic insufficiency	No change
Severe hepatic insufficiency	No change

Drug Interactions: Alcohol (disulfiram-like reaction); antiplatelet agents, heparin, thrombolytics, warfarin (↑ risk of bleeding)
Adverse Effects: Drug fever/rash, hemolytic anemia. ↑ INR due to MTT side chain, but no increase in clinical bleeding
Resistance Potential: Low
Allergic Potential: Low
Safety in Pregnancy: B
Comments: Less effective than cefoxitin against B. fragilis D.O.T strains. Na⁺ content = 3.5 mEq/g

Cerebrospinal Fluid Penetration: < 10%
Bile Penetration: 20%

REFERENCES:
Moes GS, MacPherson BR. Cefotetan-induced hemolytic anemia: A case report and a review of the literature. Arch Pathol Lab Med 124:1344-6, 2000.

Ray EK, Warkentin TE, O'Hoski PL. Delayed onset of life-threatening immune hemolysis after perioperative antimicrobial prophylaxis with cefotetan. Can J Surg 43:461-2, 2000.

Stroneck D, Procter JL, Johnson J. Drug-induced hemolysis: Cefotetan-dependent hemolytic anemia mimicking an acute intravascular immune transfusion reaction. Am J Hematol 64:67-70, 2000.

Cefoxitin (Mefoxin)

Drug Class: 2nd generation cephalosporin (Cephamycin)
Usual Dose: 2 gm (IV) q6h
Pharmacokinetic Parameters:
Peak serum level: 221 mcg/mL
Bioavailability: Not applicable
Excreted unchanged: 80%
Serum half-life (normal/ESRD): 1/21 hrs
Plasma protein binding: 75%
Volume of distribution (V_d): 0.12 L/kg
Primary Mode of Elimination: Renal
Dosage Adjustments:

CrCl ~ 40–60 mL/min	1 gm (IV) q8h
CrCl ~ 10–30 mL/min	1 gm (IV) q12h
CrCl < 10 mL/min	1 gm (IV) q24h
Post–HD dose*	1 gm (IV)
Post–PD dose	None
Post–CVVH dose*	2 gm (IV)
Moderate hepatic insufficiency	No change
Severe hepatic insufficiency	No change

Drug Interactions: None
Adverse Effects: Drug fever/rash
Resistance Potential: Low
Allergic Potential: Low

---

* Resume dosing for CrCl < 10 mL/min after supplemental dose. "Usual dose" assumes normal renal and hepatic function. CrCl = creatinine clearance; CVVH = continuous veno-venous hemofiltration; HD = hemodialysis; PD = peritoneal dialysis. See pp. 252-255 for definitions/explanations, p. 1 for abbreviations

Safety in Pregnancy: B
Comments: Effective against B. fragilis, including D.O.T. strains B. distasonis, B. ovatus, B. thetiaotamicron. Na⁺ content = 2.3 mEq/g
Cerebrospinal Fluid Penetration: < 10%
Bile Penetration: 250%

REFERENCES:
Hansen EA, Cunha BA. Cefoxitin. Antibiotics for Clinicians 5:33-41, 2001.
Donowitz GR, Mandell GL. Beta-lactam antibiotics. N Engl J Med 318:419-26 and 318:490-500, 1993.
Marshall WF Blair JE. The cephalosporins. Mayo Clin Proc 74:187-95, 1999.

Cefpodoxime (Vantin)

Drug Class: 3rd generation oral cephalosporin
Usual Dose: 200 mg (PO) q12h
Pharmacokinetic Parameters:
Peak serum level: 2.3 mcg/mL
Bioavailability: 46%
Excreted unchanged: 80%
Serum half-life (normal/ESRD): 2.3/2.6 hrs
Plasma protein binding: 20%
Volume of distribution (V_d): 0.9 L/kg
Primary Mode of Elimination: Renal
Dosage Adjustments:

CrCl ~ 40–60 mL/min	No change
CrCl ~ 10–30 mL/min	200 mg (PO) q24h
CrCl < 10 mL/min	200 mg (PO) q48h
Post-HD dose*	200 mg (PO)
Post-PD dose	None
Post-CVVH dose*	200 mg (PO)
Moderate hepatic insufficiency	No change
Severe hepatic insufficiency	No change

Drug Interactions: None
Adverse Effects: Drug fever/rash, pulmonary infiltrates with eosinophilia, hepatotoxicity
Resistance Potential: Low
Allergic Potential: High
Safety in Pregnancy: B

Comments: Only oral 3rd generation cephalosporin active against S. aureus (MSSA)
Cerebrospinal Fluid Penetration: < 10%
Bile Penetration: 100%

REFERENCES:
Adam D, Bergogne-Berezin E, Jones RN. Symposium on cefpodoxime proxetil: A new third generation oral cephalosporin. Drugs 42:1-66, 1991.
Cohen R. Clinical experience with cefpodoxime proxetil in acute otitis media. Pediatr Infect Dis J 14:S12-8, 1995.
Schatz BS, Karavokiros KT, Taeubel MA, et al. Comparison of cefprozil, cefpodoxime proxetil, loracarbef, cefixime, and ceftibuten. Ann Pharmacother 30:258-68, 1996.

Cefprozil (Cefzil)

Drug Class: 2nd generation oral cephalosporin
Usual Dose: 500 mg (PO) q12h
Pharmacokinetic Parameters:
Peak serum level: 10 mcg/mL
Bioavailability: 95%
Excreted unchanged: 65%
Serum half-life (normal/ESRD): 1.3/6 hrs
Plasma protein binding: 40%
Volume of distribution (V_d): 0.65 L/kg
Primary Mode of Elimination: Renal
Dosage Adjustments:

CrCl ~ 40–60 mL/min	No change
CrCl ~ 10–30 mL/min	500 mg (PO) q24h
CrCl < 10 mL/min	500 mg (PO) q24h
Post-HD dose*	500 mg (PO)
Post-PD dose	None
Post-CVVH dose*	500 mg (PO)
Moderate hepatic insufficiency	No change
Severe hepatic insufficiency	No change

Drug Interactions: None
Adverse Effects: Drug fever/rash
Resistance Potential: Low
Allergic Potential: Low
Safety in Pregnancy: B

---

* Resume dosing for CrCl < 10 mL/min after supplemental dose. "Usual dose" assumes normal renal and hepatic function. CrCl = creatinine clearance; CVVH = continuous venovenous hemofiltration; HD = hemodialysis; PD = peritoneal dialysis. See pp. 252-255 for definitions/explanations, p. 1 for abbreviations

Comments: Penetrates oral/respiratory secretions well
Cerebrospinal Fluid Penetration: < 10%

REFERENCES:
Cunha BA. New antibiotics for the treatment of acute exacerbations of chronic bronchitis. Adv Ther 13:313-23, 1996.
Gainer RB 2nd. Cefprozil: A new cephalosporin; its use in various clinical trials. South Med J 88:338-46, 1995.
Marshall WF Blair JE. The cephalosporins. Mayo Clin Proc 74:187-95, 1999.
Schatz BS, Karavokiros KT, Taeubel MA, et al. Comparison of cefprozil, cefpodoxime, proxetil, loracarbef, cefixime, and ceftibuten. Ann Pharmacother 30:258-68, 1996.

Ceftazidime (Fortaz, Tazicef, Tazidime)

Drug Class: 3rd generation cephalosporin
Usual Dose: 2 gm (IV) q8h
Pharmacokinetic Parameters:
Peak serum level: 120 mcg/mL
Bioavailability: Not applicable
Excreted unchanged: 85%
Serum half-life (normal/ESRD): 1.8/21 hrs
Plasma protein binding: 17%
Volume of distribution (V_d): 0.36 L/kg
Primary Mode of Elimination: Renal
Dosage Adjustments:

CrCl ~ 40–60 mL/min	1 gm (IV) q8h
CrCl ~ 10–30 mL/min	1 gm (IV) q12h
CrCl < 10 mL/min	1 gm (IV) q24h
Post–HD dose*	1 gm (IV)
Post–PD dose	None
Post–CVVH dose*	2 gm (IV)
Moderate hepatic insufficiency	No change
Severe hepatic insufficiency	No change

Drug Interactions: None
Adverse Effects: Drug fever/rash
Resistance Potential: High (Enterobacter, Klebsiella, P. aeruginosa)
Allergic Potential: High
Safety in Pregnancy: B
Comments: Incompatible in solutions containing vancomycin or aminoglycosides. Use increases prevalence of MRSA. Inducer of E. coli/Klebsiella ESBLs. Na^+ content = 2.3 mEq/g. Meningeal dose = 2 gm (IV) q8h
Cerebrospinal Fluid Penetration:
Non-inflamed meninges = 1%
Inflamed meninges = 20%
Bile Penetration: 50%

REFERENCES:
Briscoe-Dwyer L. Ceftazidime. Antibiotics for Clinicians 1:41-8, 1997.
Klein NC, Cunha BA. Third-generation cephalosporins. Med Clin North Am 79:705-19, 1995.
Marshall WF, Blair JE. The cephalosporins. Mayo Clin Proc 74:187-95, 1999.
Nicolau DP, Nightingale CH, Banevicius MA, et al. Serum bactericidal activity of ceftazidime: Continuous infusion versus intermittent injections. Antimicrob Agents Chemother 40:61-4, 1996.
Owens JC, Jr, Ambrose PG, Quintiliani R. Ceftazidime to cefepime formulary switch: Pharmacodynamic rationale. Conn Med 225-7, 1997.
Rains CP, Bryson HM, Peters DH. Ceftazidime: An update of its antibacterial activity, pharmacokinetic properties, and therapeutic efficacy. Drugs 49:577-617, 1995.

Ceftibuten (Cedax)

Drug Class: 3rd generation oral cephalosporin
Usual Dose: 400 mg (PO) q24h
Pharmacokinetic Parameters:
Peak serum level: 15 mcg/mL
Bioavailability: 80%
Excreted unchanged: 70%
Serum half-life (normal/ESRD): 2.4/22 hrs
Plasma protein binding: 65%
Volume of distribution (V_d): 0.2 L/kg
Primary Mode of Elimination: Renal
Dosage Adjustments:

CrCl ~ 40–60 mL/min	200 mg (PO) q24h
CrCl ~ 10–30 mL/min	200 mg (PO) q24h
CrCl < 10 mL/min	100 mg (PO) q24h

---

* Resume dosing for CrCl < 10 mL/min after supplemental dose. "Usual dose" assumes normal renal and hepatic function. CrCl = creatinine clearance; CVVH = continuous veno-venous hemofiltration; HD = hemodialysis; PD = peritoneal dialysis. See pp. 252-255 for definitions/explanations, p. 1 for abbreviations

Post–HD dose*	200 mg (PO)
Post–PD dose	None
Post–CVVH dose*	400 mg (PO)
Moderate hepatic insufficiency	No change
Severe hepatic insufficiency	No change

Drug Interactions: None
Adverse Effects: Drug fever/rash
Resistance Potential: High (S. pneumoniae)
Allergic Potential: High
Safety in Pregnancy: B
Comments: Least anti–S. pneumoniae activity among oral 3rd generation cephalosporins
Cerebrospinal Fluid Penetration: < 10%

REFERENCES:
Guay DR. Ceftibuten: A new expanded-spectrum oral cephalosporin. Ann Pharmacother 31:1022-33, 1997.
Owens RC Jr, Nightingale CH, Nicolau DP. Ceftibuten: An overview. Pharmacother 17:707-20, 1997.
Wiseman LR, Balfour JA. Ceftibuten: A review of its antibacterial activity, pharmacokinetic properties and clinical efficacy. Drugs 47:784-808, 1994.

Ceftizoxime (Cefizox)

Drug Class: 3rd generation cephalosporin
Usual Dose: 2 gm (IV) q8h
Pharmacokinetic Parameters:
Peak serum level: 132 mcg/mL
Bioavailability: Not applicable
Excreted unchanged: 90%
Serum half-life (normal/ESRD): 1.4/35 hrs
Plasma protein binding: 40%
Volume of distribution (V_d): 0.32 L/kg
Primary Mode of Elimination: Renal
Dosage Adjustments:

CrCl ~ 40–60 mL/min	1 gm (IV) q8h
CrCl ~ 10–30 mL/min	1 gm (IV) q12h
CrCl < 10 mL/min	1 gm (IV) q24h
Post–HD dose*	1 gm (IV)

Post–PD dose	None
Post–CVVH dose*	2 gm (IV)
Moderate hepatic insufficiency	No change
Severe hepatic insufficiency	No change

Drug Interactions: None
Adverse Effects: Drug fever/rash
Resistance Potential: Low
Allergic Potential: High
Safety in Pregnancy: B
Comments: Na+ content = 2.6 mEq/g.
Meningeal dose = 3 gm (IV) q6h
Cerebrospinal Fluid Penetration:
Non-inflamed meninges = 1%
Inflamed meninges = 10%
Bile Penetration: 50%

REFERENCES:
Klein NC, Cunha BA. Third-generation cephalosporins. Med Clin North Am 79:705-19, 1995.
Donowitz GR, Mandell GL. Beta-lactam antibiotics. N Engl J Med 318.419-26 and 318.490-500, 1993.
Marshall WF Blair JE. The cephalosporins. Mayo Clin Proc 74:187-95, 1999.

Ceftriaxone (Rocephin)

Drug Class: 3rd generation cephalosporin
Usual Dose: 1-2 gm (IV) q24h
Pharmacokinetic Parameters:
Peak serum level: 123-223 mcg/mL
Bioavailability: Not applicable
Excreted unchanged: 65%
Serum half-life (normal/ESRD): 8/18 hrs
Plasma protein binding: 90%
Volume of distribution (V_d): 0.3 L/kg
Primary Mode of Elimination: Renal/hepatic
Dosage Adjustments:

CrCl ~ 40–60 mL/min	No change
CrCl ~ 10–30 mL/min	No change
CrCl < 10 mL/min	No change
Post–HD dose	None

---

* Resume dosing for CrCl < 10 mL/min after supplemental dose. "Usual dose" assumes normal renal and hepatic function. CrCl = creatinine clearance; CVVH = continuous veno venous hemofiltration; HD = hemodialysis; PD = peritoneal dialysis. See pp. 252-255 for definitions/explanations, p. 1 for abbreviations

Post–PD dose	None
Post–CVVH dose*	2 gm (IV)
Moderate hepatic insufficiency	No change
Severe hepatic insufficiency	No change

Drug Interactions: None
Adverse Effects: Drug fever/rash, irritative diarrhea, pseudo-biliary lithiasis, may interfere with platelet aggregation
Resistance Potential: Low
Allergic Potential: High
Safety in Pregnancy: B. Avoid near term in 3rd trimester (↑ incidence of kernicterus in newborns)
Comments: May be given IV or IM. Incompatible in solutions containing vancomycin. Na+ content = 2.6 mEq/g. Meningeal dose = 2 gm (IV) q12h
Cerebrospinal Fluid Penetration:
Non-inflamed meninges = 1%
Inflamed meninges = 10%
Bile Penetration: 500%

REFERENCES:
Cunha BA, Klein NC. The selection and use of cephalosporins: A review. Adv Ther 12:83-101, 1995.
Grassi C. Ceftriaxone. Antibiotics for Clinicians 2:49-57, 1998.
Klein NC, Cunha BA. Third -generation cephalosporins. Med Clin North Am 79:705-19, 1995.
Marshall WF, Blair JE. The cephalosporins. Mayo Clin Proc 74:187-95, 1999.
Schaad UB, Suter S, Gianella-Borradori A, et al. A comparison of ceftriaxone and cefuroxime for the treatment of bacterial meningitis in children. N Engl J Med 322:141-7, 1990.

Cefuroxime (Kefurox, Zinacef, Ceftin)

Drug Class: 2nd generation IV/oral cephalosporin
Usual Dose: 1.5 gm (IV) q8h; 500 mg (PO) q12h
Pharmacokinetic Parameters:
Peak serum level: 125 (IV)/70 (PO) mcg/mL

Bioavailability: 52 %
Excreted unchanged: 90%
Serum half-life (normal/ESRD): 1.2/17 hrs
Plasma protein binding: 50%
Volume of distribution (V_d): 0.15 L/kg
Primary Mode of Elimination: Renal
Dosage Adjustments:

CrCl ~ 40–60 mL/min	750 mg (IV) q8h 250 mg (PO) q12h
CrCl ~ 10–30 mL/min	750 mg (IV) q12h 250 mg (PO) q24h
CrCl < 10 mL/min	750 mg (IV) q24h 250 mg (PO) q48h
Post–HD dose*	750 mg (IV) 250 mg (PO)
Post–PD dose	None
Post–CVVH dose*	1.5 gm (IV) 500 mg (PO)
Moderate hepatic insufficiency	No change
Severe hepatic insufficiency	No change

Drug Interactions: None
Adverse Effects: Drug fever/rash
Resistance Potential: Low
Allergic Potential: High
Safety in Pregnancy: B
Comments: Oral preparation penetrates oral/respiratory secretions well. Na+ content (IV preparation) = 2.4 mEq/g. Do not use for meningitis prophylaxis (H. influenzae bacteremia) or therapy
Cerebrospinal Fluid Penetration: < 10%

REFERENCES:
Gentry LO, Zeluff BJ, Cooley DA. Antibiotic prophylaxis in open-heart surgery: A comparison of cefamandole, cefuroxime, and cefazolin. Ann Thorac Surg 46:167-71, 1988.
Marshall WF, Blair JE. The cephalosporins. Mayo Clin Proc 74:187-95, 1999.
Perry Cm, Brogden RN. Cefuroxime axetil. A review of its antibacterial activity, pharmacokinetic properties, and therapeutic efficacy. Drugs 52:125-58, 1996.

---

* Resume dosing for CrCl < 10 mL/min after supplemental dose. "Usual dose" assumes normal renal and hepatic function. CrCl = creatinine clearance; CVVH = continuous veno-venous hemofiltration; HD = hemodialysis; PD = peritoneal dialysis. See pp. 252-255 for definitions/explanations, p. 1 for abbreviations

Cephalexin (Keflex)

Drug Class: 1st generation oral cephalosporin
Usual Dose: 500 mg (PO) q6h
Pharmacokinetic Parameters:
Peak serum level: 18 mcg/mL
Bioavailability: 99%
Excreted unchanged: 98%
Serum half-life (normal/ESRD): 0.7/16 hrs
Plasma protein binding: 10%
Volume of distribution (V_d): 0.35 L/kg
Primary Mode of Elimination: Renal
Dosage Adjustments:

CrCl ~ 40–60 mL/min	No change
CrCl ~ 10–30 mL/min	250 mg (PO) q8h
CrCl < 10 mL/min	250 mg (PO) q12h
Post–HD dose*	250 mg (PO)
Post–PD dose	None
Post–CVVH dose*	500 mg (PO)
Moderate hepatic insufficiency	No change
Severe hepatic insufficiency	No change

Drug Interactions: None
Adverse Effects: Drug fever/rash
Resistance Potential: Low
Allergic Potential: High
Safety in Pregnancy: B
Comments: Highly active against S. aureus (MSSA) and Group A streptococci. Limited activity against H. influenzae
Cerebrospinal Fluid Penetration: < 10%
Bile Penetration: 200%

REFERENCES:
Chow M, Quintiliani R, Cunha BA, et al. Pharmacokinetics of high dose oral cephalosporins. J Pharmacol 19:185-194, 1979.
Donowitz GR, Mandell GL. Beta-lactam antibiotics. N Engl J Med 318:419-26 and 318:490-500, 1993.
Marshall WF Blair JE. The cephalosporins. Mayo Clin Proc 74:187-95, 1999.
Smith GH. Oral cephalosporins in perspective. DICP 24:45-51, 1990.

Chloramphenicol (Chloromycetin)

Drug Class: Does not belong to specific class
Usual Dose: 500 mg (IV/PO) q6h
Pharmacokinetic Parameters:
Peak serum level: 9 mcg/mL
Bioavailability: 90%
Excreted unchanged: 10%
Serum half-life (normal/ESRD): 2.5/3 hrs
Plasma protein binding: 80%
Volume of distribution (V_d): 1 L/kg
Primary Mode of Elimination: Hepatic
Dosage Adjustments:

CrCl ~ 40–60 mL/min	No change
CrCl ~ 10–30 mL/min	No change
CrCl < 10 mL/min	No change
Post–HD dose	None
Post–PD dose	None
Post–CVVH dose	None
Moderate hepatic insufficiency	No change
Severe hepatic insufficiency	250 mg (IV/PO) q6h

Drug Interactions: Barbiturates (↑ barbiturate effect, ↓ chloramphenicol effect); cyclophosphamide (↑ cyclophosphamide toxicity); cyanocobalamin, iron (↓ response to interacting drug); warfarin (↑ INR); phenytoin (↑ phenytoin toxicity); rifabutin, rifampin (↓ chloramphenicol levels); sulfonylureas (↑ sulfonylurea effect, hypoglycemia)
Adverse Effects:
Dose–related bone marrow suppression
Reversible. Bone marrow aspirate shows vacuolated WBCs ("chloramphenicol effect," not toxicity). Does not precede aplastic anemia
Idiosyncratic bone marrow toxicity
Irreversible aplastic anemia. May occur after only one dose; monitoring with serial CBCs is useless. Very rare. Usually associated with IM, intraocular, or oral administration. Rarely, if

ever, with IV chloramphenicol

Resistance Potential: Low

Allergic Potential: Low

Safety in Pregnancy: C

Comments: Incompatible in solutions containing diphenylhydantoin, methylprednisone, aminophylline, ampicillin, gentamicin, erythromycin, vancomycin. Dose-related marrow suppression is common, but reversible. Hepatic toxicity related to prolonged/high doses (> 4 gm/d). Oral administration results in higher serum levels than IV administration. Do not administer IM. Chloramphenicol is inactivated in bile. Urinary concentrations are therapeutically ineffective. Na^+ content = 2.25 mEq/g.

Meningeal dose = usual dose

Cerebrospinal Fluid Penetration:

Non-inflamed meninges = 90%

Inflamed meninges = 90%

REFERENCES:

Cunha BA. New uses of older antibiotics. Postgrad Med 100:68-88, 1997.

Feder HM Jr, Osier C, Maderazo EG. Chloramphenicol: A review of its use in clinical practice. Rev Infect Dis 3:479- 91, 1981.

Kasten MJ. Clindamycin, metronidazole, and chloramphenicol. Mayo Clin Proc 74:825-33, 1999.

Smilack JD, Wilson WE, Cocerill FR 3rd. Tetracycline, chloramphenicol, erythromycin, clindamycin, and metronidazole. Mayo Clin Proc 66:1270-80, 1991.

Tunkel AR, Wispelwey B, Scheld M. Bacterial meningitis: Recent advances in pathophysiology and treatment. Ann Intern Med 112:610-23, 1990.

Ciprofloxacin (Cipro)

Drug Class: Fluoroquinolone

Usual Dose: 400 mg (IV) q12h; 500-750 mg (PO) q12h

Pharmacokinetic Parameters:

Peak serum level: 4.6 (IV)/2.8 (PO) mcg/mL

Bioavailability: 70%

Excreted unchanged: 70%

Serum half-life (normal/ESRD): 4/8 hrs

Plasma protein binding: 30%

Volume of distribution (V_d): 2.5 L/kg

Primary Mode of Elimination: Renal

Dosage Adjustments:

CrCl ~ 40–60 mL/min	200 mg (IV) q12h; 250 mg (PO) q12h
CrCl ~ 10–30 mL/min	200 mg (IV) q24h; 250 mg (PO) q24h
CrCl < 10 mL/min	200 mg (IV) q48h; 250 mg (PO) q48h
Post–HD dose	None
Post–PD dose	None
Post–CVVH dose*	200 mg (IV); 250 mg (PO)
Moderate hepatic insufficiency	No change
Severe hepatic insufficiency	No change

Drug Interactions: Al^{++}, Ca^{++}, Fe^{++}, Mg^{++}, Zn^{++} antacids, citrate/citric acid, dairy products (↓ absorption of ciprofloxacin only if taken together); caffeine, cyclosporine, theophylline (↑ interacting drug levels); cimetidine (↑ ciprofloxacin levels); foscarnet (↑ risk of seizures); insulin, oral hypoglycemics (slight ↑ or ↓ in blood glucose); NSAIDs (may ↑ risk of seizures/CNS stimulation); phenytoin (↑ or ↓ phenytoin levels); probenecid (↑ ciprofloxacin levels); warfarin (↑ INR)

Adverse Effects: Drug fever/rash, seizures, Achilles tendon rupture/tendinitis

Resistance Potential: High (P. aeruginosa, S. pneumoniae). Use increases prevalence of MRSA and extended-spectrum beta-lactamases (ESBLs)

Allergic Potential: Low

Safety in Pregnancy: C

Comments: Enteral feeding decreases ciprofloxacin absorption ≥ 30%. Avoid in patients with severe renal insufficiency or CNS/seizure disorders. Administer 2 hours before or after H_2 antagonists, omeprazole, sucralfate, calcium, iron, zinc, multivitamins, or aluminum/magnesium containing medications

Cerebrospinal Fluid Penetration:

Non-inflamed meninges = 10%

Inflamed meninges = 26%

---

* Resume dosing for CrCl < 10 mL/min after supplemental dose. "Usual dose" assumes normal renal and hepatic function. CrCl = creatinine clearance; CVVH = continuous veno-venous hemofiltration; HD = hemodialysis; PD = peritoneal dialysis. See pp. 252-255 for definitions/explanations, p. 1 for abbreviations

Bile Penetration: 3000%

REFERENCES:
Cunha BA: The fluoroquinolones in urinary tract
  infections: A review. Adv Ther 16:277-96, 1994.
Cunha BA. Ciprofloxacin resistant Streptococcus
  pneumoniae not fluoroquinolone resistant
  Streptococcus pneumoniae. Infect Dis Pract 24:30-
  31, 2000.
Davis R, Markham A, Balfour JA. Ciprofloxacin: An
  updated review of its pharmacology, therapeutic
  efficacy, and tolerability. Drugs 51:1019-74, 1996.
Sanders CC. Ciprofloxacin: In vitro activity, mechanism
  of action, resistance. Rev Infect Dis 10:516-27, 1998.
Walker RC, Wright AJ. The fluoroquinolones. Mayo
  Clin Proc 66:1249-59, 1991.

Clarithromycin (Biaxin)

Drug Class: Macrolide
Usual Dose: 500 mg (PO) q12h
Pharmacokinetic Parameters:
Peak serum level: 3 mcg/mL
Bioavailability: 50%
Excreted unchanged: 20%
Serum half-life (normal/ESRD): 4/4 hrs
Plasma protein binding: 70%
Volume of distribution (V_d): 3 L/kg
Primary Mode of Elimination: Hepatic
Dosage Adjustments:

CrCl ~ 40–60 mL/min	No change
CrCl ~ 10–30 mL/min	No change
CrCl < 10 mL/min	250 mg (PO) q12h
Post–HD dose	None
Post–PD dose	None
Post–CVVH dose	None
Moderate hepatic insufficiency	No change
Severe hepatic insufficiency	No change

Drug Interactions: Amiodarone, procainamide,
sotalol, astemizole, terfenadine, cisapride,
pimozide (may ↑ QT interval, torsade de
pointes); carbamazepine (↑ carbamazepine
levels, nystagmus, nausea, vomiting, diarrhea);

cimetidine, digoxin, ergot alkaloids, midazolam,
triazolam, phenytoin, ritonavir, tacrolimus,
valproic acid (↑ interacting drug levels);
clozapine, corticosteroids (not studied);
cyclosporine (↑ cyclosporine levels with toxicity);
efavirenz (↓ clarithromycin levels); rifabutin,
rifampin (↓ clarithromycin levels, ↑ interacting
drug levels); statins (↑ risk of rhabdomyolysis);
theophylline (↑ theophylline levels, nausea,
vomiting, seizures, apnea); warfarin (↑ INR);
zidovudine (↓ zidovudine levels)
Adverse Effects: Nausea, vomiting, GI upset,
irritative diarrhea, abdominal pain. May ↑ QT_c;
avoid with other medications that prolong the
QT_c interval and in patients with cardiac
arrhythmias/heart block
Resistance Potential: Low to moderate
(S. pneumoniae, H. influenzae)
Allergic Potential: Low
Safety in Pregnancy: C
Comments: Peculiar taste of "aluminum sand"
sensation on swallowing
Cerebrospinal Fluid Penetration: < 10%
Bile Penetration: 7000%

REFERENCES:
Alvarez-Elcoro S, Enzler MJ. The macrolides:
  Erythromycin, clarithromycin and azithromycin. Mayo
  Clin Proc 4:613- 34, 1999.
Benson CA, Williams PL, Cohn DL, and the ACTG
  196/CPCRA 009 Study Team. Clarithromycin or
  rifabutin alone or in combination for primary
  prophylaxis of Mycobacterium avium complex disease
  in patients with AIDS: A randomized, double-blinded,
  placebo-controlled trial. J Infect Dis 181(4):1289-97,
  2000.
Chaisson RE, Keiser P, Pierce M, et al. Clarithromycin
  and ethambutol with or without clofazimine for the
  treatment of bacteremic Mycobacterium avium
  complex disease in patients with HIV infection. AIDS
  11:311-317, 1997.
McConnell SA, Amsden GW. Review and comparison of
  advanced-generation macrolides clarithromycin and
  dirithromycin. Pharmacotherapy 19:404-15, 1999.
Periti P, Mazzei T. Clarithromycin: Pharmacokinetic and
  pharmacodynamic interrelationships and dosage
  regimen. J Chemother 11:11-27, 1999.
Rodvold KA. Clinical pharmacokinetics of clarithromycin.
  Clin Pharmacokinet 37:385-98, 1999.
Schlossberg D. Azithromycin and clarithromycin. Med
  Clin North Am 79:803-16, 1995.
Tartaglione TA. Therapeutic options for the
  management and prevention of Mycobacterium avium

---

* Resume dosing for CrCl < 10 mL/min after supplemental dose. "Usual dose" assumes normal renal and
hepatic function. CrCl = creatinine clearance; CVVH = continuous venovenous hemofiltration; HD =
hemodialysis; PD = peritoneal dialysis. See pp. 252-255 for definitions/explanations, p. 1 for abbreviations

complex infection in patients with acquired immunodeficiency syndrome. Pharmacotherapy 16:171-82, 1996.

Clarithromycin XL (Biaxin XL)

Drug Class: Macrolide
Usual Dose: 1 gm (PO) q24h
Pharmacokinetic Parameters:
Peak serum level: 3 mcg/mL
Bioavailability: 50%
Excreted unchanged: 20%
Serum half-life (normal/ESRD): 4/4 hrs
Plasma protein binding: 70%
Volume of distribution (V_d): 3 L/kg
Primary Mode of Elimination: Hepatic
Dosage Adjustments:

CrCl ~ 40–60 mL/min	500 mg (PO) q24h
CrCl ~ 10–30 mL/min	500 mg (PO) q24h
CrCl < 10 mL/min	500 mg (PO) q48h
Post–HD dose	None
Post–PD dose	None
Post–CVVH dose	None
Moderate hepatic insufficiency	No change
Severe hepatic insufficiency	No change

Drug Interactions: Amiodarone, procainamide, sotalol, astemizole, terfenadine, cisapride, pimozide (may ↑ QT interval, torsade de pointes); carbamazepine (↑ carbamazepine levels, nystagmus, nausea, vomiting, diarrhea); cimetidine, digoxin, ergot alkaloids, midazolam, triazolam, phenytoin, ritonavir, tacrolimus, valproic acid (↑ interacting drug levels); clozapine, corticosteroids (not studied); cyclosporine (↑ cyclosporine levels with toxicity); efavirenz (↓ clarithromycin levels); rifabutin, rifampin (↓ clarithromycin levels, ↑ interacting drug levels); statins (↑ risk of rhabdomyolysis); theophylline (↑ theophylline levels, nausea, vomiting, seizures, apnea); warfarin (↑ INR); zidovudine (↓ zidovudine levels)

Adverse Effects: Few/no GI symptoms. May ↑ QT_c; avoid with other medications that prolong the QT_c interval and in patients with cardiac arrhythmias/heart block
Resistance Potential: Low to moderate (S. pneumoniae, H. influenzae)
Allergic Potential: Low
Safety in Pregnancy: C
Comments: Two 500 mg tablets of XL preparation permits once daily dosing and decreases GI intolerance
Cerebrospinal Fluid Penetration: < 10%
Bile Penetration: 7000%

REFERENCES:
Adler JL, Jannetti W, Schneider D, et al. Phase III, randomized, double-blind study of clarithromycin extended-release and immediate-release formulations in the treatment of patients with acute exacerbation of chronic bronchitis. Clin Ther 22:1410-20, 2000.
Anzueto A, Fisher CL Jr, Busman T. Comparison of the efficacy of extended-release clarithromycin tablets and amoxicillin/clavulanate tablets in the treatment of acute exacerbation of chronic bronchitis. Clin Ther 23:72-86, 2000.
Laine L, Estrada R, Trujillo M, et al. Once-daily therapy for H. pylori infection: Randomized comparison of four regimens. Am J Gastroenterol 94:962-6, 1999.

Clindamycin (Cleocin)

Drug Class: Lincosamide
Usual Dose: 600 mg (IV) q8h; 300 mg (PO) q8h
Pharmacokinetic Parameters:
Peak serum level: 10 mcg/mL
Bioavailability: 90%
Excreted unchanged: 10%
Serum half-life (normal/ESRD): 2.4/2.4 hrs
Plasma protein binding: 90%
Volume of distribution (V_d): 1 L/kg
Primary Mode of Elimination: Hepatic
Dosage Adjustments:

CrCl ~ 40–60 mL/min	No change
CrCl ~ 10–30 mL/min	No change
CrCl < 10 mL/min	No change
Post–HD dose	None
Post–PD dose	None

---

* Resume dosing for CrCl < 10 mL/min after supplemental dose. "Usual dose" assumes normal renal and hepatic function. CrCl = creatinine clearance; CVVH = continuous veno-venous hemofiltration; HD = hemodialysis; PD = peritoneal dialysis. See pp. 252-255 for definitions/explanations, p. 1 for abbreviations

Post–CVVH dose	None
Moderate hepatic insufficiency	No change
Severe hepatic insufficiency	300 mg (IV) q8h 150 mg (PO)

Drug Interactions: Muscle relaxants, neuromuscular blockers (↑ apnea, respiratory paralysis); kaolin (↓ clindamycin absorption); theophylline (↑ theophylline levels, seizures)
Adverse Effects: C. difficile diarrhea/colitis, neuromuscular blockade
Resistance Potential: Low
Allergic Potential: Low
Safety in Pregnancy: B
Comments: C. difficile diarrhea more common with PO vs. IV clindamycin. Anti-spasmodics contraindicated in C. difficile diarrhea
Cerebrospinal Fluid Penetration: < 10%
Bile Penetration: 300%

REFERENCES:
Falagas ME, Gorbach SL. Clindamycin and metronidazole. Med Clin North Am 79:845-67, 1995.
Kasten MJ. Clindamycin, metronidazole, and chloramphenicol. Mayo Clin Proc 74:825-33, 1999.
Klepser ME, Nicolau DP, Quintiliani R, et al. Bactericidal activity of low-dose clindamycin administered at 8- and 12-hour intervals against Streptococcus pneumoniae and Bacteroides fragilis. Antimicrob Agents Chemotherap 41:630-5, 1997.

Cycloserine (Seromycin)

Drug Class: Anti-TB drug
Usual Dose: 250 mg (PO) q12h
Pharmacokinetic Parameters:
Peak serum level: 10 mcg/mL
Bioavailability: 90%
Excreted unchanged: 65%
Serum half-life (normal/ESRD): 0.5 hrs/no data
Plasma protein binding: No data
Volume of distribution (V_d): 0.2 L/kg
Primary Mode of Elimination: Renal
Dosage Adjustments:

CrCl ~ 40–60 mL/min	No change
CrCl ~ 10–30 mL/min	250 mg (PO) q24h

CrCl < 10 mL/min	250 mg (PO) q48h
Post–HD dose	None
Post–PD dose	None
Post–CVVH dose	None
Moderate hepatic insufficiency	No change
Severe hepatic insufficiency	No change

Drug Interactions: Alcohol (seizures); ethambutol, ethionamide (drowsiness, dizziness); phenytoin (↑ phenytoin levels)
Adverse Effects: Peripheral neuropathy, seizures (dose related), psychosis/delirium
Resistance Potential: Low
Allergic Potential: Low
Safety in Pregnancy: C
Comments: Avoid in patients with seizures. Ethambutol, ethionamide, or ethanol may increase CNS toxicity.
Meningeal dose = usual dose
Cerebrospinal Fluid Penetration:
Non-inflamed meninges = 90%
Inflamed meninges = 90%

REFERENCES:
Davidson PT, Le HQ. Drug treatment of tuberculosis - 1992. Drugs 43:651-73, 1992.
Drugs for tuberculosis. Med Lett Drugs Ther 35:99-101,1993.
Iseman MD. Treatment of multidrug resistant tuberculosis. N Engl J Med 329:784-91, 1993.

Dapsone

Drug Class: Antiparasitic (PABA antagonist)
Usual Dose: 100 mg (PO) q24h
Pharmacokinetic Parameters:
Peak serum level: 1.8 mcg/mL
Bioavailability: 85%
Excreted unchanged: 10%
Serum half-life (normal/ESRD): 25/30 hrs
Plasma protein binding: 80%
Volume of distribution (V_d): 1.2 L/kg
Primary Mode of Elimination: Hepatic/renal

---

* Resume dosing for CrCl < 10 mL/min after supplemental dose. "Usual dose" assumes normal renal and hepatic function. CrCl = creatinine clearance, CVVH = continuous veno venous hemofiltration; HD = hemodialysis; PD = peritoneal dialysis. See pp. 252-255 for definitions/explanations, p. 1 for abbreviations

Dosage Adjustments:

CrCl ~ 40–60 mL/min	No change
CrCl ~ 10–30 mL/min	No change
CrCl < 10 mL/min	No change
Post–HD dose	None
Post–PD dose	None
Post–CVVH dose	None
Moderate hepatic insufficiency	No change
Severe hepatic insufficiency	No information

Drug Interactions: Didanosine (↓ dapsone absorption); oral contraceptives (↓ oral contraceptive effect); pyrimethamine, zidovudine (↑ bone marrow suppression); rifabutin, rifampin (↓ dapsone levels); trimethoprim (↑ dapsone and trimethoprim levels, methemoglobinemia)
Adverse Effects: Drug fever/rash, nausea, vomiting, hemolytic anemia in G6PD deficiency, methemoglobinemia
Resistance Potential: Low
Allergic Potential: High
Safety in Pregnancy: C
Comments: Useful in sulfa (SMX) allergic patients. Avoid, if possible, in G6PD deficiency or hemoglobin M deficiency

REFERENCES:
El-Sadr WM, Murphy RI, Yurik TM, et al. Atovaquone compared with dapsone to the prevention of Pneumocystis carinii in patients with HIV infection who cannot tolerate trimethoprim, sulfonamides, or both. N Engl J Med 339:1889-95, 1998.
Medina I, Mills J, Leoung G, et al. Oral therapy for Pneumocystis carinii pneumonia in the acquired immunodeficiency syndrome. A controlled trial of trimethoprim-sulfamethoxazole versus trimethoprim-dapsone. N Engl J Med 323:776-82, 1990.
Podzamczer D, Salazar A, Jiminez J, et al. Intermittent trimethoprim-sulfamethoxazole compared with dapsone-pyrimethamine for the simultaneous primary prophylaxis of Pneumocystis pneumonia and toxoplasmosis in patients infected with HIV. Ann Intern Med 122:755-61, 1995.

Delavirdine (Rescriptor)

Drug Class: Antiretroviral NNRTI (non-nucleoside reverse transcriptase inhibitor)
Usual Dose: 400 mg (PO) q8h
Pharmacokinetic Parameters:
Peak serum level: 30 mcg/mL
Bioavailability: 85%
Excreted unchanged: 5%
Serum half-life (normal/ESRD): 5.8 hrs/no data
Plasma protein binding: 98%
Volume of distribution (V_d): 0.5 L/kg
Primary Mode of Elimination: Hepatic
Dosage Adjustments:

CrCl ~ 40–60 mL/min	No change
CrCl ~ 10–30 mL/min	No change
CrCl < 10 mL/min	No change
Post–HD dose	None
Post–PD dose	None
Post–CVVH dose	None
Moderate hepatic insufficiency	No information
Severe hepatic insufficiency	No information

Antiretroviral Dosage Adjustments:

Amprenavir	No information
Efavirenz	No information
Indinavir	Indinavir 600 mg q8h
Lopinavir/ritonavir	No information
Nelfinavir	No information (monitor for neutropenia)
Nevirapine	No information
Ritonavir	Delavirdine: no change; ritonavir: No information

---

* Resume dosing for CrCl < 10 mL/min after supplemental dose. "Usual dose" assumes normal renal and hepatic function. CrCl = creatinine clearance; CVVH = continuous veno-venous hemofiltration; HD = hemodialysis; PD = peritoneal dialysis. See pp. 252-255 for definitions/explanations, p. 1 for abbreviations

Saquinavir soft-gel	Saquinavir soft-gel 800 mg q8h (monitor transaminases)
Rifampin	Avoid combination
Rifabutin	Not recommended

Drug Interactions: Antiretrovirals, rifabutin, rifampin (see dose adjustment grid, above); astemizole, terfenadine, benzodiazepines, cisapride, H₂ blockers, proton pump inhibitors, ergot alkaloids, quinidine, statins (avoid if possible), carbamazepine, phenobarbital, phenytoin (may ↓ delavirdine levels, monitor anticonvulsant levels); clarithromycin, dapsone, nifedipine, warfarin (↑ interacting drug levels); sildenafil (do not exceed 25 mg in 48 hrs)
Adverse Effects: Drug fever/rash, Stevens–Johnson syndrome (rare), headache, nausea/vomiting, diarrhea, ↑ SGOT/SGPT
HIV Resistance Potential: Low (triple therapy); high (mono/double drug therapy)
Allergic Potential: High
Safety in Pregnancy: C
Comments: May be taken with or without food, but food decreases absorption by 20%. May disperse 100 mg tablets in > 3 oz. water to produce slurry. Separate dosing with ddI or antacids by 1 hour. Effective antiretroviral therapy consists of at least 3 antiretrovirals (same/different classes)
Cerebrospinal Fluid Penetration: 40%

REFERENCES:
Been-Tiktak AM, Boucher CA, Brun-Vezinet F, et al. Efficacy and safety of combination therapy with delavirdine and zidovudine: A European/Australian phase II trial. Intern J Antimcrob Agents 11:13-21, 1999.

Conway B. Initial therapy with protease inhibitor-sparing regimens: Evaluation of nevirapine and delavirdine. Clin Infect Dis 2:130-4, 2000.

Demeter LM, Shafer RW, Meehan PM, et al. Delavirdine susceptibilities and associated reverse transcriptase mutations in human immunodeficiency virus type 1 isolates from patients in a phase I/II trial of delavirdine monotherapy (ACTG260). Antimicrob Agents Chemother 44:794-7, 2000.

Panel on Clinical Practices for Treatment of HIV Infection. Guidelines for the use of antiretroviral agents in HIV-infected adults and adolescents.

Department of Health and Human Services. April 23, 2001. www.hivatis.org

Didanosine (Videx) ddI

Drug Class: Antiretroviral NRTI (nucleoside reverse transcriptase inhibitor)
Usual Dose: > 60 kg: 200 mg (PO) q12h; < 60 kg: 125 mg (PO) q12h (see comments)
Pharmacokinetic Parameters:
Peak serum level: 29 mcg/mL
Bioavailability: 30-40%
Excreted unchanged: 60%
Serum half-life (normal/ESRD): 1.6/4.5 hrs
Plasma protein binding: ≤ 5%
Volume of distribution (V_d): 1.1 L/kg
Primary Mode of Elimination: Renal
Dosage Adjustments for Patients > 60 kg:

CrCl ~ 40–60 mL/min	No change
CrCl ~ 10–30 mL/min	100 mg (PO) q12h
CrCl < 10 mL/min	100 mg (PO) q24h
Post–HD dose*	100 mg (PO)
Post–PD dose	None
Post–CVVH dose*	200 mg (PO)
Moderate hepatic insufficiency	No change
Severe hepatic insufficiency	100 mg (PO) q24h

Drug Interactions: Alcohol, lamivudine, pentamidine, valproic acid (↑ risk of pancreatitis); dapsone, fluoroquinolones, ketoconazole, itraconazole, tetracyclines (↓ absorption of interacting drug; give 2 hours after didanosine); dapsone, INH, metronidazole, nitrofurantoin, stavudine, vincristine, zalcitabine, neurotoxic drugs or history of neuropathy (↑ risk of peripheral neuropathy); dapsone (↓ dapsone absorption, which increases risk of PCP)
Adverse Effects: Headache, depression, nausea, vomiting, GI upset/abdominal pain, diarrhea, drug fever/rash, anemia, leukopenia, thrombocytopenia, hepatotoxicity/hepatic necrosis, pancreatitis (may be fatal),

---
* Resume dosing for CrCl < 10 mL/min after supplemental dose. "Usual dose" assumes normal renal and hepatic function. CrCl = creatinine clearance; CVVH = continuous veno-venous hemofiltration; HD = hemodialysis; PD = peritoneal dialysis. See pp. 252-255 for definitions/explanations, p. 1 for abbreviations

hypertriglyceridemia, hyperuricemia, lactic acidosis, lipoatrophy, wasting, dose-dependent (≥ 0.06 mg/kg/d) peripheral neuropathy, hyperglycemia, lactic acidosis with hepatic steatosis (rare, but potentially life-threatening toxicity with use of NRTIs; pregnant women taking didanosine + stavudine may be at increased risk)
HIV Resistance Potential: Low (triple therapy); high (mono/double drug therapy)
Allergic Potential: Low
Safety in Pregnancy: B
Comments: Available as tablets, buffered powder for oral solution, and enteric-coated extended-release capsules (Videx EC 400 mg PO q24h). Take 30 minutes before or 2 hours after meal (food decreases serum concentrations by ↓ 49%). Chew tablets thoroughly. Twice daily dosing is preferred, but once daily dosing (> 60 kg: 400 mg EC capsules; < 60 kg: 250 mg tablet or EC capsulue) may be considered for patients requiring a simplified dosing schedule. Avoid in patients with alcoholic cirrhosis/history of pancreatitis. Na^+ content = 11.5 mEq/g. Effective antiretroviral therapy consists of at least 3 antiretrovirals (same/different classes)
Cerebrospinal Fluid Penetration: 20%

REFERENCES:
Hirsch MS, D'Aquila RT. Therapy for human immunodeficiency virus infection. N Engl J Med 328:1686-95, 1993.
HIV Trialists' Collaborative Group. Zidovudine, didanosine, and zalcitabine in the treatment of HIV infection: Meta-analyses of the randomised evidence. Lancet 353:2014-2025, 1999.
Montaner JS, Reiss P, Cooper D, et al. A randomized, double-blind trial comparing combinations of nevirapine, didanosine, and zidovudine for HIV-infected patients: The INCAS trial. Italy, the Netherlands, Canada and Australia Study. J Am Med Assoc 279:930-937, 1998.
Panel on Clinical Practices for Treatment of HIV Infection. Guidelines for the use of antiretroviral agents in HIV-infected adults and adolescents. Department of Health and Human Services. April 23, 2001. www.hivatis.org
Perry CM, Balfour JA. Didanosine: An update on its antiviral activity, pharmacokinetic properties, and therapeutic efficacy in the management of HIV disease. Drugs 52:928-62, 1996.
Rathbun RC, Martin ES 3rd. Didanosine therapy in
patients intolerant of or failing zidovudine therapy. Ann Pharmacother 26:1347-51, 1992.

Doxycycline (Vibramycin, Vibra-tabs)

Drug Class: 2nd generation IV/PO tetracycline
Usual Dose: 100-200 mg (IV/PO) q12h (see comments)
Pharmacokinetic Parameters:
Peak serum level: 100/200 mg = 4/8 mcg/mL
Bioavailability: 93%
Excreted unchanged: 40%
Serum half-life (normal/ESRD): 18-22/24 hrs
Plasma protein binding: 93%
Volume of distribution (V_d): 0.75 L/kg
Primary Mode of Elimination: Hepatic
Dosage Adjustments:

CrCl ~ 40–60 mL/min	No change
CrCl ~ 10–30 mL/min	No change
CrCl < 10 mL/min	No change
Post–HD dose	None
Post–PD dose	None
Post–CVVH dose	None
Moderate hepatic insufficiency	No change
Severe hepatic insufficiency	No change

Drug Interactions: Antacids, Al^{++}, Ca^{++}, Fe^{++}, Mg^{++}, Zn^{++}, multivitamins, sucralfate (↓ doxycycline absorption); barbiturates, carbamazepine, phenytoin (↓ doxycycline half-life); bicarbonate (↓ doxycycline absorption, ↑ doxycycline clearance); warfarin (↑ INR)
Adverse Effects: Nausea if not taken with food. Phlebitis if given IV in inadequate volume. Avoid in pregnancy and children < 8 years
Resistance Potential: Low
Allergic Potential: Low
Safety in Pregnancy: D
Comments: Minimal potential for Candida overgrowth/diarrhea. Photosensitivity rare.

---

* Resume dosing for CrCl < 10 mL/min after supplemental dose. "Usual dose" assumes normal renal and hepatic function. CrCl = creatinine clearance; CVVH = continuous veno-venous hemofiltration; HD = hemodialysis; PD = peritoneal dialysis. See pp. 252-255 for definitions/explanations, p. 1 for abbreviations

Tablets better tolerated than capsules. Absorption minimally effected by iron, bismuth, milk, or antacids containing Ca^{++}, Mg^{++}, or Al^{++}. Serum half-life increases with multiple doses. For serious systemic infection, begin therapy with a loading dose of 200 mg (IV/PO) q12h x 3 days, then continue at same dose or decrease to 100 mg (IV/PO) q12h to complete therapy. Meningeal dose = 200 mg (IV/PO) q12h

Cerebrospinal Fluid Penetration:
Non-inflamed meninges = 25%
Inflamed meninges = 25%
Bile Penetration: 3000%

REFERENCES:
Cunha BA. Doxycycline. Antibiotics for Clinicians 3:21-33, 1999.
Cunha BA. Doxycycline re-revisited. Arch Intern Med 159:1006-7, 1999.
Cunha BA, Domenico PD, Cunha CB. Pharmacodynamics of doxycycline. Clin Micro Infect Dis 6:270-3, 2000.
Shea KW, Ueno Y, Abumustafa F, et al. Doxycycline activity against Streptococcus pneumoniae. Chest 107:1775-6, 1995.

Efavirenz (Sustiva)

Drug Class: Antiretroviral NNRTI (non-nucleoside reverse transcriptase inhibitor)
Usual Dose: 600 mg (PO) q24h
Pharmacokinetic Parameters:
Peak serum level: 4.5 mcg/mL
Bioavailability: No data
Excreted unchanged: 40%
Serum half-life (normal/ESRD): 40-55 hrs/no data
Plasma protein binding: 99%
Volume of distribution (V_d): No data
Primary Mode of Elimination: Hepatic
Dosage Adjustments:

CrCl ~ 40–60 mL/min	No change
CrCl ~ 10–30 mL/min	No change
CrCl < 10 mL/min	No change
Post–HD dose	None
Post–PD dose	None
Post–CVVH dose	None

Moderate hepatic insufficiency	No information
Severe hepatic	No information

Antiretroviral Dosage Adjustments:

Amprenavir	Amprenavir 1200 mg q8h as single PI, or 1200 mg q12h + ritonavir 200 mg q12h
Delavirdine	No information
Indinavir	Indinavir 1000 mg q8h
Lopinavir/ritonavir (l/r)	Consider l/r 533/133 mg q12h in PI-experienced patients
Nelfinavir	No changes
Nevirapine	No information
Ritonavir	Ritonavir 600 mg q12h (500 mg q12h for intolerance)
Saquinavir	Avoid combination
Rifampin	No changes
Rifabutin	Rifabutin 450-600 mg q24h or 600 mg 2-3x/week if not on protease inhibitor

Drug Interactions: Antiretrovirals, rifabutin, rifampin (see dose adjustment grid, above); astemizole, terfenadine, cisapride, ergotamine, midazolam, triazolam (avoid); carbamazepine, phenobarbital, phenytoin (monitor anticonvulsant levels; use with caution); caspofungin (↓ caspofungin levels, may ↓ caspofungin effect); methadone, telithromycin (↓ interacting drug levels; titrate methadone dose to effect)
Adverse Effects: Drug fever/rash, CNS symptoms (nightmares, dizziness, neuropsychiatric symptoms, difficulty concentrating, somnolence), ↑ SGOT/SGPT, E. multiforme/Stevens–Johnson syndrome (rare),

---

* Resume dosing for CrCl < 10 mL/min after supplemental dose. "Usual dose" assumes normal renal and hepatic function. CrCl = creatinine clearance; CVVH = continuous veno-venous hemofiltration; HD = hemodialysis; PD = peritoneal dialysis. See pp. 252-255 for definitions/explanations, p. 1 for abbreviations

false positive cannabinoid test
HIV Resistance Potential: Low (triple therapy); high (mono/double drug therapy)
Allergic Potential: High
Safety in Pregnancy: C
Comments: Rash/CNS symptoms usually resolve spontaneously over 2-4 weeks. Take at bedtime to minimize CNS effects. Avoid taking after high fat meals (levels ↑ 50%). Prolonged high peak serum concentrations avoids trough problems with antiretrovirals with short $t_{1/2}$. Effective antiretroviral therapy consists of at least 3 antiretrovirals (same/different classes).
Cerebrospinal Fluid Penetration: 1%

REFERENCES:
Caro JJ, O'Brien JA, Migliaccio-Walle K, et al. Economic analysis of initial HIV treatment. Efavirenz- versus indinavir- containing triple therapy. Pharmacoeconomics 19:95-104, 2001.
Go JC, Cunha BA. Efavirenz. Antibiotics for Clinicians 5:1-8, 2001.
Haas DW, Fessel WJ, Delapenha RA, et al. Therapy with efavirenz plus indinavir in patients with extensive prior nucleoside reverse-transcriptase inhibitor experience: A randomized, double-blind, placebo-controlled trial. J Infect Dis 183:392-400, 2001.
Marzolini C, Telenti A, Decosterd LA, et al. Efavirenz plasma levels can predict treatment failure and central nervous system side effects in HIV-1-infected patients. AIDS 15:71-5, 2001.
Panel on Clinical Practices for Treatment of HIV Infection. Guidelines for the use of antiretroviral agents in HIV-infected adults and adolescents. Department of Health and Human Services. April 23, 2001. www.hivatis.org
Tenorio AR, Irlanda IE, Narkiewicz E, et al. Efficacy and safety of the combination of efavirenz and abacavir in HIV-infected patients failing antiretroviral therapy. AIDS 14:1470-1, 2000.
Three new drugs for HIV infection. Med Lett Drugs Ther 40:114-6, 1998.

Ertapenem (Invanz)

Drug Class: Carbapenem
Usual Dose: 1 gm (IV/IM) q24h
Pharmacokinetic Parameters:
Peak serum level: 150 mcg/mL
Bioavailability: 92% (IM)
Excreted unchanged: 30-40%
Serum half-life (normal/ESRD): 4/14 hrs

Plasma protein binding: 6-17%
Volume of distribution (V_d): 8 L/kg
Primary Mode of Elimination: Renal
Dosage Adjustments:

CrCl ~ 40–60 mL/min	No change
CrCl ~ 10–30 mL/min	No change
CrCl < 10 mL/min	500 mg (IV) q24h
Post–HD dose	No information
Post–PD dose	No information
Post–CVVH dose	No information
Moderate hepatic insufficiency	No change
Severe hepatic insufficiency	No change

Drug Interactions: No data
Adverse Effects: Low seizure potential. Mild headache, infrequent nausea or diarrhea
Resistance Potential: Low
Allergic Potential: Low
Safety in Pregnancy: C
Comments: Dose-dependent protein binding. Compared to imipenem, ertapenem has little activity against enterococci, Acinetobacter, or P. aeruginosa, but greater activity against ESBLs
Cerebrospinal Fluid Penetration: No data
Bile Penetration: No data

REFERENCES:
Goldstein EJ, Citron DM, Vreni Merriam C, et al. Comparative in vitro activities of ertapenem (MK-0826) against 1,001 anaerobes isolated from human intra-abdominal infections. Antimicrob Agents Chemother 44:2389-94, 2000.
Wexler HM, Molitoris D, Finegold SM. In vitro activities of MK-826 (L-749, 345) against 363 strains of anaerobic bacteria. Antimicrob Agents Chemother 44:2222-4, 2000.

Erythromycin lactobionate, base (various)

Drug Class: Macrolide
Usual Dose: 1 gm (IV) q6h; 500 mg (PO) q6h
Pharmacokinetic Parameters:

---

* Resume dosing for CrCl < 10 mL/min after supplemental dose. "Usual dose" assumes normal renal and hepatic function. CrCl = creatinine clearance; CVVH = continuous veno-venous hemofiltration; HD = hemodialysis; PD = peritoneal dialysis. See pp. 252-255 for definitions/explanations, p. 1 for abbreviations

Peak serum level: 12 (IV);1.2 (PO) mcg/mL
Bioavailability: 50%
Excreted unchanged: 15%
Serum half-life (normal/ESRD): 1.4/5.4 hrs
Plasma protein binding: 80%
Volume of distribution (V_d): 1 L/kg
Primary Mode of Elimination: Hepatic
Dosage Adjustments:

CrCl ~ 40–60 mL/min	No change
CrCl ~ 10–30 mL/min	No change
CrCl < 10 mL/min	No change
Post–HD dose	None
Post–PD dose	None
Post–CVVH dose	None
Moderate hepatic insufficiency	No change
Severe hepatic insufficiency	500 mg (IV) q12h

Drug Interactions: Amiodarone, procainamide, sotalol, astemizole, terfenadine, cisapride, pimozide (may ↑ QT interval, torsade de pointes); carbamazepine (↑ carbamazepine levels, nystagmus, nausea, vomiting, diarrhea; avoid combination); cimetidine, digoxin, ergot alkaloids, felodipine, midazolam, triazolam, phenytoin, ritonavir, tacrolimus, valproic acid (↑ interacting drug levels); clozapine (↑ clozapine levels; CNS toxicity); corticosteroids (↑ corticosteroid effect); cyclosporine (↑ cyclosporine levels with toxicity); efavirenz (↓ erythromycin levels); rifabutin, rifampin (↓ erythromycin levels, ↑ interacting drug levels); statins (↑ risk of rhabdomyolysis); theophylline (↑ theophylline levels, nausea, vomiting, seizures, apnea); warfarin (↑ INR); zidovudine (↓ zidovudine levels)
Adverse Effects: Nausea, vomiting, GI upset, irritative diarrhea, abdominal pain, phlebitis. May ↑ QT_c; avoid with other medications that prolong the QT_c interval and in patients with cardiac arrhythmias/heart block
Resistance Potential: Low to moderate (S. pneumoniae, S. aureus [MSSA], H. influenzae,

Group A streptococci)
Allergic Potential: Low
Safety in Pregnancy: B
Comments: Do not mix erythromycin with B/C vitamins, glucose solutions, cephalothin, tetracycline, chloramphenicol, heparin, or warfarin. Increases GI motility. Monitor potential hepatotoxicity with serial SGOTs/SGPTs
Cerebrospinal Fluid Penetration: < 10%

REFERENCES:
Alvarez-Elcoro S, Enzler MJ. The macrolides: Erythromycin, clarithromycin and azithromycin. Mayo Clin Proc 74:613-34, 1999.
Amsden GW. Erythromycin, clarithromycin, and azithromycin: Are the differences real? Clinical Therapeutics 18:572, 1996.
Cunha BA. The virtues of doxycycline and the evils of erythromycin. Adv Ther 14:172-80, 1997.
Smilack JD, Wilson WE, Cocerill FR 3rd. Tetracycline, chloramphenicol, erythromycin, clindamycin, and metronidazole. Mayo Clin Proc 66:1270-80, 1991.

Ethambutol (Myambutol) EMB

Drug Class: Anti–TB drug
Usual Dose: 15 mg/kg (PO) q24h
Pharmacokinetic Parameters:
Peak serum level: 2 mcg/mL
Bioavailability: 80%
Excreted unchanged: 80%
Serum half-life (normal/ESRD): 4/10 hrs
Plasma protein binding: 20%
Volume of distribution (V_d): 2 L/kg
Primary Mode of Elimination: Renal/hepatic
Dosage Adjustments:

CrCl ~ 40–60 mL/min	No change
CrCl ~ 10–30 mL/min	No change
CrCl < 10 mL/min	15 mg/kg (PO) q48h
Post–HD dose*	400 mg (PO)
Post–PD dose	None
Post–CVVH dose*	800 mg (PO)
Moderate hepatic insufficiency	No change

---
* Resume dosing for CrCl < 10 mL/min after supplemental dose. "Usual dose" assumes normal renal and hepatic function. CrCl = creatinine clearance; CVVH = continuous veno-venous hemofiltration; HD = hemodialysis; PD = peritoneal dialysis. See pp. 252-255 for definitions/explanations, p. 1 for abbreviations

Severe hepatic insufficiency	15 mg/kg (PO) q48h

Drug Interactions: Aluminum salts, didanosine buffer (↓ ethambutol and interacting drug absorption)

Adverse Effects: Drug fever/rash, ↓ visual acuity, central scotomata, color blindness (red–green), metallic taste, mental confusion, peripheral neuropathy, ↑ uric acid

Resistance Potential: Low

Allergic Potential: Low

Safety in Pregnancy: B

Comments: Optic neuritis may occur with high doses (≥ 15 mg/kg/day).
Meningeal dose = 25 mg/kg (PO) q24h

Cerebrospinal Fluid Penetration:
Non-inflamed meninges = 1%
Inflamed meninges = 40%

REFERENCES:
Chaisson RE, Keiser P, Pierce M, et al. Clarithromycin and ethambutol with or without clofazimine for the treatment of bacteremic Mycobacterium avium complex disease in patients with HIV infection. AIDS 11:311-317, 1997.
Davidson PT, Le HQ. Drug treatment of tuberculosis 1992. Drugs 43:651-73, 1992.
Drugs for tuberculosis. Med Lett Drugs Ther 35:99-101,1993.
Van Scoy RE, Wilkowske CJ. Antituberculous agents. Mayo Clin Proc 67:179-87, 1992.

Ethionamide (Trecator)

Drug Class: Anti–TB drug
Usual Dose: 500 mg (PO) q12h
Pharmacokinetic Parameters:
Peak serum level: 20 mcg/mL
Bioavailability: 80%
Excreted unchanged: 1%
Serum half-life (normal/ESRD): 4/9 hrs
Plasma protein binding: 10%
Volume of distribution (V_d): No data
Primary Mode of Elimination: Renal/hepatic
Dosage Adjustments:

CrCl ~ 40–60 mL/min	No change
CrCl ~ 10–30 mL/min	No change

CrCl < 10 mL/min	500 mg (PO) q24h
Post–HD dose	No information
Post–PD dose	No information
Post–CVVH dose	No information
Moderate hepatic insufficiency	No change
Severe hepatic insufficiency	500 mg (PO) q24h

Drug Interactions: Cycloserine (↑ neurologic toxicity); ethambutol (↑ GI distress, neuritis, hepatotoxicity); INH (peripheral neuritis, hepatotoxicity); pyrazinamide, rifampin (hepatotoxicity)

Adverse Effects: ↑ SGOT/SGPT, headache, nausea/vomiting, abdominal pain, tremor, olfactory abnormalities, alopecia, gynecomastia, hypoglycemia, impotence, neurotoxicity (central/peripheral neuropathy)

Resistance Potential: Low

Allergic Potential: Low

Safety in Pregnancy: C

Comments: Additive toxicity with thiacetazone

Cerebrospinal Fluid Penetration: 100%

REFERENCES:
Davidson PT, Le HQ. Drug treatment of tuberculosis 1992. Drugs 43:651-73, 1992.
Drugs for tuberculosis. Med Lett Drugs Ther 35:99-101,1993.
Iseman MD. Treatment of multidrug resistant tuberculosis. N Engl J Med 329:784-91, 1993.

Famciclovir (Famvir)

Drug Class: Antiviral
Usual Dose: <u>HSV</u>: 500 mg (PO) q12h; <u>VZV</u>: 500 mg (PO) q8h
Pharmacokinetic Parameters:
Peak serum level: 3.3 mcg/mL
Bioavailability: 75%
Excreted unchanged: 60%
Serum half-life (normal/ESRD): 2.5/20 hrs
Plasma protein binding: 20%
Volume of distribution (V_d): 1.5 L/kg
Primary Mode of Elimination: Renal

---

* Resume dosing for CrCl < 10 mL/min after supplemental dose. "Usual dose" assumes normal renal and hepatic function. CrCl = creatinine clearance; CVVH = continuous veno-venous hemofiltration; HD = hemodialysis; PD = peritoneal dialysis. See pp. 252-255 for definitions/explanations, p. 1 for abbreviations

Dosage Adjustments for HSV/VZV:

CrCl ~ 40–60 mL/min	500 mg (PO) q24h/ 500 mg (PO) q12h
CrCl ~ 10–30 mL/min	500 mg (PO) q36h/ 500 mg (PO) q24h
CrCl < 10 mL/min	250 mg (PO) q24h/ 250 mg (PO) q24h
Post–HD dose	None
Post–PD dose	None
Post–CVVH dose	None
Moderate hepatic insufficiency	No change
Severe hepatic insufficiency	No change

Drug Interactions: Digoxin (↑ digoxin levels)
Adverse Effects: Headache, seizures/tremors (dose related), nausea
Resistance Potential: Low
Allergic Potential: Low
Safety in Pregnancy: B
Comments: 99% converted to penciclovir in liver/GI tract.
Meningeal dose = VZV dose
Cerebrospinal Fluid Penetration: 50%

REFERENCES:

Alrabiah FA, Sacks SL. New anti-herpesvirus agents. Their targets and therapeutic potential. Drugs 52:17-32, 1996.

Bassett KL, Green CJ, Wright JM. Famciclovir and postherpetic neuralgia. Ann Intern Med 131:712-3, 1999.

Luber AD, Flaherty JF Jr. Famciclovir for treatment of herpesvirus infections. Ann Pharmacother 30:978-85, 1996.

Rayes N, Seehofer D, Hopf U, et al. Comparison of famciclovir and lamivudine in the long-term treatment of hepatitis B infection after liver transplantation. Transplantation 71:96-101, 2001.

Tyring S, Belanger R, Bezwoda W, et al. A randomized, double-blind trial of famciclovir versus acyclovir for the treatment of localized dermatomal herpes zoster in immunocompromised patients. Cancer Invest 19:13-22, 2001.

Fluconazole (Diflucan)

Drug Class: Antifungal
Usual Dose: 400 mg (IV/PO) x 1 dose, then 200 mg (IV/PO) q24h (see comments)
Pharmacokinetic Parameters:
Peak serum level: 6.7 mcg/mL
Bioavailability: 95%
Excreted unchanged: 70%
Serum half-life (normal/ESRD): 27/100 hrs
Plasma protein binding: 12%
Volume of distribution (V_d): 0.7 L/kg
Primary Mode of Elimination: Renal
Dosage Adjustments:

CrCl ~ 40–60 mL/min	No change
CrCl ~ 10–30 mL/min	No change
CrCl < 10 mL/min	200 mg (IV/PO) q48h
Post–HD dose*	200 mg (IV/PO)
Post–PD dose*	100 mg (IV/PO)
Post–CVVH dose*	200 mg (IV/PO)
Moderate hepatic insufficiency	No change
Severe hepatic insufficiency	No change

Drug Interactions: Astemizole, cisapride, terfenadine (may ↑ QT interval, torsades de pointes); cyclosporine, oral hypoglycemics, tacrolimus, theophylline, zidovudine (↑ interacting drug levels with possible toxicity); hydrochlorothiazide (↑ fluconazole levels); phenytoin, rifabutin, rifampin (↓ fluconazole levels, ↑ interacting drug levels); warfarin (↑ INR)
Adverse Effects: ↑ SGOT/SGPT, hypokalemia
Resistance Potential: Moderate (C. albicans)
Allergic Potential: Low
Safety in Pregnancy: C
Comments: Usual dose for candidemia (C. albicans) = 400 mg (IV/PO) q24h after loading dose of 800 mg (IV/PO).
Meningeal dose = 400 mg (IV/PO) q24h
Cerebrospinal Fluid Penetration:
Non-inflamed meninges: = 80%
Inflamed meninges: = 80%

---

* Resume dosing for CrCl < 10 mL/min after supplemental dose. "Usual dose" assumes normal renal and hepatic function. CrCl = creatinine clearance, CVVH = continuous veno venous hemofiltration; HD = hemodialysis; PD = peritoneal dialysis. See pp. 252-255 for definitions/explanations, p. 1 for abbreviations

REFERENCES:

Goa KL, Barradell LB. Fluconazole: An update of its pharmacodynamics and pharmacokinetic properties and therapeutic use in major superficial and systemic mycoses in immunocompromised patients. Drugs 50:658-90, 1995.

Kauffman CA, Carver PL. Antifungal agents in the 1990s: Current status and future developments. Drugs 53:539-49, 1997.

Kowalsky SF, Dixon DM. Fluconazole: A new antifungal agent. Clin Pharmacol 10:179-94, 1991.

Owens RC, Ambrose PG. Fluconazole. Antibiotics for Clinicians 1:109-117, 1997.

Terrell CL. Antifungal agents: Part II. The azoles. Mayo Clin Proc 74:78-100, 1999.

Flucytosine (Ancobon) 5-FC

Drug Class: Antifungal
Usual Dose: 500 mg (PO) q6h
Pharmacokinetic Parameters:
Peak serum level: 3.5 mcg/mL
Bioavailability: 95%
Excreted unchanged: 90%
Serum half-life (normal/ESRD): 4/100 hrs
Plasma protein binding: 40%
Volume of distribution (V_d): 0.6 L/kg
Primary Mode of Elimination: Renal
Dosage Adjustments:

CrCl ~ 40–60 mL/min	500 mg (PO) q12h
CrCl ~ 10–30 mL/min	500 mg (PO) q18h
CrCl < 10 mL/min	500 mg (PO) q24h
Post–HD dose*	500 mg (PO)
Post–PD dose*	500 mg (PO)
Post–CVVH dose*	500 mg (PO)
Moderate hepatic insufficiency	No change
Severe hepatic insufficiency	No change

Drug Interactions: Cytarabine (↓ flucytosine effect); zidovudine (neutropenia)
Adverse Effects: Leukopenia, anemia, thrombocytopenia, nausea, vomiting, abdominal pain, ↑ SGOT/SGPT, drug fever/rashes
Resistance Potential: High (C. albicans)

Allergic Potential: High
Safety in Pregnancy: C
Comments: Always use in combination with amphotericin B for cryptococcal meningitis.
Na^+ content = 37.5 mEq/g.
Meningeal dose = usual dose
Cerebrospinal Fluid Penetration:
Non-inflamed meninges = 100%
Inflamed meninges = 100%

REFERENCES:

Lyman CA, Walsh TJ. Systemically administered antifungal agents. A review of their clinical pharmacology and therapeutic applications: Part I. Amphotericin B preparations and flucytosine. Mayo Clin Proc 73:1205-25, 1998.

Wintermeyer SM, Mahata MC. Stability of flucytosine in an extemporaneously compounded oral liquid. Am J Health Syst Pharm 53:407-9, 1996.

Foscarnet (Foscavir)

Drug Class: Antiviral (HSV,CMV)
Usual Dose: HSV: 40 mg/kg (IV) q12h x 2-3 weeks; CMV: 90 mg/kg (IV) q12h x 2-3 weeks (induction dose), then 90 mg/kg (IV) q24h (maintenance dose) for life-long suppression
Pharmacokinetic Parameters:
Peak serum level: 150 mcg/mL
Bioavailability: Not applicable
Excreted unchanged: 85%
Serum half-life (normal/ESRD): 3/100 hrs
Plasma protein binding: 17%
Volume of distribution (V_d): 0.5 L/kg
Primary Mode of Elimination: Renal /hepatic
Dosage Adjustments:

Induction (mg/kg)		
CrCl (mL/min/kg)	HSV	CMV
> 1.4	40 q8h	90 q12h
> 1.0 - 1.4	30 q8h	70 q12h
> 0.8 - 1.0	35 q12h	50 q12h
> 0.6 - 0.8	25 q12h	80 q24h
> 0.5 - 0.6	40 q24h	60 q24h
≥ 0.4 - 0.5	35 q24h	50 q24h

---

* Resume dosing for CrCl < 10 mL/min after supplemental dose. "Usual dose" assumes normal renal and hepatic function. CrCl = creatinine clearance; CVVH = continuous veno-venous hemofiltration; HD = hemodialysis; PD = peritoneal dialysis. See pp. 252-255 for definitions/explanations, p. 1 for abbreviations

< 0.4	Not recommended	
CMV maintenance range (mg/kg)*		
CrCl > 1.4	90 q24h	120 q24h
> 1.0 - 1.4	70 q24h	90 q24h
> 0.8 - 1.0	50 q24h	65 q24h
> 0.6 - 0.8	80 q48h	105 q48h
> 0.5 - 0.6	60 q48h	80 q48h
≥ 0.4 - 0.5	50 q48h	65 q48h
< 0.4	Not recommended	
Post–HD dose*	45 mg/kg (IV)	
Post–PD dose	No information	
Post–CVVH dose	No information	
Mod. hepatic insufficiency	No change	
Severe hepatic insufficiency	No change	

Infusion pump must be used. Adequate hydration is recommended to prevent renal toxicity
* Higher doses may be considered for early reinduction due to progression of CMV retinitis, and for patients showing excellent tolerance

Drug Interactions: Ciprofloxacin (↑ risk of seizures); amphotericin B, aminoglycosides, cis-platinum, cyclosporine, other nephrotoxic drugs (↑ nephrotoxicity); pentamidine IV (severe hypocalcemia reported; do not combine); zidovudine (↑ incidence/severity of anemia)
Adverse Effects: Major side effects include nephrotoxicity and tetany (from ↓ Ca^{++}). Others include nausea, vomiting, GI upset, headache, seizures, peripheral neuropathy, hallucinations, tremors, nephrogenic DI, ↓ Ca^{++}, ↓ Mg^{++}, ↓ PO$_4^-$, oral/genital ulcers
Resistance Potential: Low
Allergic Potential: Low
Safety in Pregnancy: C
Comments: Renal failure prevented/minimized by adequate hydration. Administer by IV slow

infusion ≤ 1 mg/kg/min using an infusion pump
Meningeal dose = usual dose
Cerebrospinal Fluid Penetration:
Non-inflamed meninges = 90%
Inflamed meninges = 100%

REFERENCES:
Chrisp P, Clissold SP. Foscarnet: A review of its antiviral activity, pharmacokinetic properties, and therapeutic use in immunocompromised patients with cytomegalovirus retinitis. Drugs 41:104-29, 1991.
Derary G, Martinez F, Katlama C, et al. Foscarnet nephrotoxicity: Mechanism, Incidence and prevention. Am J Nephrol 9:316-21, 1989.
Whitley RJ, Jacobson MA, Friedberg DN, et al. Guidelines for the treatment of cytomegalovirus diseases in patients with AIDS in the era of potent antiretroviral therapy. Arch Intern Med 158:957-69, 1998.

Fosfomycin (Monurol)

Drug Class: Urinary antiseptic
Usual Dose: 3 gm (PO) q24h
Pharmacokinetic Parameters:
Peak serum level: 26 mcg/mL
Bioavailability: 40%
Excreted unchanged: 80%
Serum half-life (normal/ESRD): 5.7/50 hrs
Plasma protein binding: 3%
Volume of distribution (V_d): 2 L/kg
Primary Mode of Elimination: Renal
Dosage Adjustments:

CrCl ~ 40–60 mL/min	No change
CrCl ~ 10–30 mL/min	Avoid
CrCl < 10 mL/min	Avoid
Post–HD dose	Avoid
Post–PD dose	Avoid
Post–CVVH dose	Avoid
Moderate hepatic insufficiency	No change
Severe hepatic insufficiency	No change

Drug Interactions: Antacids, metoclopramide (↓ fosfomycin effect)

---
* Resume dosing for CrCl < 10 mL/min after supplemental dose. "Usual dose" assumes normal renal and hepatic function. CrCl = creatinine clearance, CVVH = continuous veno-venous hemofiltration; HD = hemodialysis; PD = peritoneal dialysis. See pp. 252-255 for definitions/explanations, p. 1 for abbreviations

Adverse Effects: Nausea, vomiting, GI upset, diarrhea, ↑ SGOT/SGPT, thrombocytosis, eosinophilia
Resistance Potential: Low
Allergic Potential: Low
Safety in Pregnancy: B
Comments: May be taken with or without food. Useful only for cystitis, not pyelonephritis/urosepsis. Treat UTIs x 3 days in males, as single dose in females

REFERENCES:
Gosden PE, Reeves DS. Fosfomycin. Antibiotics for Clinicians 2:121-28, 1998.
Patel SS, Balfour JA, Bryson HM. Fosfomycin tromethamine: Pharmacokinetic properties and therapeutic efficacy as a single-dose oral treatment for acute uncomplicated low urinary tract infections. Drugs 53:637-56, 1997.

Ganciclovir (Cytovene)

Drug Class: Antiviral, nucleoside inhibitor/analogue
Usual Dose: 5 mg/kg (IV) q12h x 3-6 weeks (induction), then 5 mg/kg (IV) q24h or 1 gm (PO) q8h (maintenance) for CMV retinitis (see comments)
Pharmacokinetic Parameters:
Peak serum level: 8.3 mcg/mL
Bioavailability: 5%
Excreted unchanged: 90%
Serum half-life (normal/ESRD): 3.6/28 hrs
Plasma protein binding: 1%
Volume of distribution (V_d): 15.3 L/kg
Primary Mode of Elimination: Renal/hepatic
Dosage Adjustments:

CrCl ~ 40–60 mL/min	2.5 mg/kg (IV) q12h (induction), then 2.5 mg/kg (IV) q24h or 1500 mg (PO) q24h or 500 mg (PO) q12h (maintenance)
CrCl ~ 10–30 mL/min	1.25 mg/kg (IV) q24h (induction), then 0.625 mg/kg (IV) q24h or 500 mg (PO) q24h (maintenance)
CrCl < 10 mL/min	1.25 mg/kg (IV) q24h (induction), then 0.625 mg/kg (IV) q24h or 500 mg (PO) q24h (maintenance)
Post–HD dose*	1.25 mg/kg (IV), then 0.625 mg/kg (IV) or 500 mg (PO)
Post–PD dose	None
Post–CVVH dose*	5 mg/kg (IV)
Moderate hepatic insufficiency	No change
Severe hepatic insufficiency	No change

Drug Interactions: Cytotoxic drugs (may produce additive toxicity: stomatitis, bone marrow depression, alopecia); imipenem (↑ risk of seizures); probenecid (↑ ganciclovir levels); zidovudine (↓ ganciclovir levels, ↑ zidovudine levels, possible neutropenia)
Adverse Effects: Headaches, hallucinations, seizures/tremor (dose related), drug fever/rash, diarrhea, nausea/vomiting, GI upset, leukopenia, thrombocytopenia, anemia, retinal detachment
Resistance Potential: Low
Allergic Potential: High
Safety in Pregnancy: C
Comments: Induction doses are always given IV. Maintenance doses may be given IV or PO. For CMV encephalitis, use same dosing regimen as for CMV retinitis (CNS penetration = 70%). For CMV pneumonitis, give 2.5 mg/kg (IV) q8h x 20 doses plus IVIG 500 mg/kg (IV) q48h x 10 doses; then follow with 5 mg/kg (IV) 3-5x/week x 20 doses plus IVIG 500 mg/kg (IV) 2x/week x 8 doses. For CMV colitis/esophagitis, use same dose for CMV retinitis induction x 3-6 weeks. Continue maintenance doses for CMV retinitis, encephalitis, and colitis/esophagitis until CD_4 cell count > 100–200. Bioavailability increased with food: 5% fasting; 6-9% with food; 28-31% with fatty food. Na^+ content = 4.0 mEq/g. Meningeal dose = CMV retinitis dose
Cerebrospinal Fluid Penetration: 41%

---

* Resume dosing for CrCl < 10 mL/min after supplemental dose. "Usual dose" assumes normal renal and hepatic function. CrCl = creatinine clearance; CVVH = continuous veno-venous hemofiltration; HD = hemodialysis; PD = peritoneal dialysis. See pp. 252-255 for definitions/explanations, p. 1 for abbreviations

REFERENCES:
Alrabiah FA, Sacks SL. New antiherpesvirus agents: Their targets and therapeutic potential. Drugs 52:17-32,1996.
Komanduri KV, Viswanathan MB, Wieder ED, et al. Restoration of cytomegalovirus-specific CD4+ T-lymphocyte responses after ganciclovir and highly active antiretroviral therapy in individuals infected with HIV-1. Nat Med 4:953-956, 1998.
Matthews T, Boehme R. Antiviral activity and mechanism of action of ganciclovir. Rev Infect Dis 10:490-4, 1988.
Whitley RJ, Jacobson MA, Friedberg DN, et al. Guidelines for the treatment of cytomegalovirus diseases in patients with AIDS in the era of potent antiretroviral therapy. Arch Intern Med 158:957-69, 1998.

Gatifloxacin (Tequin)

Drug Class: Fluoroquinolone
Usual Dose: 400 mg (IV/PO) q24h
Pharmacokinetic Parameters:
Peak serum level: 5.5 (IV)/3.8 (PO) mcg/mL
Bioavailability: 96%
Excreted unchanged: 70%
Serum half-life (normal/ESRD): 7/36 hrs
Plasma protein binding: 20%
Volume of distribution (V_d): 2 L/kg
Primary Mode of Elimination: Renal
Dosage Adjustments:

CrCl ~ 40–60 mL/min	No change
CrCl ~ 10–30 mL/min	200 mg (IV/PO) q24h
CrCl < 10 mL/min	200 mg (IV/PO) q24h
Post–HD dose*	200 mg (IV/PO)
Post–PD dose	None
Post–CVVH dose*	400 mg (IV/PO)
Moderate hepatic insufficiency	No change
Severe hepatic insufficiency	No change

Drug Interactions: Al^{++}, Fe^{++}, Mg^{++}, Zn^{++} antacids, citrate/citric acid, dairy products (↓ absorption of gatifloxacin only if taken together); amiodarone, procainamide, sotalol (may ↑ QT interval, torsade de pointes); digoxin (↑ digoxin levels 18-56%, ↑ digoxin effects); insulin, oral hypoglycemics (hypoglycemia); probenecid (↑ gatifloxacin levels); NSAIDs (CNS stimulation)
Adverse Effects: Headache, dizziness, nausea, diarrhea, vomiting, vaginitis, hyperglycemia. May ↑ QT_c; avoid with medications that prolong the QT_c interval and in patients with cardiac arrhythmias/heart block
Resistance Potential: Low
Allergic Potential: Low
Safety in Pregnancy: C
Comments: Nausea most common GI side effect. Take 4 hours or after before aluminum/magnesium-containing antacids; not affected by calcium-containing antacids. Caution in diabetics receiving anti-diabetic agents
Cerebrospinal Fluid Penetration: 36%

REFERENCES:
Fish DN, North DS. Gatifloxacin, an advanced 8-methoxy fluoroquinolone. Pharmacotherapy 21:35-59, 2001.
Gatifloxacin and moxifloxacin: Two new fluoroquinolones. Med Lett Drugs Ther 42:1072:15, 2000.
Perry CM, Barman Balfour JA, Lamb HM. Gatifloxacin. Drugs 58:683-96, 1999.

Gemifloxacin (Factiv)

Drug Class: Fluoroquinolone
Usual Dose: 320 mg (PO) q24h
Pharmacokinetic Parameters:
Peak serum level: 1.5 mcg/mL
Bioavailability: 70%
Excreted unchanged: 35%
Serum half-life (normal/ESRD): 8/10 hrs
Plasma protein binding: 60%
Volume of distribution (V_d): 2 L/kg
Primary Mode of Elimination: Renal
Dosage Adjustments:

CrCl ~ 40–60 mL/min	No change
CrCl ~ 10–30 mL/min	160 mg (PO) q24h
CrCl < 10 mL/min	160 mg (PO) q48h
Post–HD dose	No information

Post–PD dose	No information
Post–CVVH dose	No information
Moderate hepatic insufficiency	No change
Severe hepatic insufficiency	No change

Drug Interactions: No data
Adverse Effects: Severe rash, severe hypersensitivity hepatitis
Resistance Potential: Low
Allergic Potential: Low
Safety in Pregnancy: C
Comments: Take 4 hours before or after calcium/magnesium containing antacids. Use another quinolone
Cerebrospinal Fluid Penetration: < 10%

REFERENCES:
Goldstein EJ. Review of the in vitro activity of gemifloxacin against gram-positive and gram-negative anaerobic pathogens. J Antimicrob Chemother 45:55-65, 2000.
Hammerschlag MR. Activity of gemifloxacin and other new quinolones against Chlamydia pneumoniae: A review. J Antimicrob Chemother 45:35-9, 2000.
Lower MD, Lamb HMN. Gemifloxacin. Drugs 59:1137-47, 2000.

Gentamicin (Garamycin)

Drug Class: Aminoglycoside
Usual Dose: 5 mg/kg (IV) q24h or 240 mg (IV) q24h (preferred over q8h dosing)
Pharmacokinetic Parameters:
Peak serum levels: 4-8 mcg/mL (q8h dosing); 16-24 mcg/mL (q24h dosing)
Bioavailability: Not applicable
Excreted unchanged: 95%
Serum half-life (normal/ESRD): 2.5/48 hrs
Plasma protein binding: < 5%
Volume of distribution (V_d): 0.25 L/kg
Primary Mode of Elimination: Renal
Dosage Adjustments:

CrCl ~ 40–60 mL/min	2.5 mg/kg (IV) q24h or 120 mg (IV) q24h

CrCl ~ 10–30 mL/min	2.5 mg/kg (IV) q48h or 120 mg (IV) q48h
CrCl < 10 mL/min	1.25 mg/kg (IV) q48h or 60 mg (IV) q48h
Post–HD dose*	1.25 mg/kg (IV) or 80 mg (IV)
Post–PD dose*	0.6 mg/kg (IV) or 40 mg (IV)
Post–CVVH dose*	1.42 mg/kg (IV) or 100 mg (IV)
Moderate hepatic insufficiency	No change
Severe hepatic insufficiency	No change

Drug Interactions: Amphotericin B, cephalothin, cyclosporine, enflurane, methoxyflurane, NSAIDs, polymyxin B, radiographic contrast, vancomycin (↑ nephrotoxicity); cis-platinum (↑ nephrotoxicity, ↑ ototoxicity); loop diuretics (↑ ototoxicity); neuromuscular blocking agents, magnesium sulfate (↑ apnea, prolonged paralysis); non-polarizing muscle relaxants (↑ apnea)
Adverse Effects: Neuromuscular blockade with rapid infusion/absorption. Nephrotoxicity only with prolonged/extremely high serum trough levels; may cause reversible non-oliguric renal failure (ATN). Ototoxicity associated with prolonged/extremely high peak serum levels (usually irreversible): Cochlear toxicity (1/3 of ototoxicity) manifests as decreased high frequency hearing, but deafness is unusual. Vestibular toxicity (2/3 of ototoxicity) develops before ototoxicity, and typically manifests as tinnitus
Resistance Potential: High (P. aeruginosa)
Allergic Potential: Low
Safety in Pregnancy: C
Comments: Dose for synergy = 2.5 mg/kg (IV) q24h or 120 mg (IV) q24h. Single daily dosing greatly reduces nephrotoxic/ototoxic potential. Incompatible with solutions containing β–lactams, erythromycin, chloramphenicol, furosemide, sodium bicarbonate. IV infusion

---

* Resume dosing for CrCl < 10 mL/min after supplemental dose. "Usual dose" assumes normal renal and hepatic function. CrCl = creatinine clearance; CVVH = continuous veno-venous hemofiltration; HD = hemodialysis; PD = peritoneal dialysis. See pp. 252-255 for definitions/explanations, p. 1 for abbreviations

should be given slowly over 1 hour. May be given IM. Avoid intraperitoneal infusion due to risk of neuromuscular blockade. Avoid intratracheal/aerosolized intrapulmonary instillation, which predisposes to antibiotic resistance. V_d increases with edema/ascites, trauma, burns, cystic fibrosis; may require ↑ dose. V_d decreases with dehydration, obesity; may require ↓ dose. Renal cast counts are the best indicator of aminoglycoside nephrotoxicity, not serum creatinine. Dialysis removes ~ 1/3 of gentamicin from serum

Therapeutic Serum Concentrations:
Peak (q24h/q8h dosing) = 16-24/8-10 mcg/mL
Trough (q24h/q8h dosing) = 0/1-2 mcg/mL
Intrathecal (IT) dose = 5 mg (IT) q24h

Cerebrospinal Fluid Penetration:
Non-inflamed meninges = 0%
Inflamed meninges = 20%

Bile Penetration: 30%

REFERENCES:
Cunha BA. Aminoglycosides: Current role in antimicrobial therapy. Pharmacotherapy 8:334-50, 1988.
Edson RS, Terrell CL. The aminoglycosides. Mayo Clin Proc 74:519-28, 1999.
Freeman CD, Nicolau DP, Belliveau PP, et al. Once-daily dosing of aminoglycosides: Review and recommendations for clinical practice. J Antimicrob Chemother 39:677-86, 1997.

Grepafloxacin (Raxar)

Drug Class: Fluoroquinolone
Usual Dose: 400 mg (PO) q24h
Pharmacokinetic Parameters:
Peak serum level: 1.4 mcg/mL
Bioavailability: 70%
Excreted unchanged: No data
Serum half-life (normal/ESRD): 15/15 hrs
Plasma protein binding: No data
Volume of distribution (V_d): No data
Primary Mode of Elimination: Hepatic
Dosage Adjustments:

CrCl ~ 40–60 mL/min	No change
CrCl ~ 10–30 mL/min	No change
CrCl < 10 mL/min	No change

Post–HD dose	No information
Post–PD dose	No information
Post–CVVH dose	No information
Moderate hepatic insufficiency	No information
Severe hepatic insufficiency	No information

Drug Interactions: No data
Adverse Effects: Drug fever/rash, GI upset, hepatotoxicity. May ↑ QT_c; avoid with other medications that prolong the QT_c interval and in patients with cardiac arrhythmias/heart block.
Resistance Potential: Low
Allergic Potential: Low
Safety in Pregnancy: C
Comments: Take 4 hours before or after calcium/magnesium containing antacids. Hepatotoxic. Use another quinolone

REFERENCES:
Efthymiopoulos C. Pharmacokinetics of grepafloxacin. J Antimicrob Chemother 40:35-43, 1997.
Lode H, Vogel F, Elies W. Grepafloxacin: A review of its safety profile based on clinical trials and postmarketing surveillance. Clinical Therapeutics 21:61-74, 1999.
Stahlmann R, Schwabe R. Safety profile of grepafloxacin compared with other fluoroquinolones. J Antimicrob Chemother 40:83-92, 1997.
Wagstaff AJ, Balfour JA. Grepafloxacin. Drugs 53:817-24, 1997.
Wiedemann B, Heisig P. Antibacterial activity of grepafloxacin. J Antimicrob Chemother 40:19-35, 1997.

Griseofulvin (Fulvicin, Grifulvin, Ultra, Gris-PEG, Grisactin)

Drug Class: Antifungal
Usual Dose: 500 mg–1 gm (PO) q24h (microsize); 330 mg (PO) q24h (ultramicrosize)
Pharmacokinetic Parameters:
Peak serum level: 1-2 mcg/mL
Bioavailability: 50%
Excreted unchanged: 1%

Serum half-life (normal/ESRD): 9/22 hrs
Plasma protein binding: 84%
Volume of distribution (V_d): No data
Primary Mode of Elimination: Hepatic
Dosage Adjustments:

CrCl ~ 40–60 mL/min	No change
CrCl ~ 10–30 mL/min	No change
CrCl < 10 mL/min	No change
Post–HD dose	None
Post–PD dose	None
Post–CVVH dose	None
Moderate hepatic insufficiency	No change
Severe hepatic insufficiency	No change

Drug Interactions: Alcohol (↑ griseofulvin toxicity); barbiturates (↓ griseofulvin levels); oral contraceptives, warfarin (↓ interacting drug levels)
Adverse Effects: Photosensitivity reactions, headache, nausea, vomiting, diarrhea, angular stomatitis, glossitis, leukopenia
Resistance Potential: Low
Allergic Potential: Moderate
Safety in Pregnancy: C
Comments: May exacerbate SLE/acute intermittent porphyria. Take microsize griseofulvin with fatty meal to ↑ absorption to ~ 70%. Ultramicrosize griseofulvin is absorbed 1.5 times better than microsize griseofulvin

REFERENCES:
Trepanier EF, Amsden GW. Current issues in onychomycosis. Ann Pharmacotherapy 32:204-14, 1998.

Imipenem (Primaxin)

Drug Class: Carbapenem
Usual Dose: 1 gm (IV) q6h
Pharmacokinetic Parameters:
Peak serum level: 60 mcg/mL
Bioavailability: Not applicable

Excreted unchanged: 60%
Serum half-life (normal/ESRD): 1/4 hrs
Plasma protein binding: 20%
Volume of distribution (V_d): 0.2 L/kg
Primary Mode of Elimination: Renal
Dosage Adjustments:

CrCl ~ 40–60 mL/min	500 mg (IV) q6h
CrCl ~ 10–30 mL/min	500 mg (IV) q12h
CrCl < 10 mL/min	250 mg (IV) q12h
Post–HD dose*	250 mg (IV)
Post–PD dose	None
Post–CVVH dose*	500 mg (IV)
Moderate hepatic insufficiency	No change
Severe hepatic insufficiency	No change

Drug Interactions: Cyclosporine (↑ cyclosporine levels); ganciclovir (↑ risk of seizures); probenecid (↑ imipenem levels)
Adverse Effects: Seizures, phlebitis
Resistance Potential: High (P. aeruginosa)
Allergic Potential: Low
Safety in Pregnancy: C
Comments: Incompatible in solutions containing vancomycin or metronidazole. Seizures more likely in renal insufficiency/high doses. No cross allergenicity with penicillins, β–lactams; safe to use in penicillin allergic patients. Inhibits endotoxin release from gram-negative bacilli. Na^+ content = 3.2 mEq/gm
Cerebrospinal Fluid Penetration:
Non-inflamed meninges = 10%
Inflamed meninges = 15%
Bile Penetration: 1%

REFERENCES:
Balfour JA, Bryson HM, Brogden RN. Imipenem/cilastatin: An update of its antibacterial activity, pharmacokinetics, and therapeutic efficacy in the treatment of serious infections. Drugs 51:99-136, 1996

Barza M. Imipenem: First of a new class of beta-lactam antibiotics. Ann Intern Med 103:552-60, 1985.

Cunha BA. Cross allergenicity of penicillin with

carbapenems and monobactams. J Crit Illness 13:344, 1998.

Helinger WC, Brewer NS. Carbapenems and monobactams: Imipenem, meropenem, and aztreonam. Mayo Clin Proc 74:420-34, 1999.

Indinavir (Crixivan)

Drug Class: Antiretroviral protease inhibitor
Usual Dose: 800 mg (PO) q8h
Pharmacokinetic Parameters:
Peak serum level: 252 mcg/mL
Bioavailability: 65% (77% with food)
Excreted unchanged: 10%
Serum half-life (normal/ESRD): 2 hrs/no data
Plasma protein binding: 60 %
Volume of distribution (V_d): No data
Primary Mode of Elimination: Hepatic
Dosage Adjustments:

CrCl ~ 40–60 mL/min	No change
CrCl ~ 10–30 mL/min	No change
CrCl < 10 mL/min	No change
Post–HD dose	None
Post–PD dose	None
Post–CVVH dose	None
Moderate hepatic insufficiency	600 mg (PO) q8h
Severe hepatic insufficiency	400 mg (PO) q8h

Antiretroviral Dosage Adjustments:

Amprenavir	No changes
Delavirdine	Indinavir 600 mg q8h
Efavirenz	Indinavir 1000 mg q8h
Lopinavir/ritonavir	Indinavir 600 mg q12h
Nelfinavir	Limited data for indinavir 1200 mg q12h + nelfinavir 1250 mg q12h
Nevirapine	Indinavir 1000 mg q8h
Ritonavir	Indinavir 800 mg q12h + ritonavir 100-200 mg q12h, or 400 mg q12h of each drug
Saquinavir	No information
Rifampin	Avoid combination
Rifabutin	Indinavir 1000 mg q8h; rifabutin 150 mg q24h or 300 mg 2-3x/week

Drug Interactions: Antiretrovirals, rifabutin, rifampin (see dose adjustment grid, above); astemizole, terfenadine, benzodiazepines, cisapride, ergot alkaloids, statins, St. John's wort (avoid if possible); calcium channel blockers (↑ calcium channel blocker levels); carbamazepine, phenobarbital, phenytoin (↓ indinavir levels, ↑ anticonvulsant levels; monitor); clarithromycin, erythromycin, telithromycin (↑ indinavir and macrolide levels); didanosine (administer indinavir on empty stomach 2 hours apart); ethinyl estradiol, norethindrone (↑ interacting drug levels; no dosage adjustment); grapefruit juice (↓ indinavir levels); itraconazole, ketoconazole (↑ indinavir levels; sildenafil (↑ or ↓ sildenafil levels; do not exceed 25 mg in 48 hrs); theophylline (↓ theophylline levels)

Adverse Effects: Nausea, vomiting, diarrhea, anemia, leukopenia, headache, insomnia, nephrolithiasis, hyperglycemia (including worsening diabetes, new-onset diabetes, DKA), ↑ SGOT/SGPT, ↑ indirect bilirubin (2° to drug-induced Gilbert's syndrome; inconsequential), fat redistribution, lipid abnormalities (evaluate risk of coronary disease/pancreatitis), abdominal pain, possible ↑ bleeding in hemophilia

HIV Resistance Potential: Low (triple therapy); high (mono/double drug therapy)
Allergic Potential: Low
Safety in Pregnancy: C
Comments: Renal stone formation may be prevented/minimized by adequate hydration; ↑ risk of nephrolithiasis with alcohol. Take 1 hour

---

before or 2 hours after meals (may take with skim milk or low fat meal). Separate dosing with ddI by 1 hour. Effective antiretroviral therapy consists of at least 3 antiretrovirals (same/different classes)
Cerebrospinal Fluid Penetration: 16%

REFERENCES:

Acosta EP, Henry K, Baken L, et al. Indinavir concentrations and antiviral effect. Pharmacotherapy 19:708-712, 1999.

Deeks SG, Smith M, Holodniy M, et al. HIV-1 protease inhibitors: A review for clinicians. JAMA 277:145-53, 1997.

Go J, Cunha BA. Indinavir: A review. Antibiotics for Clinicians 3:81-87, 1999.

McDonald CK, Kuritzkes DR. Human immunodeficiency virus type 1 protease inhibitors. Arch Intern Med 157:951-9, 1997.

Panel on Clinical Practices for Treatment of HIV Infection. Guidelines for the use of antiretroviral agents in HIV-infected adults and adolescents. Department of Health and Human Services. April 23, 2001. www.hivatis.org

Isoniazid (INH)

Drug Class: Anti–TB drug
Usual Dose: 300 mg (PO) q24h
Pharmacokinetic Parameters:
Peak serum level: 7 mcg/mL
Bioavailability: 90%
Excreted unchanged: 25%
Serum half-life (normal/ESRD): 1/1 hr
Plasma protein binding: 15%
Volume of distribution (V_d): 0.75 L/kg
Primary Mode of Elimination: Hepatic
Dosage Adjustment:

CrCl ~ 40–60 mL/min	No change
CrCl ~ 10–30 mL/min	No change
CrCl < 10 mL/min	No change
Post–HD dose	None
Post–PD dose	None
Post–CVVH dose	None
Moderate hepatic insufficiency	No change

Severe hepatic insufficiency	100 mg (PO) q24h

Drug Interactions: Alcohol, rifampin (↑ risk of hepatic injury); alfentanil (↑ duration of alfentanil effect); aluminum salts (↓ isoniazid absorption); carbamazepine, phenytoin (↑ interacting drug levels); itraconazole (↓ itraconazole levels); warfarin (↑ INR)
Adverse Effects: ↑ SGOT/SGPT, drug fever/rash, age-dependent hepatotoxicity (after age 40), ↑ hepatotoxicity in slow acetylators, drug–induced ANA/SLE, hemolytic anemia
Resistance Potential: Low
Allergic Potential: Low
Safety in Pregnancy: C
Comments: Administer with 50 mg of pyridoxine daily to prevent peripheral neuropathy. Increased blood pressure/rash with tyramine–containing products, e.g., cheese/wine.
Meningeal dose = usual dose
Cerebrospinal Fluid Penetration:
Non-inflamed meninges = 90%
Inflamed meninges = 90%

REFERENCES:

Davidson PT, Le HQ. Drug treatment of tuberculosis 1992. Drugs 43:651-73, 1992. Drugs for tuberculosis. Med Lett Drugs Ther 35:99- 101,1993.

Van Scoy RE, Wilkowske CJ. Antituberculous agents. Mayo Clin Proc 67:179-87, 1992.

Itraconazole (Sporanox)

Drug Class: Antifungal
Usual Dose: 200 mg (IV/PO) q24h; 200 mg capsules/solution (PO) q24h (see comments)
Pharmacokinetic Parameters:
Peak serum level: 2 mcg/mL
Bioavailability: 55%
Excreted unchanged: 35%
Serum half-life (normal/ESRD): 35/35 hrs
Plasma protein binding: 99%
Volume of distribution (V_d): 10 L/kg
Primary Mode of Elimination: Hepatic
Dosage Adjustments:

CrCl ~ 40–60 mL/min	No change

---

* Resume dosing for CrCl < 10 mL/min after supplemental dose. "Usual dose" assumes normal renal and hepatic function. CrCl = creatinine clearance; CVVH = continuous veno-venous hemofiltration; HD = hemodialysis; PD = peritoneal dialysis. See pp. 252-255 for definitions/explanations, p. 1 for abbreviations

CrCl ~ 10–30 mL/min	No change
CrCl < 10 mL/min	No change
Post–HD dose	None
Post–PD dose	None
Post–CVVH dose	None
Moderate hepatic insufficiency	No change
Severe hepatic insufficiency	No change

Drug Interactions: Astemizole, cisapride, terfenadine (may ↑ QT interval, torsades de pointes); carbamazepine, INH (↓ itraconazole levels); cimetidine, famotidine, nizatidine, ranitidine, omeprazole, INH (↓ itraconazole absorption); cyclosporine, digoxin, loratadine, tacrolimus (↑ interacting drug levels with possible toxicity); didanosine (↓ itraconazole levels); midazolam, triazolam (↑ interacting drug levels, ↑ sedative effects); oral hypoglycemics (severe hypoglycemia); phenytoin, rifabutin, rifampin (↓ itraconazole levels, ↑ interacting drug levels); statins (↑ statin levels; rhabdomyolysis reported); warfarin (↑ INR)
Adverse Effects: Nausea, vomiting, diarrhea, ↑ SGOT/SGPT
Resistance Potential: Low
Allergic Potential: Low
Safety in Pregnancy: C
Comments: Requires gastric acidity for absorption. Solution better absorbed without food; capsules better absorbed with food. (Capsule bioavailability is food dependent: 40% fasting/90% post-prandial.) Give antacids/H₂ blockers 2 hours following itraconazole dose. Risk of hypoaldosteronism with doses ≥ 600 mg/day. Begin itraconazole for acute/severe infections with a loading regimen of 200 mg (IV) q12h x 2 days, then give 200 mg (IV or PO) q24h maintenance dose. For oral therapy, 10 mL of solution without food has equivalent bioavailability to 100 mg capsule with food
Cerebrospinal Fluid Penetration: < 10%

REFERENCES:
Cleary JD, Taylor JW, Chapman SW. Itraconazole in antifungal therapy. Ann Pharmacother 26:502-9, 1992.
Go J, Cunha BA. Itraconazole. Antibiotics for Clinicians 3:61-70, 1999.
Grant SM, Clissold SP. Itraconazole: A review of its pharmacodynamic and pharmacokinetic properties, and therapeutic use in superficial and systemic mycoses. Drugs 37:310-44, 1989.
Kauffman CA, Carver PL. Antifungal agents in the 1990s: Current status and future developments. Drugs 53:539- 49, 1997.
Klein NC, Cunha BA. Antifungal therapy of the pulmonary mycoses. Chest 110:525-30, 1999.
Lyman CA, Walsh TJ. Systemically administered antifungal agents : A review of their clinical pharmacology and therapeutic applications. Drugs 44:9-35, 1992.
Terrell CL. Antifungal agents Part II. The azoles. Mayo Clin Proc 74:78-100, 1999.

Ketoconazole (Nizoral)

Drug Class: Antifungal
Usual Dose: 200 mg (PO) q24h
Pharmacokinetic Parameters:
Peak serum level: 1.5 mcg/mL
Bioavailability: 82%
Excreted unchanged: 70%
Serum half-life (normal/ESRD): 6/20 hrs
Plasma protein binding: 96%
Volume of distribution (V_d): 0.83 L/kg
Primary Mode of Elimination: Hepatic
Dosage Adjustments:

CrCl ~ 40–60 mL/min	No change
CrCl ~ 10–30 mL/min	No change
CrCl < 10 mL/min	No change
Post–HD dose	None
Post–PD dose	None
Post–CVVH dose	None
Moderate hepatic insufficiency	No change
Severe hepatic insufficiency	100 mg (PO) q24h

Drug Interactions: Astemizole, cisapride,

terfenadine (may ↑ QT interval, torsades de pointes); carbamazepine, INH (↓ ketoconazole levels); cimetidine, famotidine, nizatidine, ranitidine, omeprazole, INH (↓ ketoconazole absorption); cyclosporine, digoxin, loratadine, tacrolimus (↑ interacting drug levels with possible toxicity); didanosine (↓ ketoconazole levels); midazolam, triazolam (↑ interacting drug levels, ↑ sedative effects); oral hypoglycemics (severe hypoglycemia); phenytoin, rifabutin, rifampin (↓ ketoconazole levels, ↑ interacting drug); statins (↑ statin levels; rhabdomyolysis reported); warfarin (↑ INR)

Adverse Effects: Nausea, vomiting, abdominal pain, pruritus
Resistance Potential: High (C. albicans)
Allergic Potential: Low
Safety in Pregnancy: C
Comments: Dose-dependent reduction in gonadal (androgenic) function. Decreased cortisol production with doses ≥ 800 mg/day, but does not result in adrenal insufficiency
Cerebrospinal Fluid Penetration: < 10%

REFERENCES:
Allen LV. Ketoconazole oral suspension. US Pharm 18:98-9, 1993.
Como JA, Dismukes WE. Oral azole drugs as systemic antifungal therapy. N Engl J Med 330:263-72, 1993.
Lyman CA, Walsh TJ. Systemically administered antifungal agents : A review of their clinical pharmacology and therapeutic applications. Drugs 44:9-35, 1992.
Terrell CL. Antifungal agents: Part II. The azoles. Mayo Clin Proc 74:78-100, 1999.

Lamivudine (Epivir) 3TC

Drug Class: Antiretroviral NRTI (nucleoside reverse transcriptase inhibitor); Antiviral (HBV)
Usual Dose: 150 mg (PO) q12h
Pharmacokinetic Parameters:
Peak serum level: 1.5 mcg/mL
Bioavailability: 86%
Excreted unchanged: 90%
Serum half-life (normal/ESRD): 3-6/20 hrs
Plasma protein binding: 36%
Volume of distribution (V_d): 1.3 L/kg
Primary Mode of Elimination: Renal

Dosage Adjustments:

CrCl ~ 40–60 mL/min	No change
CrCl ~ 10–30 mL/min	150 mg (PO) q24h
CrCl < 10 mL/min	50 mg (PO) q24h
Post–HD dose*	100 mg (PO)
Post–PD dose*	50 mg (PO)
Post–CVVH dose*	150 mg (PO)
Moderate hepatic insufficiency	No change
Severe hepatic insufficiency	No change

Drug Interactions: Didanosine, zalcitabine (↑ risk of pancreatitis); TMP-SMX (↑ lamivudine levels); zidovudine (↑ zidovudine levels)
Adverse Effects: Drug fever/rash, abdominal pain/diarrhea, nausea, vomiting, anemia, leukopenia, photophobia, depression, cough, nasal complaints, headache, dizziness, peripheral neuropathy, pancreatitis, myalgias, lactic acidosis with hepatic steatosis (rare, but potentially life-threatening toxicity with NRTIs)
HIV Resistance Potential: Low (triple therapy); high (mono/double drug therapy)
Allergic Potential: Low
Safety in Pregnancy: C
Comments: Potential cross resistance with didanosine. Prevents development of AZT resistance and restores AZT susceptibility. May be taken with or without food. Effective against HBV in HIV patients with 3-6 months of therapy, but HBV may reactivate after lamivudine therapy is stopped. Also a component of Combivir and Trizivir. Effective antiretroviral therapy consists of at least 3 antiretrovirals (same/different classes)
Cerebrospinal Fluid Penetration: 15%

REFERENCES:
Eron JJ, Benoit SL, Jemsek J, et al. Treatment with lamivudine, zidovudine, or both in HIV-positive patients with 200 to 500 CD4 cells per cubic millimeter. N Engl J Med 333:1662-9, 1995.
Lai CI, Chien RN. Leung NW, et al. A one-year trial of lamivudine for chronic hepatitis B. N Engl J Med 339:61-8, 1998.

---

* Resume dosing for CrCl < 10 mL/min after supplemental dose. "Usual dose" assumes normal renal and hepatic function. CrCl = creatinine clearance; CVVH = continuous veno-venous hemofiltration; HD = hemodialysis; PD = peritoneal dialysis. See pp. 252-255 for definitions/explanations, p. 1 for abbreviations

Murphy RL, Brun S, Hicks C, et al. ABT-378/ritonavir plus stavudine and lamivudine for the treatment of antiretroviral-naive adults with HIV-1 infection: 48-week results. AIDS 15:F1-9, 2001.

Panel on Clinical Practices for Treatment of HIV Infection. Guidelines for the use of antiretroviral agents in HIV-infected adults and adolescents. Department of Health and Human Services. April 23, 2001. www.hivatis.org

Perry CM, Faulds D. Lamivudine. A review of its antiviral activity, pharmacokinetic properties and therapeutic efficacy in the management of HIV infection. Drugs 53:657-80, 1997.

Staszewski S, Morales-Ramirez J, Trashima KT, et al. Efavirenz plus zidovudine and lamivudine, efavirenz plus indinavir, and indinavir plus zidovudine and lamivudine in the treatment of HIV-1 infection in adults. N Engl J Med 341:1865-1873, 1999.

Lamivudine + zidovudine (Combivir)

Drug Class: Antiretroviral NRTIs combination
Usual Dose: Combivir tablet = 150 mg lamivudine + 300 mg zidovudine. Usual dose = 1 tablet (PO) q12h
Pharmacokinetic Parameters:
Peak serum level: 1.5/1.2 mcg/mL
Bioavailability: 82/6%
Excreted unchanged: 90/16%
Serum half-life (normal/ESRD): [6/1]/[20/1.4] hrs
Plasma protein binding: 36/20%
Volume of distribution (V_d): 1.3/1.6 L/kg
Primary Mode of Elimination: Renal
Dosage Adjustments:

CrCl ~ 40–60 mL/min	No change
CrCl ~ 10–30 mL/min	1 tablet (PO) q24h
CrCl < 10 mL/min	1 tablet (PO) q48h
Post–HD dose*	1 tablet (PO)
Post–PD dose	None
Post–CVVH dose*	1 tablet (PO)
Moderate hepatic insufficiency	No change
Severe hepatic insufficiency	No change

Drug Interactions: Acetaminophen (↑ Combivir toxicity); acyclovir (↑ lethargy, fatigue); amprenavir, atovaquone (↑ zidovudine levels); cidofovir (↑ zidovudine levels, flu-like symptoms); clarithromycin (↓ zidovudine levels); dapsone, doxorubicin (neutropenia); TMP-SMX (↑ lamivudine and zidovudine levels)
Adverse Effects: Headache, nausea, malaise, cough/nasal congestion, lipodystrophy, pancreatitis, steatosis, leukopenia, anemia, myopathy, neuropathy
HIV Resistance Potential: Low (triple therapy); high (mono/double drug therapy)
Allergic Potential: Low
Safety in Pregnancy: C
Comments: Avoid if history of pancreatitis. Effective antiretroviral therapy consists of at least 3 antiretrovirals (same/different classes)
Cerebrospinal Fluid Penetration: Lamivudine = 12%; zidovudine = 60%

REFERENCES:

Drugs for AIDS and associated infections. Med Lett Drug Ther 35:79-86, 1993.

Hirsch MS, D'Aquila RT. Therapy for human immunodeficiency virus infection. N Engl J Med 328:1685-95, 1993.

McLeod GX, Hammer SM. Zidovudine: Five years later. Ann Intern Med 117:487-510, 1992.

Panel on Clinical Practices for Treatment of HIV Infection. Guidelines for the use of antiretroviral agents in HIV-infected adults and adolescents. Department of Health and Human Services. April 23, 2001. www.hivatis.org

Staszewski S, Morales-Ramirez J, Trashima KT, et al. Efavirenz plus zidovudine and lamivudine, efavirenz plus indinavir, and indinavir plus zidovudine and lamivudine in the treatment of HIV-1 infection in adults. N Engl J Med 341:1865-1873, 1999.

Levofloxacin (Levaquin)

Drug Class: Fluoroquinolone
Usual Dose: 500 mg (IV/PO) q24h
Pharmacokinetic Parameters:
Peak serum level: 6.2 mcg/mL
Bioavailability: 99%
Excreted unchanged: 80%

---

* Resume dosing for CrCl < 10 mL/min after supplemental dose. "Usual dose" assumes normal renal and hepatic function. CrCl = creatinine clearance; CVVH = continuous veno venous hemofiltration; HD = hemodialysis; PD = peritoneal dialysis. See pp. 252-255 for definitions/explanations, p. 1 for abbreviations

Serum half-life (normal/ESRD): 7/8.2 hrs
Plasma protein binding: 30%
Volume of distribution (V_d): 1.3 L/kg
Primary Mode of Elimination: Renal
Dosage Adjustments:

CrCl ~ 40–60 mL/min	250 mg (IV/PO) q24h
CrCl ~ 10–30 mL/min	250 mg (IV/PO) q48h
CrCl < 10 mL/min	250 mg (IV/PO) q48h
Post–HD dose	None
Post–PD dose	None
Post–CVVH dose*	500 mg (IV/PO)
Moderate hepatic insufficiency	No change
Severe hepatic insufficiency	No change

Drug Interactions: Al^{++}, Ca^{++}, Fe^{++}, Mg^{++}, Zn^{++} antacids, citrate/citric acid, dairy products (↓ absorption of levofloxacin only if taken together); NSAIDs (CNS stimulation); probenecid (↑ levofloxacin levels); warfarin (↑ INR)
Adverse Effects: Drug fever/rash, mild nausea
Resistance Potential: Low
Allergic Potential: Low
Safety in Pregnancy: C
Comments: Lowest incidence of GI side effects among fluoroquinolones. Take 2 hours before or after calcium/magnesium containing antacids. Does not lower seizure potential. Does not increase digoxin concentrations. Use 750 mg (IV/PO) q24h for nosocomial pneumonia or complicated skin/soft tissue infections. Only quinolone indicated for highly penicillin-resistant S. pneumoniae
Cerebrospinal Fluid Penetration: 16%

REFERENCES:
Cunha BA. Community-acquired pneumonia: Diagnostic and therapeutic considerations. Med Clin North Am 85:43-77. 2001.
Cunha BA. Quinolones: Clinical aspects. Antibiotics for Clinicians 2:129-35, 1998.
Drago L, DeVecchi E, Mombelli L, et al. Activity of levofloxacin and ciprofloxacin against urinary pathogens. J. Antimicrobial Chemo 48: 37-45, 2001.
Nightingale CH, Grant EM, Quintiliani R. Pharmacodynamics and pharmacokinetics of levofloxacin. Chemotherapy 46:6-14, 2000.
Thornsberry C, Karlowsky JA, Sahm DF. Levofloxacin-resistant Streptococcus pneumoniae: Second look. Antimicrob Agents Chemother 45:2183-83, 2001.

Linezolid (Zyvox)

Drug Class: Oxazolidinone
Usual Dose: 600 mg (IV/PO) q12h
Pharmacokinetic Parameters:
Peak serum level: 16 mcg/mL
Bioavailability: 100%
Excreted unchanged: 30%
Serum half-life (normal/ESRD): 5.5/5.5 hrs
Plasma protein binding: 31%
Volume of distribution (V_d): 0.64 L/kg
Primary Mode of Elimination: Hepatic/metabolized
Dosage Adjustments:

CrCl ~ 40–60 mL/min	No change
CrCl ~ 10–30 mL/min	No change
CrCl < 10 mL/min	No change
Post–HD dose*	200 mg (IV/PO)
Post–PD dose	None
Post–CVVH dose*	200 mg (IV/PO)
Moderate hepatic insufficiency	No change
Severe hepatic insufficiency	No change

Drug Interactions: Pseudoephedrine, tyramine-containing foods (↑ risk of hypertensive crisis); serotonergic agents, e.g., SSRI's, tricyclic antidepressants (↑ risk of serotonin syndrome)
Adverse Effects: Mild, readily reversible thrombocytopenia, anemia, or leukopenia may occur after ≥ 2 weeks of therapy
Resistance Potential: Low
Allergic Potential: Low
Safety in Pregnancy: C
Comments: May be taken with or without food. Ideal for IV-to-PO switch programs. Unlike

---

vancomycin, linezolid does not increase VRE prevalence and is available orally for MRSA, MRSE, and E. faecalis infections. Unlike quinupristin/dalfopristin, linezolid is active against E. faecalis and is available orally for MRSA, MRSE, and E. faecium (VRE) infections. Meningeal dose = usual dose
Cerebrospinal Fluid Penetration: 70%

REFERENCES:

Cercenado E, Garcia-Garrote F, Bouza E. In vitro activity of linezolid against multiple resistant gram-positive clinical isolates. J Antimicrob Chemother 47:77-81, 2001.

Go J, Cunha BA. Linezolid: A review. Antibiotics for Clinicians 4:82-88, 2000.

Green SL, Maddox JC, Huttenbach ED. Linezolid and reversible myelosuppression. JAMA 285:1291, 2001.

Hamel JC, Stapert D, Moerman JK, et al. Linezolid, critical characteristics. Infection 28:60-4, 2000.

Plouffe JF. Emerging therapies for serious gram-positive bacterial infections: a focus on linezolid. Clin Infect Dis 4:144-9, 2000.

Lopinavir + ritonavir (Kaletra)

Drug Class: Antiretroviral protease inhibitor combination
Usual Dose: Kaletra capsule = 133.3 mg lopinavir + 33.3 mg ritonavir. Oral solution (per ml) = 80 mg lopinavir + 20 mg ritonavir. Usual dose = 3 capsules or 5 mL (PO) q12h with food
Pharmacokinetic Parameters:
Peak serum level: 9.6/≤ 1 mcg/mL
Bioavailability: No data
Excreted unchanged: 3%
Serum half-life (normal/ESRD): 5-6/5-6 hrs
Plasma protein binding: 99%
Volume of distribution (V_d): No data
Primary Mode of Elimination: Hepatic
Dosage Adjustments:

CrCl ~ 40-60 mL/min	No change
CrCl ~ 10-30 mL/min	No change
CrCl < 10 mL/min	No change
Post-HD dose	None
Post-PD dose	None
Post-CVVH dose	None
Moderate hepatic insufficiency	No change
Severe hepatic insufficiency	3 capsules (PO) q24h or 5 mL (PO) q24h

Antiretroviral Dosage Adjustments:

Amprenavir	Amprenavir 600-750 mg q12h
Delavirdine	No information
Efavirenz	Consider lopinavir/ritonavir 533/133 mg q12h in PI-experienced patients
Indinavir	Indinavir 600 mg q12h
Nelfinavir	No information
Nevirapine	Consider lopinavir/ritonavir 533/133 mg q12h in PI-experienced patients
Saquinavir	Saquinavir 800 mg q12h

Drug Interactions: Antiretrovirals, rifabutin, rifampin (see dose adjustment grid, above); astemizole, terfenadine, benzodiazepines, cisapride, ergotamine, flecainide, pimozide, propafenone, statins, St. John's wort (avoid if possible). Insufficient data on other drug interactions listed for ritonavir alone
Adverse Effects: Diarrhea (very common), headache, nausea, vomiting, asthenia, ↑ SGOT/SGPT, abdominal pain, pancreatitis, paresthesias, hyperglycemia (including worsening diabetes, new-onset diabetes, DKA), ↑ cholesterol/triglycerides (evaluate risk for coronary disease, pancreatitis), ↑ CPK, ↑ uric acid, fat redistribution, possible increased bleeding in hemophilia. Oral solution contains

---

* Resume dosing for CrCl < 10 mL/min after supplemental dose. "Usual dose" assumes normal renal and hepatic function. CrCl = creatinine clearance, CVVH = continuous veno-venous hemofiltration; HD = hemodialysis; PD = peritoneal dialysis. See pp. 252-255 for definitions/explanations, p. 1 for abbreviations

42.4% alcohol
HIV Resistance Potential: Low (triple therapy); high (mono/double drug therapy)
Allergic Potential: Low
Safety in Pregnancy: C
Comments: Lopinavir serum concentrations with moderately fatty meals are increased 43% (capsules)/54% (oral solution). Refrigerated capsules stable until date on label; if stored at room temperature, capsules stable x 2 months. Ritonavir 100 mg is not an effective anti-HIV dose. Although Kaletra is a double drug combination, it should be regarded as equivalent to lopinavir monotherapy, requiring 2 additional antiretroviral agents for effective antiretroviral therapy

REFERENCES:
Fischl MA. Antiretroviral therapy in 1999 for antiretroviral-naive individuals with HIV infection. AIDS 13:49-59, 1999.
Havlir DV. Lange JM. New antiretrovirals and new combinations. AIDS 12:165-74, 1998.
Horowitz HW, Telzak EE, Sepkowitz KA, et al. Human immunodeficiency virus infection. Disease-A-Month 44:677-716, 1998.
Panel on Clinical Practices for Treatment of HIV Infection. Guidelines for the use of antiretroviral agents in HIV-infected adults and adolescents. Department of Health and Human Services. April 23, 2001. www.hivatis.org

Loracarbef (Lorabid)

Drug Class: 2nd generation oral cephalosporin
Usual Dose: 400 mg (PO) q12h
Pharmacokinetic Parameters:
Peak serum level: 14 mcg/mL
Bioavailability: 90%
Excreted unchanged: 90%
Serum half-life (normal/ESRD): 1.2/32 hrs
Plasma protein binding: 25%
Volume of distribution (V_d): 0.35 L/kg
Primary Mode of Elimination: Renal
Dosage Adjustments:

CrCl ~ 40–60 mL/min	200 mg (PO) q12h
CrCl ~ 10–30 mL/min	200 mg (PO) q24h
CrCl < 10 mL/min	200 mg (PO) q48h

Post–HD dose*	200 mg (PO)
Post–PD dose	None
Post–CVVH dose*	400 mg (PO)
Moderate hepatic insufficiency	No change
Severe hepatic insufficiency	No change

Drug Interactions: None
Adverse Effects: Drug fever/rash, diarrhea
Resistance Potential: Low
Allergic Potential: Low
Safety in Pregnancy: B
Comments: Take 1 hour before or 2 hours after meals
Cerebrospinal Fluid Penetration: < 10%

REFERENCES:
Bandak SI, Turnak MR, Allen BS, et al. Assessment of the susceptibility of Streptococcus pneumoniae to cefaclor and loracarbef in 13 cases. J Chemother 12:299-305, 2000.
Gooch WM 3rd, Adelglass J, Kelsey DK, et al. Loracarbef versus clarithromycin in children with acute otitis media with effusion. Clin her 21:711-22, 1999.
Paster RZ, McAdoo MA, Keyserling CH. A comparison of a five-day regimen of cefdinir with a seven-day regimen of loracarbef for the treatment of acute exacerbations of chronic bronchitis. Int J Clin Pract 64:293-9, 2000.

Meropenem (Merrem)

Drug Class: Carbapenem
Usual Dose: 1 gm (IV) q8h
Pharmacokinetic Parameters:
Peak serum level: 62 mcg/mL
Bioavailability: Not applicable
Excreted unchanged: 70%
Serum half-life (normal/ESRD): 1/7 hrs
Plasma protein binding: 2%
Volume of distribution (V_d): 0.35 L/kg
Primary Mode of Elimination: Renal
Dosage Adjustments:

CrCl ~ 40–60 mL/min	1 gm (IV) q12h
CrCl ~ 10–30 mL/min	500 mg (IV) q12h

---

* Resume dosing for CrCl < 10 mL/min after supplemental dose. "Usual dose" assumes normal renal and hepatic function. CrCl = creatinine clearance; CVVH = continuous veno-venous hemofiltration; HD = hemodialysis; PD = peritoneal dialysis. See pp. 252-255 for definitions/explanations, p. 1 for abbreviations

CrCl < 10 mL/min	500 mg (IV) q24h
Post–HD dose*	500 mg (IV)
Post–PD dose	None
Post–CVVH dose*	1 gm (IV)
Moderate hepatic insufficiency	No change
Severe hepatic insufficiency	No change

Drug Interactions: Probenecid (↑ meropenem half-life by 40%)
Adverse Effects: Rarely, mild infusion site inflammation
Resistance Potential: Low
Allergic Potential: Low
Safety in Pregnancy: B
Comments: No adverse effects with 2 gm (IV) q8h regimen. No cross allergenicity with penicillins/β–lactams; safe to use in penicillin allergic patients. Meropenem (1 gm) may be given by rapid IV infusion over 15-30 minutes (C_{max} = 49 mcg/mL) or as a bolus IV injection over 3-5 minutes (C_{max} = 112 mcg/mL). Inhibits endotoxin release from gram-negative bacilli. Na^+ content = 3.92 mEq/g.
Meningeal dose = 2 gm (IV) q8h
Cerebrospinal Fluid Penetration:
Non-inflamed meninges = 10%
Inflamed meninges = 15%

REFERENCES:
Cunha BA. Cross allergenicity of penicillin with carbapenems and monobactams. J Crit Illness 13:344,1998.
Cunha BA: The safety of meropenem in elderly and renally impaired patients. Intern J Antimcrob Ther 10:109-117, 1998.
Cunha BA. The use of meropenem in critical care. Antibiotics for Clinicians 4:59-66, 2000.
Fish DN, Singletary TJ. Meropenem: A new carbapenem antibiotic. Pharmacotherapy 17:644-69, 1997.
Hellinger WC, Brewer NS. Carbapenems and monobactams: Imipenem, meropenem, and aztreonam. Mayo Clin Proc 74:420-34, 1999.

Methenamine hippurate (Hiprex, Urex)
Methenamine mandelate (Mandelamine)

Drug Class: Urinary antiseptic
Usual Dose: 1 gm (PO) q6h (hippurate); 1 gm (PO) q6h (mandelate)
Pharmacokinetic Parameters:
Peak serum level: Not applicable
Bioavailability: 90%
Excreted unchanged: 90%
Serum half-life (normal/ESRD): 4 hrs/no data
Plasma protein binding: Not applicable
Volume of distribution (V_d): Not applicable
Primary Mode of Elimination: Renal
Dosage Adjustments:

CrCl ~ 40–60 mL/min	500 mg (PO) q12h
CrCl ~ 10–30 mL/min	Avoid
CrCl < 10 mL/min	Avoid
Post–HD dose	Avoid
Post–PD dose	Avoid
Post–CVVH dose	Avoid
Moderate hepatic insufficiency	No change
Severe hepatic insufficiency	No change

Drug Interactions: Acetazolamide, sodium bicarbonate, thiazide diuretics (↓ antibacterial effect due to ↑ urinary pH ≥ 5.5)
Adverse Effects: GI upset
Resistance Potential: Low
Allergic Potential: Low
Safety in Pregnancy: C
Comments: Take with food to decrease GI upset. Effectiveness depends on maintaining an acid urine (pH ≤ 5.5) with acidifying agents (e.g., ascorbic acid). Useful mainly for catheter–associated bacteriuria, not UTIs. Forms formaldehyde in acid urine; resistance does not develop

---

* Resume dosing for CrCl < 10 mL/min after supplemental dose. "Usual dose" assumes normal renal and hepatic function. CrCl = creatinine clearance; CVVH = continuous veno-venous hemofiltration; HD = hemodialysis; PD = peritoneal dialysis. See pp. 252-255 for definitions/explanations, p. 1 for abbreviations

REFERENCES:

Cunha BA, Comer JB. Pharmacokinetic considerations in the treatment of urinary tract infections. Conn Med 43:347-53, 1979.

Klinge D, Mannisto P, Mantyla R, et al. Pharmacokinetics of methenamine in healthy volunteers. J Antimicrob Chemother 9:209-16, 1982.

Musher DM, Griggith DP. Generation of formaldehyde from methenamine: Effect of pH and concentration, and antibacterial effect. Antimicobr Agents Chemother 6:708-11, 1974.

Musher DM, Griffith DP, Templeton GB. Further observations of the potentiation of the antibacterial effect of methenamine by acetohydroxamic acid. J Infect Dis 133:564-67, 1976.

Metronidazole (Flagyl)

Drug Class: Nitroimidazole antiparasitic/antibiotic
Usual Dose: 1 gm (IV) q24h; 500 mg (PO) q12h
Pharmacokinetic Parameters:
Peak serum level: 26 mcg/mL
Bioavailability: 90%
Excreted unchanged: 20%
Serum half-life (normal/ESRD): 8/14 hrs
Plasma protein binding: 20%
Volume of distribution (V_d): 0.85 L/kg
Primary Mode of Elimination: Hepatic
Dosage Adjustments:

CrCl ~ 40–60 mL/min	No change
CrCl ~ 10–30 mL/min	No change
CrCl < 10 mL/min	No change
Post–HD dose	None
Post–PD dose	None
Post–CVVH dose	None
Moderate hepatic insufficiency	No change
Severe hepatic insufficiency	500 mg (IV/PO) q24h

Drug Interactions: Alcohol (disulfiram-like reaction); disulfiram (acute toxic psychosis); warfarin (↑ INR); phenobarbital, phenytoin (↑ metronidazole metabolism)
Adverse Effects: Disulfiram reaction

(tachycardia/flushing) with alcohol, nausea, vomiting, GI upset, metallic taste
Resistance Potential: Low
Allergic Potential: Low
Safety in Pregnancy: B (avoid in 1st trimester)
Comments: Q12h dosing is preferred to q6h dosing because of long half-life. May discolor urine brown. For C. difficile diarrhea, use 250 mg (PO) q6h. For C. difficile colitis, use 500 mg (IV or PO) q12h or 1 gm (IV) q24h.
Na^+ content = 28 mEq/g.
Meningeal dose = usual dose
Cerebrospinal Fluid Penetration:
Non-inflamed meninges = 30%
Inflamed meninges = 100%

REFERENCES:

Falagas ME, Gorbach SL. Clindamycin and metronidazole. Med Clin North Am 79:845-67, 1995.

Freeman CD, Klutman NE. Metronidazole: A therapeutic review and update. Drugs 54:679-708, 1997.

Kasten MJ. Clindamycin, metronidazole, and chloramphenicol. Mayo Clin Proc 74:825-33, 1999.

Mezlocillin (Mezlin)

Drug Class: Antipseudomonal penicillin
Usual Dose: 3 gm (IV) q6h
Pharmacokinetic Parameters:
Peak serum level: 300 mcg/mL
Bioavailability: Not applicable
Excreted unchanged: 65%
Serum half-life (normal/ESRD): 1.1 hrs/no data
Plasma protein binding: 30%
Volume of distribution (V_d): 0.18 L/kg
Primary Mode of Elimination: Renal
Dosage Adjustments:

CrCl ~ 40–60 mL/min	1.5 gm (IV) q6h
CrCl ~ 10–30 mL/min	1.5 gm (IV) q8h
CrCl < 10 mL/min	1.5 gm (IV) q12h
Post–HD dose*	3 gm (IV)
Post–PD dose*	1.5 gm (IV)
Post–CVVH dose*	3 gm (IV)
Moderate hepatic insufficiency	No change

---

* Resume dosing for CrCl < 10 mL/min after supplemental dose. "Usual dose" assumes normal renal and hepatic function. CrCl = creatinine clearance; CVVH = continuous veno-venous hemofiltration; HD = hemodialysis; PD = peritoneal dialysis. See pp. 252-255 for definitions/explanations, p. 1 for abbreviations

Severe hepatic insufficiency	No information

Drug Interactions: Aminoglycosides (inactivation of mezlocillin in renal failure); warfarin (↑ INR); oral contraceptives (↓ oral contraceptive effect); cefoxitin (↓ mezlocillin effect)

Adverse Effects: Drug fever/rash, E. multiforme/Stevens–Johnson syndrome, anaphylactic reactions (hypotension, laryngospasm, bronchospasm), hives; serum sickness. Dose-dependent inhibition of platelet aggregation is minimal/absent (usual dose is less than carbenicillin)

Resistance Potential: Low
Allergic Potential: Low
Safety in Pregnancy: B
Comments: Dose-dependent half-life ($t_{1/2}$). Na^+ content = 1.8 mEq/g
Cerebrospinal Fluid Penetration: < 10%

REFERENCES:
Donowitz GR, Mandell GL. Beta-lactam antibiotics. N Engl J Med 318.419-26 and 318:490-500, 1993.
Wright AJ. The penicillins. Mayo Clin Proc 74:290-307, 1999.
Wright AJ, Wirkowske CJ. The penicillins. Mayo Clin Proc 66:1047-63, 1991.

Minocycline (Minocin)

Drug Class: 2nd generation tetracycline
Usual Dose: 100 mg (IV/PO) q12h
Pharmacokinetic Parameters:
Peak serum level: 4 mcg/mL
Bioavailability: 95%
Excreted unchanged: 10%
Serum half-life (normal/ESRD): 18/22 hrs
Plasma protein binding: 75%
Volume of distribution (V_d): 1.5 L/kg
Primary Mode of Elimination: Hepatic
Dosage Adjustments:

CrCl ~ 40–60 mL/min	No change
CrCl ~ 10–30 mL/min	No change
CrCl < 10 mL/min	No change
Post–HD dose	None

Post–PD dose	None
Post–CVVH dose	None
Moderate hepatic insufficiency	No change
Severe hepatic insufficiency	100 mg (IV/PO) q24h

Drug Interactions: Antacids, Al^{++}, Ca^{++}, Fe^{++}, Mg^{++}, Zn^{++}, multivitamins, sucralfate (↓ minocycline absorption); isotretinoin (pseudotumor cerebri); warfarin (↑ INR)

Adverse Effects: Nausea, GI upset if not taken with food, hyperpigmentation of skin with prolonged use, vestibular toxicity (dizziness), photosensitivity rare

Resistance Potential: Low
Allergic Potential: Low
Safety in Pregnancy: X
Comments: Infuse slowly over 1 hour. Dizziness due to high inner ear levels.
Meningeal dose = usual dose
Cerebrospinal Fluid Penetration:
Non-inflamed meninges = 50%
Inflamed meninges = 50%
Bile Penetration: 1000%

REFERENCES:
Cunha BA: Minocycline vs. doxycycline for the antimicrobial therapy of lyme neuroborreliosis. Clin Infect Dis 30:237-238, 2000.
Jonas M, Cunha BA. Therapeutic Drug Monitoring 4:137-45, 1982.
Klein NC, Cunha BA. New uses for older antibiotics. Med Clin North Am 85:125-32, 2001.
Smilack JD, Wilson WE, Cocerill FR 3rd. Tetracycline, chloramphenicol, erythromycin, clindamycin, and metronidazole. Mayo Clin Proc 66:1270-80, 1991.

Moxifloxacin (Avelox)

Drug Class: Fluoroquinolone
Usual Dose: 400 mg (IV/PO) q24h
Pharmacokinetic Parameters:
Peak serum level: 4.5 mcg/mL
Bioavailability: 90%
Excreted unchanged: 20%
Serum half-life (normal/ESRD): 12/12 hrs
Plasma protein binding: 50%

Volume of distribution (V_d): 2 L/kg
Primary Mode of Elimination: Hepatic
Dosage Adjustments:

CrCl ~ 40–60 mL/min	No change
CrCl ~ 10–30 mL/min	No change
CrCl < 10 mL/min	No change
Post–HD dose	None
Post–PD dose	None
Post–CVVH dose	None
Moderate hepatic insufficiency	No change
Severe hepatic insufficiency	400 mg (IV/PO) q48h

Drug Interactions: Al^{++}, Fe^{++}, Mg^{++}, Zn^{++} antacids, citrate/citric acid, dairy products (↓ absorption of fluoroquinolones only if taken together); amiodarone, procainamide, sotalol (may ↑ QT interval, torsade de pointes)
Adverse Effects: May ↑ QT_c interval; avoid taking with other medications that prolong the QT_c interval, and in patients with cardiac arrhythmias/heart block
Resistance Potential: Low
Allergic Potential: Low
Safety in Pregnancy: C
Comments: Only quinolone with anti–B. fragilis activity. Take 4 hours before or 8 hours after calcium/magnesium containing antacids
Cerebrospinal Fluid Penetration: < 10%

REFERENCES:
Balfour JA, Wiseman LR. Moxifloxacin. Drugs 57:363-73, 1999.
Blondeau JM. Expanded activity and utility of the new fluoroquinolones: A review. Clinical Therapeutics 21:3-40, 1999.
Klutman NE, Culley CM, Lacy ME, et al. Moxifloxacin. Antibiotics for Clinicians. 5:17-27, 2001.
Gatifloxacin and Moxifloxacin: Two new fluoroquinolones. Med Lett Drugs 1072:15, 2000.

Nafcillin (Unipen)

Drug Class: Antistaphylococcal penicillin

Usual Dose: 2 gm (IV) q4h
Pharmacokinetic Parameters:
Peak serum level: 80 mcg/mL
Bioavailability: Not applicable
Excreted unchanged: 35%
Serum half-life (normal/ESRD): 0.5/1.2 hrs
Plasma protein binding: 90%
Volume of distribution (V_d): 0.35 L/kg
Primary Mode of Elimination: Hepatic
Dosage Adjustments:

CrCl ~ 40–60 mL/min	No change
CrCl ~ 10–30 mL/min	No change
CrCl < 10 mL/min	No change
Post–HD dose	None
Post–PD dose	None
Post–CVVH dose	None
Moderate hepatic insufficiency	No change
Severe hepatic insufficiency	1 gm (IV) q4h

Drug Interactions: Cyclosporine (↓ cyclosporine levels); nifedipine, warfarin (↓ interacting drug effect)
Adverse Effects: Drug fever/rash, leukopenia
Resistance Potential: Low
Allergic Potential: High
Safety in Pregnancy: B
Comments: Avoid oral formulation (not well absorbed/erratic serum levels). Na^+ content = 3.1 mEq/g. Meningeal dose = usual dose
Cerebrospinal Fluid Penetration:
Non-inflamed meninges = 1%
Inflamed meninges = 20%
Bile Penetration: 100%

REFERENCES:
Donowitz GR, Mandell GL. Beta-lactam antibiotics. N Engl J Med 318:419-26 and 318:490-500, 1993.
Lestico MR, Vick KE, Hetsko CM. Hepatic and renal dysfunction following nafcillin administration. Annals Pharmacol 26:985-90, 1992.
Wright AJ. The penicillins. Mayo Clin Proc 74:290-307, 1999.

---

* Resume dosing for CrCl < 10 mL/min after supplemental dose. "Usual dose" assumes normal renal and hepatic function. CrCl = creatinine clearance; CVVH = continuous veno-venous hemofiltration; HD = hemodialysis; PD = peritoneal dialysis. See pp. 252-255 for definitions/explanations, p. 1 for abbreviations

Nelfinavir (Viracept)

Drug Class: Antiretroviral protease inhibitor
Usual Dose: 750 mg (PO) q8h or 1250 mg (PO) q12h
Pharmacokinetic Parameters:
Peak serum level: 35 mcg/mL
Bioavailability: 20-80%
Excreted unchanged: 23%
Serum half-life (normal/ESRD): 4 hrs/no data
Plasma protein binding: 98%
Volume of distribution (V_d): 5 L/kg
Primary Mode of Elimination: Hepatic
Dosage Adjustments:

CrCl ~ 40–60 mL/min	No change
CrCl ~ 10–30 mL/min	No change
CrCl < 10 mL/min	No change
Post–HD dose	None
Post-PD dose	None
Post-CVVH dose	None
Moderate hepatic insufficiency	No change
Severe hepatic insufficiency	Avoid

Antiretroviral Dosage Adjustments:

Amprenavir	No information
Delavirdine	No information (monitor for neutropenia)
Efavirenz	No changes
Indinavir	Limited data for nelfinavir 1250 mg q12h + indinavir 1200 mg q12h
Lopinavir/ritonavir	No information
Nevirapine	No changes
Ritonavir	Nelfinavir 500-750 mg q12h + ritonavir 400 mg q12h
Saquinavir soft-gel	Saquinavir soft-gel 800 mg q8h or 1200 mg q12h
Rifampin	Avoid combination
Rifabutin	Nelfinavir 1000 mg q8h; rifabutin 150 mg q24h or 300 mg 2-3x/week

Drug Interactions: Antiretrovirals, rifabutin, rifampin (see dose adjustment grid, above); amiodarone, quinidine, astemizole, terfenadine, benzodiazepines, cisapride, ergot alkaloids, statins, St. John's wort (avoid if possible); carbamazepine, phenytoin, phenobarbital (↓ nelfinavir levels, ↑ anticonvulsant levels; monitor); caspofungin (↓ caspofungin levels, may ↓ caspofungin effect); clarithromycin, erythromycin, telithromycin (↑ nelfinavir and macrolide levels); didanosine (dosing conflict with food; give nelfinavir with food 2 hours before or 1 hour after didanosine); itraconazole, ketoconazole (↑ nelfinavir levels); lamivudine (↑ lamivudine levels); methadone (may require ↑ methadone dose); oral contraceptives, zidovudine (↓ zidovudine levels); sildenafil (↑ or ↓ sildenafil levels; do not exceed 25 mg in 48 hrs)
Adverse Effects: Impaired concentration, nausea, abdominal pain, secretory diarrhea, ↑ SGOT/SGPT, rash, ↑ cholesterol/triglycerides (evaluate risk for coronary disease/pancreatitis), fat redistribution, hyperglycemia (including worsening diabetes, new-onset diabetes, DKA), possible increased bleeding in hemophilia
HIV Resistance Potential: Low (triple therapy); high (mono/double drug therapy)
Allergic Potential: Low
Safety in Pregnancy: B
Comments: Take with food (absorption increased 300%). Effective antiretroviral therapy consists of at least 3 antiretrovirals (same/different classes)
Cerebrospinal Fluid Penetration: < 10%

---

* Resume dosing for CrCl < 10 mL/min after supplemental dose. "Usual dose" assumes normal renal and hepatic function. CrCl = creatinine clearance; CVVH = continuous veno-venous hemofiltration; HD = hemodialysis; PD = peritoneal dialysis. See pp. 252-255 for definitions/explanations, p. 1 for abbreviations

REFERENCES:
Deeks SG, Smith M, Holodniy M, et al. HIV-1 protease
    inhibitors: A review for clinicians. JAMA 277:145-53,
    1997.
Go J, Cunha BA. Nelfinavir: A review. Antibiotics for
    Clinicians 4:17-23, 2000.
Kaul DR, Cinti SK, Carver PL, et al. HIV protease
    inhibitors: Advances in therapy and adverse reactions,
    including metabolic complications. Pharmacotherapy
    19:281-98, 1999.
Panel on Clinical Practices for Treatment of HIV
    Infection. Guidelines for the use of antiretroviral
    agents in HIV-infected adults and adolescents.
    Department of Health and Human Services. April 23,
    2001. www.hivatis.org
Perry CM, Benfield P. Nelfinavir. Drugs 54:81-7, 1997.

Nevirapine (Viramune)

Drug Class: Antiretroviral NNRTI (non-nucleoside reverse transcriptase inhibitor)
Usual Dose: 200 mg (PO) q24h x 2 weeks, then 200 mg (PO) q12h
Pharmacokinetic Parameters:
Peak serum level: 2.2 mcg/mL
Bioavailability: 90%
Excreted unchanged: 3%
Serum half-life (normal/ESRD): 30 hrs/no data
Plasma protein binding: 60%
Volume of distribution (V_d): 1.3 L/kg
Primary Mode of Elimination: Hepatic
Dosage Adjustments:

CrCl ~ 40–60 mL/min	No change
CrCl ~ 10–30 mL/min	No change
CrCl < 10 mL/min	No change
Post–HD dose	None
Post–PD dose	None
Post–CVVH dose	None
Moderate hepatic insufficiency	No information
Severe hepatic insufficiency	No information

Antiretroviral Dosage Adjustments:

Amprenavir	No information
Delavirdine	No information
Efavirenz	No information
Indinavir	Indinavir 1000 mg q8h
Lopinavir/ritonavir (l/r)	Consider l/r 533/133 mg q12h in PI-experienced patients
Nelfinavir	No changes
Ritonavir	No changes
Saquinavir	No information
Rifampin	Not recommended
Rifabutin	No changes for non-PI-containing regimens

Drug Interactions: Antiretrovirals, rifabutin, rifampin (see dose adjustment grid, above); carbamazepine, phenobarbital, phenytoin (monitor anticonvulsant levels); caspofungin (↓ caspofungin levels, may ↓ caspofungin effect); ethinyl estradiol (↓ ethinyl estradiol levels; use additional/alternative method); ketoconazole (avoid); methadone (↓ metadone levels; titrate methadone dose to effect); tacrolimus (↓ tacrolimus levels)
Adverse Effects: Drug fever/rash (may be severe; usually occurs within 6 weeks), Stevens–Johnson syndrome, ↑ SGOT/SGPT, fatal hepatitis, headache, diarrhea, leukopenia, stomatitis, peripheral neuropathy, paresthesias
HIV Resistance Potential: Low (triple therapy); high (mono/double drug therapy)
Allergic Potential: High
Safety in Pregnancy: C
Comments: Absorption not affected by food. Effective antiretroviral therapy consists of at least 3 antiretrovirals (same/different classes)
Cerebrospinal Fluid Penetration: 45%

REFERENCES:
D'Aquila RT, Hughes MD, Johnson VA, et al.
    Nevirapine, zidovudine, and didanosine compared
    with zidovudine and didanosine in patients with HIV-1
    infection. Ann Intern Med 124:1019-30, 1996.
Hammer SM, Kessler HA, Saag MS. Issues in

---

* Resume dosing for CrCl < 10 mL/min after supplemental dose. "Usual dose" assumes normal renal and hepatic function. CrCl = creatinine clearance; CVVH = continuous veno-venous hemofiltration; HD = hemodialysis; PD = peritoneal dialysis. See pp. 252-255 for definitions/explanations, p. 1 for abbreviations

combination antiretroviral therapy: A review. J Acquired Immune Defic Syndr 7:24-37, 1994.

Havlir DV. Lange JM. New antiretrovirals and new combinations. AIDS 12:165-74, 1998.

Montaner JS, Reiss P, Cooper D, et al. A randomized, double-blind trial comparing combinations of nevirapine, didanosine, and zidovudine for HIV-infected patients: The INCAS trial. Italy, the Netherlands, Canada and Australia Study. J Am Med Assoc 279:930-937, 1998.

Panel on Clinical Practices for Treatment of HIV Infection. Guidelines for the use of antiretroviral agents in HIV-infected adults and adolescents. Department of Health and Human Services. April 23, 2001. www.hivatis.org

Weverling GJ, Lange JM, Jurriaans S, et al. Alternative multidrug regimen provides improved suppression of HIV-1 replication over triple therapy. AIDS 12:117-22, 1998.

Nitrofurantoin (Macrodantin, Macrobid)

Drug Class: Urinary antiseptic
Usual Dose: 100 mg (PO) q12h
Pharmacokinetic Parameters:
Peak serum level: 1 mcg/mL
Bioavailability: 80%
Excreted unchanged: 40%
Serum half-life (normal/ESRD): 0.5/1 hrs
Plasma protein binding: 40%
Volume of distribution (V_d): 0.8 L/kg
Primary Mode of Elimination: Renal
Dosage Adjustments:

CrCl ~ 40–60 mL/min	100 mg (PO) q24h
CrCl ~ 10–30 mL/min	Avoid
CrCl < 10 mL/min	Avoid
Post–HD dose	Not applicable
Post–PD dose	Not applicable
Post–CVVH dose	Not applicable
Moderate hepatic insufficiency	No change
Severe hepatic insufficiency	No change

Drug Interactions: Antacids, magnesium (↓ nitrofurantoin absorption); probenecid (↑ nitrofurantoin levels)
Adverse Effects:
Acute hypersensitivity reactions (reversible): pneumonitis
Chronic reactions (irreversible): chronic hepatitis, peripheral neuropathy, interstitial fibrosis
Resistance Potential: Low
Allergic Potential: Moderate
Safety in Pregnancy: B
Comments: For UTIs only, not systemic infection. GI upset minimal with microcrystalline preparations. No transplacental transfer. Chronic toxicities associated with prolonged use/renal insufficiency; avoid in severe renal insufficiency. Preferred antimicrobial for VRE catheter-associated bacteriuria

REFERENCES:
Cunha BA. Nitrofurantoin: A review. Adv Ther 6:213-36, 1989.
Cunha BA. Nitrofurantoin: An update. OB/GYN 44:399-406, 1989.
Cunha BA. Nitrofurantoin: Bioavailability and therapeutic equivalence. Adv Ther 5:54-63, 1988.
Klein NC, Cunha BA. New uses for older antibiotics. Med Clin North Am 85:125-32, 2001.

Ofloxacin (Oflox)

Drug Class: Fluoroquinolone
Usual Dose: 400 mg (IV/PO) q12h
Pharmacokinetic Parameters:
Peak serum level: 4.6 mcg/mL
Bioavailability: 95%
Excreted unchanged: 90%
Serum half-life (normal/ESRD): 6/40 hrs
Plasma protein binding: 20%
Volume of distribution (V_d): 3 L/kg
Primary Mode of Elimination: Renal
Dosage Adjustments:

CrCl ~ 40–60 mL/min	200 mg (IV/PO) q12h
CrCl ~ 10–30 mL/min	200 mg (IV/PO) q24h
CrCl < 10 mL/min	100 mg (IV/PO) q24
Post–HD dose	None
Post–PD dose	None

---

* Resume dosing for CrCl < 10 mL/min after supplemental dose. "Usual dose" assumes normal renal and hepatic function. CrCl = creatinine clearance; CVVH = continuous veno-venous hemofiltration; HD = hemodialysis; PD = peritoneal dialysis. See pp. 252-255 for definitions/explanations, p. 1 for abbreviations

Post–CVVH dose*	200 mg (IV/PO)
Moderate hepatic insufficiency	No change
Severe hepatic insufficiency	No change

Drug Interactions: Al^{++}, Ca^{++}, Fe^{++}, Mg^{++}, Zn^{++} antacids, citrate/citric acid, dairy products (↓ absorption of ofloxacin only if taken together); cimetidine (↑ ofloxacin levels); cyclosporine (↑ cyclosporine levels); NSAIDs (CNS stimulation); probenecid (↑ ofloxacin levels); warfarin (↑ INR)
Adverse Effects: Drug fever/rash, mild neuroexcitatory symptoms
Resistance Potential: Low
Allergic Potential: Low
Safety in Pregnancy: C
Comments: H_2 antagonist increases half–life by ~ 30%. Levofloxacin has improved pharmacokinetics/pharmacodynamics and greater antimicrobial activity. Take ofloxacin 2 hours before or after calcium/magnesium containing antacids
Cerebrospinal Fluid Penetration: < 10%
Bile Penetration: 1500%

REFERENCES:
Absalon J, Domenico PD, Ortega AM, Cunha, BA. The antibacterial activity of ofloxacin versus ciprofloxacin against Pseudomonas aeruginosa in human urine. Adv Ther 13:191-4, 1996.
Hooper DC, Wolfson JS. Fluoroquinolone antimicrobial agents. N Engl J Med. 324:384-94, 1991.
Monk JP, Campoli-Richards DM. Ofloxacin: A review of its antibacterial activity, pharmacokinetics properties, and therapeutic use. Drugs 33:346-91, 1987.
Walker RC, Wright AJ. The fluoroquinolones. Mayo Clin Proc 66:1249-59, 1991.

Oxacillin (Prostaphlin)

Drug Class: Antistaphylococcal penicillin
Usual Dose: 2 gm (IV) q4h
Pharmacokinetic Parameters:
Peak serum level: 140 mcg/mL
Bioavailability: 30%
Excreted unchanged: 96%
Serum half-life (normal/ESRD): 0.5/1 hrs
Plasma protein binding: 94%

Volume of distribution (V_d): 0.2 L/kg
Primary Mode of Elimination: Renal
Dosage Adjustments:

CrCl ~ 40–60 mL/min	1 gm (IV) q4h
CrCl ~ 10–30 mL/min	1 gm (IV) q8h
CrCl < 10 mL/min	1 gm (IV) q12h
Post–HD dose	None
Post–PD dose	None
Post–CVVH dose	None
Moderate hepatic insufficiency	No change
Severe hepatic insufficiency	No change

Drug Interactions: Cyclosporine (↓ cyclosporine levels); nifedipine, warfarin (↓ interacting drug effect)
Adverse Effects: Drug fever/rash, leukopenia, ↑ SGOT/SGPT, interstitial nephritis
Resistance Potential: Low
Allergic Potential: High
Safety in Pregnancy: B
Comments: Avoid oral formulation (not well absorbed/erratic serum levels). Na^+ content = 3.1 mEq/g. Meningeal dose = usual dose
Cerebrospinal Fluid Penetration:
Non-inflamed meninges = 1%
Inflamed meninges = 10%
Bile Penetration: 25%

REFERENCES:
Donowitz GR, Mandell GL. Beta-lactam antibiotics. N Engl J Med 318:419-26 and 318:490-500, 1993.
Wright AJ. The penicillins. Mayo Clin Proc 74:290-307, 1999.

Penicillin G (various)

Drug Class: Natural penicillin
Usual Dose: 2-4 mu (IV) q4h
Pharmacokinetic Parameters:
Peak serum level: 20-40 mcg/mL
Bioavailability: Not applicable
Excreted unchanged: 80%

---
* Resume dosing for CrCl < 10 mL/min after supplemental dose. "Usual dose" assumes normal renal and hepatic function. CrCl = creatinine clearance; CVVH = continuous veno-venous hemofiltration; HD = hemodialysis; PD = peritoneal dialysis. See pp. 252-255 for definitions/explanations, p. 1 for abbreviations

Serum half-life (normal/ESRD): 0.5/5.1 hrs
Plasma protein binding: 65%
Volume of distribution (V_d): 0.3 L/kg
Primary Mode of Elimination: Renal
Dosage Adjustment:

CrCl ~ 40–60 mL/min	1–2 mu (IV) q4h
CrCl ~ 10–30 mL/min	1–2 mu (IV) q6h
CrCl < 10 mL/min	2 mu (IV) q12h
Post–HD dose*	2 mu (IV)
Post–PD dose*	1 mu (IV)
Post–CVVH dose*	2 mu (IV)
Moderate hepatic insufficiency	No change
Severe hepatic insufficiency	No change

Drug Interactions: Probenecid (↑ penicillin G levels)
Adverse Effects: Drug fever/rash, E. multiforme/Stevens–Johnson syndrome; anaphylactic reactions (hypotension, laryngospasm, bronchospasm), hives, serum sickness
Resistance Potential: Moderate (S. pneumoniae, S. aureus, N. gonorrhoeae)
Allergic Potential: High
Safety in Pregnancy: B
Comments: Incompatible in solutions containing erythromycin, aminoglycosides, calcium bicarbonate, or heparin. Jarisch–Herxheimer reactions when treating spirochetal infections, e.g., Lyme disease, syphilis, yaws. Penicillin G (potassium): K^+ content = 1.7 mEq/g; Na^+ content = 0.3 mEq/g. Penicillin G (sodium): Na^+ content = 2 mEq/g. Meningeal dose = 4 mu (IV) q4h
Cerebrospinal Fluid Penetration:
Non-inflamed meninges ≤ 1%
Inflamed meninges = 5%
Bile Penetration: 500%

REFERENCES:
Donowitz GR, Mandell GL. Beta-lactam antibiotics. N Engl J Med 318:419-26 and 318:490-500, 1993. Wright AJ. The penicillins. Mayo Clin Proc 74:290-307, 1999.

Penicillin V (various)

Drug Class: Natural penicillin
Usual Dose: 500 mg (PO) q6h
Pharmacokinetic Parameters:
Peak serum level: 5 mcg/mL
Bioavailability: 60%
Excreted unchanged: 80%
Serum half-life (normal/ESRD): 0.5/8 hrs
Plasma protein binding: 70%
Volume of distribution (V_d): 0.5 L/kg
Primary Mode of Elimination: Renal
Dosage Adjustments:

CrCl ~ 40–60 mL/min	500 mg (PO) q6h
CrCl ~ 10–30 mL/min	250 mg (PO) q6h
CrCl < 10 mL/min	250 mg (PO) q6h
Post–HD dose*	250 mg (PO)
Post–PD dose	None
Post–CVVH dose*	500 mg (PO)
Moderate hepatic insufficiency	No change
Severe hepatic insufficiency	No change

Drug Interactions: Probenecid (↑ penicillin V levels)
Adverse Effects: Drug fever/rash, E. multiforme/Stevens-Johnson syndrome, anaphylactic reactions (hypotension, laryngospasm, bronchospasm), hives, serum sickness
Resistance Potential: Moderate (S. pneumoniae, S. aureus, N. gonorrhoeae)
Allergic Potential: High
Safety in Pregnancy: B
Comments: Jarisch–Herxheimer reactions when treating spirochetal infections, e.g., Lyme disease, syphilis, yaws. Take 1 hour before or 2 hours after meals. K^+ content = 2.8 mEq/g
Cerebrospinal Fluid Penetration: < 10%

---

* Resume dosing for CrCl < 10 mL/min after supplemental dose. "Usual dose" assumes normal renal and hepatic function. CrCl = creatinine clearance; CVVH = continuous veno-venous hemofiltration; HD = hemodialysis; PD = peritoneal dialysis. See pp. 252-255 for definitions/explanations, p. 1 for abbreviations

REFERENCES:
Donowitz GR, Mandell GL. Beta-lactam antibiotics. N Engl J Med 318:419-26 and 318:490-500, 1993.
Wright AJ. The penicillins. Mayo Clin Proc 74:290-307, 1999.

Pentamidine (Pentam 300, NebuPent)

Drug Class: Antiparasitic
Usual Dose: 4 mg/kg (IV) q24h
Pharmacokinetic Parameters:
Peak serum level: 1.5 mcg/mL
Bioavailability: Not applicable
Excreted unchanged: 50%
Serum half-life (normal/ESRD): 6.4/90 hrs
Plasma protein binding: 69%
Volume of distribution (V_d): 3.9 L/kg
Primary Mode of Elimination: Metabolized
Dosage Adjustments:

CrCl ~ 40–60 mL/min	4 mg/kg (IV) q24h
CrCl ~ 10–30 mL/min	4 mg/kg (IV) q36h
CrCl < 10 mL/min	4 mg/kg (IV) q48h
Post–HD dose	None
Post–PD dose	None
Post–CVVH dose	None
Moderate hepatic insufficiency	No change
Severe hepatic insufficiency	No change

Drug Interactions: Alcohol, valproic acid (↑ risk of pancreatitis); foscarnet (severe hypocalcemia reported; do not combine); amphotericin B, aminoglycosides, capreomycin, cis-platinum, colistin, methoxyflurane, polymyxin B, vancomycin, other nephrotoxic drugs (↑ nephrotoxicity)
Adverse Effects: Rash, hypotension, hypocalcemia, hypoglycemia, ↑ creatinine, pancreatitis, local injection site reactions, severe leukopenia, anemia, thrombocytopenia, may ↑ QT_c interval with IV administration
Resistance Potential: Low

Allergic Potential: High
Safety in Pregnancy: C
Comments: Well absorbed IM, but painful. Administer IV slowly in D_5W over 1 hour, not saline. Inhaled pentamidine isethionate (NebuPent) 300 mg monthly via Respirgard II nebulizer can be used for PCP prophylaxis, but is less effective than IV/IM pentamidine and is not effective against extrapulmonary P. carinii. Adverse effects with aerosolized pentamidine include chest pain, arrhythmias, dizziness, wheezing, coughing, dyspnea, headache, anorexia, nausea, diarrhea, rash, pharyngitis. If PCP patient also has pulmonary TB, aerosolized pentamidine treatments may expose medical personnel to TB via droplet inhalation
Cerebrospinal Fluid Penetration: < 10%

REFERENCES:
Chan C, Montaner J, LeFebvre BA, et al. Atovaquone suspension compared with aerosolized pentamidine for prevention of Pneumocystis carinii pneumonia in human immunodeficiency virus infected subsets intolerant of trimethoprim or sulfamethoxazole. J Infect Dis 180:369-376, 1999.
Goa KL, Campoli-Richards DM. Pentamidine isethionate: A review of its antiprotozoal activity, pharmacokinetic properties and therapeutic use in Pneumocystis carinii pneumonia. Drugs 33:242-58, 1987.
Monk JP, Benfield P. Inhaled pentamidine: An overview of its pharmacological properties and a review of its therapeutic use in Pneumocystis carinii pneumonia. Drugs 39:741-56, 1990.
Sattler FR, Cowam R. Nielsen DM, et al. Trimethoprim-sulfamethoxazole compared with pentamidine for treatment of Pneumocystis carinii pneumonia in the acquired immunodeficiency syndrome. Ann Intern Med 109:280-7, 1988.

Piperacillin (Pipracil)

Drug Class: Antipseudomonal penicillin
Usual Dose: 4 gm (IV) q8h
Pharmacokinetic Parameters:
Peak serum level: 400 mcg/mL
Bioavailability: Not applicable
Excreted unchanged: 80%
Serum half-life (normal/ESRD): 1/3 hrs
Plasma protein binding: 22%
Volume of distribution (V_d): 0.24 L/kg
Primary Mode of Elimination: Renal

---

* Resume dosing for CrCl < 10 mL/min after supplemental dose. "Usual dose" assumes normal renal and hepatic function. CrCl = creatinine clearance; CVVH = continuous veno-venous hemofiltration; HD = hemodialysis; PD = peritoneal dialysis. See pp. 252-255 for definitions/explanations, p. 1 for abbreviations

Dosage Adjustments:

CrCl ~ 40–60 mL/min	2 gm (IV) q8h
CrCl ~ 10–30 mL/min	3 gm (IV) q12h
CrCl < 10 mL/min	2 gm (IV) q12h
Post–HD dose*	2 gm (IV)
Post–PD dose	None
Post–CVVH dose*	4 gm (IV)
Moderate hepatic insufficiency	No change
Severe hepatic insufficiency	No change

Drug Interactions: Aminoglycosides (inactivation of piperacillin in renal failure); warfarin (↑ INR); oral contraceptives (↓ oral contraceptive effect); cefoxitin (↓ piperacillin effect)

Adverse Effects: Drug fever/rash, anaphylactic reactions (hypotension, laryngospasm, bronchospasm), hives, serum sickness, leukopenia

Resistance Potential: Low

Allergic Potential: High

Safety in Pregnancy: B

Comments: 75% absorbed when given IM. Do not mix/administer with aminoglycosides. Most active antipseudomonal penicillin against P. aeruginosa. Na$^+$ content = 1.8 mEq/g. Meningeal dose = usual dose

Cerebrospinal Fluid Penetration:
Non-inflamed meninges = 1%
Inflamed meninges = 30%

Bile Penetration: 1000%

REFERENCES:
Donowitz GR, Mandell GL. Beta-lactam antibiotics. N Engl J Med 318:419-26 and 318:490 500, 1993.
Tan JS, File TM, Jr. Antipseudomonal penicillins. Med Clin North Am 79:679-93, 1995.
Wright AJ. The penicillins. Mayo Clin Proc 74:290-307, 1999.

Piperacillin/tazobactam (Zosyn)

Drug Class: Antipseudomonal penicillin
Usual Dose: 4.5 gm (IV) q8h
Pharmacokinetic Parameters:
Peak serum level: 400 mcg/mL
Bioavailability: Not applicable
Excreted unchanged: 60/15%
Serum half-life (normal/ESRD): [1.5/8] / [1/7] hrs
Plasma protein binding: 30/32%
Volume of distribution (V_d): 0.3/0.21 L/kg
Primary Mode of Elimination: Renal
Dosage Adjustments:

CrCl ~ 40–60 mL/min	3.375 gm (IV) q8h
CrCl ~ 10–30 mL/min	2.25 gm (IV) q8h
CrCl < 10 mL/min	2.25 gm (IV) q12h
Post–HD dose*	2.25 gm (IV)
Post–PD dose	None
Post–CVVH dose*	4.5 gm (IV)
Moderate hepatic insufficiency	No change
Severe hepatic insufficiency	No change

Drug Interactions: Aminoglycosides (↓ aminoglycoside levels); vecuronium (↑ vecuronium effect)

Adverse Effects: Drug fever/rash, leukopenia, insomnia, headache, constipation, nausea, hypertension

Resistance Potential: Low

Allergic Potential: High

Safety in Pregnancy: B

Comments: Dose–dependent kinetics permit 4.5 gm (IV) q8h dosing; effective against P. aeruginosa (MIC$_{90}$ = 16 mg/ml). Do not mix with Ringers lactate. Prevents/reduces incidence of C. difficile diarrhea. Na$^+$ content = 2.4 mEq/g

Cerebrospinal Fluid Penetration:
Non-inflamed meninges = 1%
Inflamed meninges = 30%

Bile Penetration: 6000%

---

* Resume dosing for CrCl < 10 mL/min after supplemental dose. "Usual dose" assumes normal renal and hepatic function. CrCl = creatinine clearance; CVVH = continuous veno venous hemofiltration; HD = hemodialysis; PD = peritoneal dialysis. See pp. 252-255 for definitions/explanations, p. 1 for abbreviations

REFERENCES:
Minnaganti VR, Cunha BA. Piperacillin/tazobactam. Antibiotics for Clinicians 3:101-8, 1999.
Piperacillin/tazobactam. Med Lett Drugs Ther 36:7-9, 1994.
Sanders WE Jr, Sanders CC. Piperacillin/tazobactam: A critical review of the evolving clinical literature. Clin Infect Dis 22:107-23, 1996.
Schoonover LL, Occhipinti DJ, Rodvold KA, et al. Piperacillin/tazobactam: A new beta-lactam/beta-lactamase inhibitor combination. Ann Pharmacother 29:501-14, 1995.

Polymyxin B

Drug Class: Phospholipid cell membrane-altering antibiotic
Usual Dose: 1.25 mg/kg (IV) q12h (1 mg = 10,000 units)
Pharmacokinetic Parameters:
Peak serum level: 8 mcg/mL
Bioavailability: Not applicable
Excreted unchanged: 60%
Serum half-life (normal/ESRD): 6/48 hrs
Plasma protein binding: < 10%
Volume of distribution (V_d): No data
Primary Mode of Elimination: Renal
Dosage Adjustments:

CrCl ~ 40–60 mL/min	No change
CrCl ~ 10–30 mL/min	No change
CrCl < 10 mL/min	0.633 mg/kg (IV) q12h
Post–HD dose	None
Post–PD dose	None
Post–CVVH dose	None
Moderate hepatic insufficiency	No change
Severe hepatic insufficiency	No change

Drug Interactions: Amphotericin B, amikacin, gentamicin, tobramycin, vancomycin (↑ nephrotoxicity)
Adverse Effects: Neurotoxicity associated with very prolonged/high serum levels;

neuromuscular blockade potential with renal failure/neuromuscular disorders
Resistance Potential: Low
Allergic Potential: Low
Safety in Pregnancy: B
Comments: Inhibits endotoxin release from gram-negative bacilli. Avoid intraperitoneal infusion due to risk of neuromuscular blockade. Increased risk of reversible non–oliguric renal failure (ATN) when used with other nephrotoxic drugs. No ototoxic potential. May be given IM with procaine, but painful. Intrathecal (IT) polymyxin B dose = 5 mg (50,000 u) q24h x 3 days, then q48h x 2 weeks. Dissolve 50 mg (500,000 u) into 10 mL for IT administration
Cerebrospinal Fluid Penetration: < 10%

REFERENCES:
Evans ME, Feola DJ, Rapp RP. Polymyxin B sulfate and colistin: Old antibiotics for emerging multiresistant gram-negative bacteria. Ann Pharmacother 33:960-7, 1999.
Horton J, Pankey GA. Polymyxin B. Med Clin North Am 66:134-42, 1995.
Menzies D, Minnaganti VR, Cunha BA. Polymyxin B. Antibiotics for Clinicians 4:33-40, 2000.
Segal-Maurer S, Mariano N, Qavi A, et al. Successful treatment of ceftazidime-resistant Klebsiella pneumoniae ventriculitis with intravenous meropenem and intraventricular polymyxin B: Case report and review. Clin Infect Dis 28:1134-8, 1999.

Pyrazinamide (PZA)

Drug Class: Anti–TB drug
Usual Dose: 25 mg/kg (PO) q24h (max. 2 gm)
Pharmacokinetic Parameters:
Peak serum level: 4 mcg/mL
Bioavailability: 90%
Excreted unchanged: 10%
Serum half-life (normal/ESRD): 9/26 hrs
Plasma protein binding: 50%
Volume of distribution (V_d): 0.9 L/kg
Primary Mode of Elimination: Hepatic
Dosage Adjustments:

CrCl ~ 40–60 mL/min	No change
CrCl ~ 10–30 mL/min	No change
CrCl < 10 mL/min	1 gm (PO) q24h

Post–HD dose*	1 gm (PO)
Post–PD dose	None
Post–CVVH dose	No information
Moderate hepatic insufficiency	500 mg (PO) q24h
Severe hepatic insufficiency	Avoid

Drug Interactions: INH, rifabutin, rifampin (may ↑ risk of hepatoxicity)
Adverse Effects: Drug fever/rash, malaise, nausea, vomiting, anorexia, ↑ SGOT/SGPT, ↑ uric acid, sideroblastic anemia
Resistance Potential: Low
Allergic Potential: Low
Safety in Pregnancy: C
Comments: Avoid in patients with gout (may precipitate acute attacks). May be administered as 4 gm (PO) 2x/week or 3 gm (PO) 3x/week. Meningeal dose = usual dose
Cerebrospinal Fluid Penetration: 100%

REFERENCES:
Davidson PT, Le HQ. Drug treatment of tuberculosis 1992. Drugs 43:651-73, 1992.
Drugs for tuberculosis. Med Lett Drugs Ther 35:99-101,1993.
Havlir DV, Barnes PF. Tuberculosis in patients with human immunodeficiency virus infection. N Engl J Med 340:367-73, 1999.
Iseman MD. Treatment of multidrug-resistant tuberculosis. N Engl J Med 329:784-91, 1993.
Van Scoy RE, Wilkowske CJ. Antituberculous agents. Mayo Clin Proc 67:179-87, 1992.

Pyrimethamine (Daraprim)

Drug Class: Antiparasitic
Usual Dose: 75 mg (PO) q24h (toxoplasmosis)
Pharmacokinetic Parameters:
Peak serum level: 0.4 mcg/mL
Bioavailability: 90%
Excreted unchanged: 25%
Serum half-life (normal/ESRD): 96 hrs/no data
Plasma protein binding: 87%
Volume of distribution (V_d): 2.5 L/kg
Primary Mode of Elimination: Hepatic
Dosage Adjustments:

CrCl ~ 40–60 mL/min	No change
CrCl ~ 10–30 mL/min	No change
CrCl < 10 mL/min	No change
Post–HD dose	None
Post–PD dose	None
Post–CVVH dose	None
Moderate hepatic insufficiency	No change
Severe hepatic insufficiency	25 mg (PO) q24h

Drug Interactions: Folic acid (↓ pyrimethamine effect); lorazepam (↑ risk of hepatotoxicity); sulfamethoxazole, trimethoprim, TMP-SMX (↑ risk of thrombocytopenia, anemia, leukopenia)
Adverse Effects: Megaloblastic anemia, leukopenia, thrombocytopenia, ataxia, tremors, seizures
Resistance Potential: Low
Allergic Potential: Low
Safety in Pregnancy: C
Comments: Antacids decrease absorption. Give folinic acid 50 mg (PO) q24h with pyrimethamine to prevent folic acid depletion
Cerebrospinal Fluid Penetration: No data

REFERENCES:
Drugs for Parasitic Infections. Med Lett Drugs Ther 40.1-12, 2000.
Podzamczer D, Salazar A, Jiminez J, et al. Intermittent trimethoprim-sulfamethoxazole compared with dapsone-pyrimethamine for the simultaneous primary prophylaxis of Pneumocystis pneumonia and toxoplasmosis in patients infected with HIV. Ann Intern Med 122:755-61, 1995.
Porter SB, Sande MA. Toxoplasmosis of the central nervous system in the acquired-immunodeficiency syndrome. N Engl J Med 327:1643-8, 1992.

Quinine sulfate

Drug Class: Antimalarial
Usual Dose: 650 mg (PO) q8h
Pharmacokinetic Parameters:
Peak serum level: 3.8 mcg/mL

---

* Resume dosing for CrCl < 10 mL/min after supplemental dose. "Usual dose" assumes normal renal and hepatic function. CrCl = creatinine clearance; CVVH = continuous veno venous hemofiltration; HD = hemodialysis; PD = peritoneal dialysis. See pp. 252-255 for definitions/explanations, p. 1 for abbreviations

Bioavailability: 80%
Excreted unchanged: 5%
Serum half-life (normal/ESRD): 7/14 hrs
Plasma protein binding: 90%
Volume of distribution (V_d): 3 L/kg
Primary Mode of Elimination: Renal/hepatic
Dosage Adjustments:

CrCl ~ 40–60 mL/min	No change
CrCl ~ 10–30 mL/min	650 mg (PO) q12h
CrCl < 10 mL/min	650 mg (PO) q24h
Post–HD dose	None
Post–PD dose	None
Post–CVVH dose	None
Moderate hepatic insufficiency	325 mg (PO) q8h
Severe hepatic insufficiency	325 mg (PO) q12h

Drug Interactions: Aluminum-based antacids (↓ quinidine absorption); astemizole, cisapride, terfenadine (↑ interacting drug levels, torsade de pointes; avoid); cimetidine, ritonavir (↑ quinidine toxicity: headache, deafness, blindness, tachycardia); cyclosporine (↓ cyclosporine levels); digoxin (↑ digoxin levels); dofetilide, flecainide (arrhythmias); mefloquine (seizures, may ↑ QT interval, torsade de pointes, cardiac arrest, ↓ mefloquine efficacy); metformin (↑ risk of lactic acidosis); pancuronium, succinylcholine, tubocurarine (neuromuscular blockade); warfarin (↑ INR)
Adverse Effects: Drug fever/rash, ↑ QT_c interval, arrhythmias, drug-induced SLE, lightheadedness, diarrhea, abdominal discomfort, nausea, vomiting, cinchonism with chronic use. Avoid in patients with G6PD deficiency
Resistance Potential: Low
Allergic Potential: High
Safety in Pregnancy: C
Comments: Tablets (sulfate salt) (100 mg, 200 mg, 300 mg)
Cerebrospinal Fluid Penetration: No data

REFERENCES:
Drugs for Parasitic Infections. Med Letter. March, 2000.
Panisko DM, Keystone JS. Treatment of malaria. Drugs 39:160-89, 1990.
Wyler DJ. Malaria: Overview and update. Clin Infect Dis 16:449-56, 1993.

Quinupristin/dalfopristin (Synercid)

Drug Class: Streptogramin
Usual Dose: 7.5 mg/kg (IV) q8h
Pharmacokinetic Parameters:
Peak serum level: 3.2/8 mcg/mL
Bioavailability: Not applicable
Excreted unchanged: 15/19%
Serum half-life (normal/ESRD): [3.1/1]/[3.1/1] hrs
Plasma protein binding: 55/15%
Volume of distribution (V_d): 0.45/0.24 L/kg
Primary Mode of Elimination: Hepatic
Dosage Adjustment:

CrCl ~ 40–60 mL/min	No change
CrCl ~ 10–30 mL/min	No change
CrCl < 10 mL/min	No change
Post–HD dose	None
Post–PD dose	None
Post–CVVH dose	None
Moderate hepatic insufficiency	No change
Severe hepatic insufficiency	No information

Drug Interactions: Amlodipine (↑ amlodipine toxicity); astemizole, cisapride (may ↑ QT interval, torsades de pointes); carbamazepine (↑ carbamazepine toxicity: ataxia, nystagmus, diplopia, headache, seizures); cyclosporine, delavirdine, indinavir, nevirapine (↑ interacting drug levels); diazepam, midazolam (↑ interacting drug effect); diltiazem, felodipine, isradipine (↑ interacting drug toxicity: dizziness, hypotension, headache, flushing); disopyramide (↑ disopyramide toxicity: arrhythmias, hypotension,

---

syncope); docetaxel (↑ interacting drug toxicity: neutropenia, anemia, neuropathy); lidocaine (↑ lidocaine toxicity: neurotoxicity, arrhythmias, seizures); methylprednisolone (↑ methylprednisolone toxicity: myopathy, diabetes mellitus, cushing's syndrome); nicardipine, nifedipine, nimodipine (↑ interacting drug toxicity: dizziness, hypotension, flushing, headache); statins (↑ risk of rhabdomyolysis)

Adverse Effects: Pain, inflammation, and swelling at infusion site, severe/prolonged myalgias, hyperbilirubinemia. Hepatic insufficiency increases concentration (AUC) of metabolites by 180%/50%

Resistance Potential: Low

Allergic Potential: Low

Safety in Pregnancy: B

Comments: Administer in D_5W or sterile water, not in saline. Does not cover E. faecalis

Cerebrospinal Fluid Penetration: < 10%

REFERENCES:
Bryson HM, Spencer CM. Quinupristin/dalfopristin. Drugs 52:406-15, 1996.
Chant C, Ryback MH. Quinupristin/dalfopristin (RP 59500): A new streptogramin antibiotic. Ann Pharmacother 29:1022-7, 1995.
Griswold MW, Lomaestro BM, Briceland LL. Quinupristin-dalfopristin (RP 59500): An injectable streptogramin combination. Am J Health Syst Pharm. 53:2045-53, 1996.
Kim MK, Nicolau DP, Nightingale CH, et al. Quinupristin/dalfopristin: A treatment option for vancomycin-resistant enterococci. Conn Med 64:209-12, 2000.
Nadler H, Dowzicky MJ, Feger C, et al. Quinupristin/dalfopristin: A novel selective-spectrum antibiotic for the treatment of multi-resistant and other gram-positive pathogens. Clin Microbiol Newslett 21:103-12, 1999.

Ribavirin (Virazole)

Drug Class: Antiviral
Usual Dose: 200 mg (PO) q8h
Pharmacokinetic Parameters:
Peak serum level: 0.28 mcg/mL
Bioavailability: 64%
Excreted unchanged: 40%
Serum half-life (normal/ESRD): 30 hrs/no data
Plasma protein binding: 0%

Volume of distribution (V_d): 10 L/kg
Primary Mode of Elimination: Hepatic
Dosage Adjustments:

CrCl ~ 40–60 mL/min	No change
CrCl ~ 10–30 mL/min	Avoid
CrCl < 10 mL/min	Avoid
Post–HD dose	Avoid
Post–PD dose	Avoid
Post–CVVH dose	Avoid
Moderate hepatic insufficiency	No change
Severe hepatic insufficiency	No change

Drug Interactions: Zidovudine (↓ zidovudine efficacy)

Adverse Effects: Drug fever/rash, nausea, vomiting, GI upset, leukopenia, hyperbilirubinemia, hemolytic anemia, ↑ uric acid

Resistance Potential: Low

Allergic Potential: Low

Safety in Pregnancy: X

Comments: For chronic HCV patients ≥ 75 kg, give 600 mg (PO) q12h; for patients < 75 kg, give 1 gm (PO) q24h in 2 divided doses. Administer with interferon alpha-2b (Intron) 3 mu (IM/SC) 3x/week

Cerebrospinal Fluid Penetration: No data

REFERENCES:
Davis GL, Esteban-Mur R, Rustgi V, et al. Interferon Alfa-2b alone or in combination with ribavirin for the treatment of relapse of chronic hepatitis C: International hepatitis interventional therapy group. N Engl J Med 339:1493-9, 1998.
Keating MR. Antiviral agents. Mayo Clin Proc 67:160-78, 1992.
McHutchison JG, Gordon SC, Schiff ER, et al. Interferon Alfa-2b alone or in combination with ribavirin as initial treatment for chronic hepatitis C. International therapy group. N Engl J Med 339:1485-92, 1998.
Ottolini MG, Hemming VG. Prevention and treatment recommendations for respiratory syncytial virus infection: Background and clinical experience 40 years after discovery. Drugs 54:867-84, 1997.

---

* Resume dosing for CrCl < 10 mL/min after supplemental dose. "Usual dose" assumes normal renal and hepatic function. CrCl = creatinine clearance; CVVH = continuous veno venous hemofiltration; HD = hemodialysis; PD = peritoneal dialysis. See pp. 252-255 for definitions/explanations, p. 1 for abbreviations

324   Antibiotic Essentials

Rifabutin (Mycobutin)

Drug Class: Anti-MAI drug
Usual Dose: 300 mg (PO) q24h
Pharmacokinetic Parameters:
Peak serum level: 0.38 mcg/mL
Bioavailability: 20%
Excreted unchanged: 10%
Serum half-life (normal/ESRD): 45/45 hrs
Plasma protein binding: 85%
Volume of distribution (V_d): 9.3 L/kg
Primary Mode of Elimination: Hepatic
Dosage Adjustments:

CrCl ~ 40–60 mL/min	No change
CrCl ~ 10–30 mL/min	No change
CrCl < 10 mL/min	No change
Post–HD dose	None
Post–PD dose	None
Post–CVVH dose	None
Moderate hepatic insufficiency	No change
Severe hepatic insufficiency	150 mg (PO) q24h

Drug Interactions: Atovaquone, amprenavir, indinavir, nelfinavir, ritonavir, clarithromycin, erythromycin, telithromycin, fluconazole, itraconazole, ketoconazole (↓ interacting drug levels, ↑ rifabutin levels); beta-blockers, clofibrate, cyclosporine, enalapril, oral contraceptives, quinidine, sulfonylureas, tocainide, warfarin (↓ interacting drug effect); corticosteroids (↑ corticosteroid requirement); delavirdine (↓ delavirdine levels, ↑ rifabutin levels; avoid); digoxin, phenytoin, propafenone, theophylline, zidovudine (↓ interacting drug levels); methadone (↓ methadone levels, withdrawal); mexiletine (↑ mexiletine clearance); protease inhibitors (↓ protease inhibitor levels, ↑ rifabutin levels; caution)
Adverse Effects: Brown/orange discoloration of body fluids, ↑ SGOT/SGPT, leukopenia, anemia, thrombocytopenia, drug fever, rash, headache, nausea, vomiting

Resistance Potential: Low
Allergic Potential: High
Safety in Pregnancy: C
Comments: Avoid in leukopenic patients with WBC ≤ 1000 cells/mm³. Always used as part of a multi-drug regimen, never as monotherapy. Meningeal dose = usual dose
Cerebrospinal Fluid Penetration: 50%

REFERENCES:
Benson CA, Williams PL, Cohn DL, and the ACTG 196/CPCRA 009 Study Team. Clarithromycin or rifabutin alone or in combination for primary prophylaxis of Mycobacterium avium complex disease in patients with AIDS: A randomized, double-blinded, placebo-controlled trial. J Infect Dis 181(4):1289-97, 2000.

Centers for Disease Control and Prevention. Notice to readers: Updated guidelines for the use of rifabutin or rifampin for the treatment and prevention of tuberculosis among HIV-infected patients taking protease inhibitors or nonnucleoside reverse transcriptase inhibitors. MMWR 49:183-189, 2000.

Drugs for AIDS and associated infections. Med Lett Drug Ther 35:79-86, 1993.

Hoy J, Mijch A, Sandland M, et al. Quadruple-drug therapy for Mycobacterium avium-intracellulare bacteremia in AIDS patients. J Infect Dis 161:801-5, 1990.

Nightingale SD, Cameron DW, Gordin FM, et al. Two controlled trials of rifabutin prophylaxis against Mycobacterium avium complex infection in AIDS. N Engl J Med 329:828-33, 1993.

Panel on Clinical Practices for Treatment of HIV Infection. Guidelines for the use of antiretroviral agents in HIV-infected adults and adolescents. Department of Health and Human Services. April 23, 2001. www.hivatis.org

Rifampin (Rifadin, Rimactane)

Drug Class: Antibiotic/anti-TB drug
Usual Dose: 600 mg (PO) q24h
Pharmacokinetic Parameters:
Peak serum level: 7 mcg/mL
Bioavailability: 95%
Excreted unchanged: 90%
Serum half-life (normal/ESRD): 3.5/11 hrs
Plasma protein binding: 80%
Volume of distribution (V_d): 0.93 L/kg
Primary Mode of Elimination: Hepatic

---

* Resume dosing for CrCl < 10 mL/min after supplemental dose. "Usual dose" assumes normal renal and hepatic function. CrCl = creatinine clearance; CVVH = continuous veno-venous hemofiltration; HD = hemodialysis; PD = peritoneal dialysis. See pp. 252-255 for definitions/explanations, p. 1 for abbreviations

Dosage Adjustments:

CrCl ~ 40–60 mL/min	No change
CrCl ~ 10–30 mL/min	No change
CrCl < 10 mL/min	No change
Post–HD dose	None
Post–PD dose	None
Post–CVVH dose	None
Moderate hepatic insufficiency	No change
Severe hepatic insufficiency	300 mg (PO) q24h

Drug Interactions: Amprenavir, indinavir, nelfinavir (↑ rifampin levels); beta-blockers, clofibrate, cyclosporine, oral contraceptives, quinidine, sulfonylureas, tocainamide, warfarin (↓ interacting drug effect); caspofungin (↓ caspofungin levels, may ↓ caspofungin effect); clarithromycin, ketoconazole (↑ rifampin levels, ↓ interacting drug levels); corticosteroids (↑ corticosteroid requirement); delavirdine (↑ rifampin levels, ↓ delavirdine levels; avoid); disopyramide, itraconazole, phenytoin, propafenone, theophylline, methadone, nelfinavir, ritonavir, tacrolimus, drugs whose metabolism is induced by rifampin, e.g., ACE inhibitors, dapsone, diazepam, digoxin, diltiazem, doxycycline, fluconazole, fluvastatin, haloperidol, nifedipine, progestins, triazolam, tricyclics, zidovudine (↓ interacting drug levels); fluconazole, TMP-SMX (↑ rifampin levels); INH (INH converted into toxic hydrazine); mexiletine (↑ mexiletine clearance); nevirapine (↓ nevirapine levels; avoid)
Adverse Effects: Red/orange discoloration of body secretions, flu-like symptoms, ↑ SGOT/SGPT, drug fever, rash, thrombocytopenia
Resistance Potential: High (Enterobacteriaceae) with monotherapy; low if used as part of combination regimen
Allergic Potential: Moderate
Safety in Pregnancy: Probably safe
Comments: For anti–TB therapy, monitor potential hepatotoxicity with serial SGOT/SGPTs

weekly x 3, then monthly x 3. Take 1 hour before or 2 hours after meals. As an anti-staphylococcal drug (with another anti-staph antibiotic), give as 300 mg (PO) q12h. Meningeal dose = usual dose
Cerebrospinal Fluid Penetration:
Non-inflamed meninges = 50%
Inflamed meninges = 50%
Bile Penetration: 7000%

REFERENCES:
Centers for Disease Control and Prevention. Notice to readers: Updated guidelines for the use of rifabutin or rifampin for the treatment and prevention of tuberculosis among HIV-infected patients taking protease inhibitors or nonnucleoside reverse transcriptase inhibitors. MMWR 49:183-189, 2000.
Davidson PT, Le HQ. Drug treatment of tuberculosis 1992. Drugs 43:651-73, 1992.
Havlir DV, Barnes PF. Tuberculosis in patients with human immunodeficiency virus infection. N Engl J Med 340:367-73, 1999.
Lundstrom TS, Sobel JD. Vancomycin, trimethoprim - sulfamethoxazole, and rifampin. Infect Dis Clin North Am 91:747-67, 1995.
Panel on Clinical Practices for Treatment of HIV Infection. Guidelines for the use of antiretroviral agents in HIV-infected adults and adolescents. Department of Health and Human Services. April 23, 2001. www.hivatis.org
Van Scoy RE, Wilkowske CJ. Antituberculous agents. Mayo Clin Proc 67:179-87, 1992.
Vesely JJ, Pien FD, Pien BC. Rifampin, a useful drug for nonmycobacterial infections. Pharmacotherapy 18:345-57, 1998.

Rimantadine (Flumadine)

Drug Class: Antiviral
Usual Dose: 200 mg (PO) q24h
Pharmacokinetic Parameters:
Peak serum level: 0.6 mcg/mL
Bioavailability: 90%
Excreted unchanged: 25%
Serum half-life (normal/ESRD): 2.5/4 hrs
Plasma protein binding: 60%
Volume of distribution (V_d): 4.5 L/kg
Primary Mode of Elimination: Hepatic
Dosage Adjustments:

CrCl ~ 40–60 mL/min	No change
CrCl ~ 10–30 mL/min	No change

---

* Resume dosing for CrCl < 10 mL/min after supplemental dose. "Usual dose" assumes normal renal and hepatic function. CrCl = creatinine clearance; CVVH = continuous veno-venous hemofiltration; HD = hemodialysis; PD = peritoneal dialysis. See pp. 252-255 for definitions/explanations, p. 1 for abbreviations

CrCl < 10 mL/min	100 mg (PO) q24h
Post–HD dose	None
Post–PD dose	None
Post–CVVH dose	None
Moderate hepatic insufficiency	No change
Severe hepatic insufficiency	100 mg (PO) q12h

Drug Interactions: Alcohol (↑ CNS effects); benztropine, trihexyphenidyl, scopolamine (↑ interacting drug effect: dry mouth, ataxia, blurred vision, slurred speech, toxic psychosis); cimetidine (↓ rimantadine clearance); CNS stimulants (additive stimulation); digoxin (↑ digoxin levels); trimethoprim (↑ rimantadine and trimethoprim levels)
Adverse Effects: Dizziness, headache, insomnia, anticholinergic effects (blurry vision, dry mouth, orthostatic hypotension, urinary retention, constipation)
Resistance Potential: Low
Allergic Potential: Low
Safety in Pregnancy: C
Comments: Less anticholinergic side effects than amantadine. Patients ≥ 60 years old or with a history of seizures should receive 100 mg (PO) q24h
Cerebrospinal Fluid Penetration: No data

REFERENCES:
Dolin R, Reichman RC, Madore HP, et al. A controlled trial of amantadine and rimantadine in the prophylaxis of Influenza A infection. N Engl J Med 307:580-4, 1982.
Keating MR. Antiviral agents. Mayo Clin Proc 67:160-78, 1992.
Wintermeyer SM, Nahata MC. Rimantadine: A clinical perspective. Ann Pharmacotherapy 29:299-310, 1995.

Ritonavir (Norvir)

Drug Class: Antiretroviral protease inhibitor
Usual Dose: 600 mg (PO) q12h (see comments)
Pharmacokinetic Parameters:
Peak serum level: 5 mcg/mL

Bioavailability: No data
Excreted unchanged: 3.5%
Serum half-life (normal/ESRD): 4 hrs/no data
Plasma protein binding: 99%
Volume of distribution (V_d): 0.4 L/kg
Primary Mode of Elimination: Hepatic
Dosage Adjustments:

CrCl ~ 40–60 mL/min	No change
CrCl ~ 10–30 mL/min	No change
CrCl < 10 mL/min	No change
Post–HD dose	None
Post–PD dose	None
Post–CVVH dose	None
Moderate hepatic insufficiency	No change
Severe hepatic insufficiency	300 mg (PO) q12h

Antiretroviral Dosage Adjustments:

Amprenavir	Limited data for ritonavir 100-200 mg q12h + amprenavir 600-1200 mg q12h
Delavirdine	Delavirdine: no change; ritonavir: No information
Efavirenz	Ritonavir 600 mg q12h (500 mg q12h for intolerance)
Indinavir	Ritonavir 100-200 mg q12h + indinavir 800 mg q12h, or 400 mg q12h of each drug
Nelfinavir	Ritonavir 400 mg q12h + nelfinavir 500-750 mg q12h
Nevirapine	No changes

---

* Resume dosing for CrCl < 10 mL/min after supplemental dose. "Usual dose" assumes normal renal and hepatic function. CrCl = creatinine clearance; CVVH = continuous veno-venous hemofiltration; HD = hemodialysis; PD = peritoneal dialysis. See pp. 252-255 for definitions/explanations, p. 1 for abbreviations

Saquinavir	Ritonavir 400 mg q12h + saquinavir 400 mg q12h
Ketoconazole	Caution; do not exceed ketoconazole 200 mg q24h
Rifampin	No information; ↑ liver toxicity possible
Rifabutin	Rifabutin 150 mg q48h or 3x/week

Drug Interactions: Antiretrovirals, rifabutin, rifampin (see dose adjustment grid, above); alprazolam, diazepam, estazolam, flurazepam, midazolam, triazolam, zolpidem, meperidine, propoxyphene, piroxicam, quinidine, amiodarone, encainide, flecainide, propafenone, astemizole, bepridil, bupropion, cisapride, clorazepate, clozapine, pimozide, St. John's wort, terfenadine (avoid); alfentanil, fentanyl, hydrocodone, tramadol, disopyramide, lidocaine, mexiletine, erythromycin, clarithromycin, warfarin, dronabinol, ondansetron, metoprolol, pindolol, propranolol, timolol, amlodipine, diltiazem, felodipine, isradipine, nicardipine, nifedipine, nimodipine, nisoldipine, nitrendipine, verapamil, etoposide, paclitaxel, tamoxifen, vinblastine, vincristine, loratadine, tricyclic antidepressants, paroxetine, nefazodone, sertraline, trazodone, fluoxetine, venlafaxine, fluvoxamine, cyclosporine, tacrolimus, chlorpromazine, clonazepam, perphenazine, risperidone, thioridazine, clozapine, pimozide, methamphetamine (↑ interacting drug levels); telithromycin (↑ ritonavir levels); codeine, hydromorphone, methadone, morphine, ketoprofen, ketorolac, naproxen, diphenoxylate, oral contraceptives, theophylline (↓ interacting drug levels); carbamazepine, phenytoin, phenobarbital, clonazepam, dexamethasone, prednisone (↓ ritonavir levels, ↑ interacting drug levels; monitor anticonvulsant levels); metronidazole (disulfiram-like reaction); tobacco (↓ ritonavir levels); sildenafil (↑ or ↓ sildenafil levels; do not exceed 25 mg in 48 hrs)
Adverse Effects: Anorexia, anemia, leukopenia, hyperglycemia (including worsening diabetes, new-onset diabetes, DKA), ↑ cholesterol/triglycerides (evaluate risk for coronary disease/pancreatitis), fat redistribution, ↑ CPK, nausea, vomiting, diarrhea, abdominal pain, circumoral/extremity paresthesias, ↑ SGOT/SGPT, pancreatitis, taste perversion, possible increased bleeding in hemophilia
HIV Resistance Potential: Low (triple therapy); high (mono/double drug therapy)
Allergic Potential: Low
Safety in Pregnancy: B
Comments: GI intolerance decreases over time. Take with food if possible (serum levels increase 15%, fewer GI side effects). Dose escalation regimen: day 1-2 (300 mg q12h), day 3-5 (400 mg q12h), day 6-13 (500 mg q12h), day 14 (600 mg q12h). Separate dosing from ddI by 2 hours. Refrigerate capsules, not oral solution. Effective antiretroviral therapy consists of at least 3 antiretrovirals (same/different classes)
Cerebrospinal Fluid Penetration: < 10%

REFERENCES:
Cameron DW, Japour AJ, Xu Y, et al. Ritonavir and saquinavir combination therapy for the treatment of HIV infection. AIDS 13:213-224, 1999.
Deeks SG, Smith M, Holodniy M, et al. HIV-1 protease inhibitors: A review for clinicians. JAMA 277:145-53, 1997.
Kaul DR, Cinti SK, Carver PL, et al. HIV protease inhibitors: Advances in therapy and adverse reactions, including metabolic complications. Pharmacotherapy 19:281-98, 1999.
Lea AP, Faulds D. Ritonavir. Drugs 52:541-6, 1996.
McDonald CK, Kuritzkes DR. Human immunodeficiency virus type 1 protease inhibitors. Arch Intern Med 157:951-9, 1997.
Panel on Clinical Practices for Treatment of HIV Infection. Guidelines for the use of antiretroviral agents in HIV-infected adults and adolescents. Department of Health and Human Services. April 23, 2001. www.hivatis.org

Saquinavir (Invirase/Fortovase)

Drug Class: Antiretroviral protease inhibitor
Usual Dose: Saquinavir hard-gel capsule (Invirase): 400 mg (PO) q12h with ritonavir (not recommended unless unable to take soft-gel capsule); Saquinavir soft-gel capsule (Fortovase): 1200 mg (PO) q8h

---

* Resume dosing for CrCl < 10 mL/min after supplemental dose. "Usual dose" assumes normal renal and hepatic function. CrCl = creatinine clearance; CVVH = continuous veno-venous hemofiltration; HD = hemodialysis; PD = peritoneal dialysis. See pp. 252-255 for definitions/explanations, p. 1 for abbreviations

Pharmacokinetic Parameters:
Peak serum level: 0.07 mcg/mL
Bioavailability: Hard-gel 4% / soft-gel 15%
Excreted unchanged: 3%
Serum half-life (normal/ESRD): 1-2 hrs/no data
Plasma protein binding: 98%
Volume of distribution (V_d): 10 L/kg
Primary Mode of Elimination: Hepatic
Dosage Adjustments:

CrCl ~ 40–60 mL/min	No change
CrCl ~ 10–30 mL/min	No change
CrCl < 10 mL/min	No change
Post–HD dose	None
Post–PD dose	None
Post–CVVH dose	None
Moderate hepatic insufficiency	No change
Severe hepatic insufficiency	Fortovase: 600 mg (PO) q8h; Invirase:

Antiretroviral Dosage Adjustments:

Amprenavir	No information
Delavirdine	Saquinavir soft-gel 800 mg q8h (monitor transaminases)
Efavirenz	Avoid combination
Indinavir	No information
Lopinavir/ritonavir	Saquinavir 800 mg q12h
Nelfinavir	Saquinavir soft-gel 800 mg q8h or 1200 mg q12h
Nevirapine	No information
Ritonavir	Saquinavir soft-gel or hard-gel 400 mg q12h + ritonavir 400 mg q12h

Rifampin	Avoid unless given with ritonavir, then use rifampin 600 mg q24h or 2-3x/week
Rifabutin	No changes unless given with ritonavir, then give rifabutin 150 mg 2-3x/week

Drug Interactions: Antiretrovirals, rifabutin, rifampin (see dose adjustment grid, above); astemizole, terfenadine, benzodiazepines, cisapride, ergotamine, statins, St. John's wort (avoid if possible); carbamazepine, phenytoin, phenobarbital, dexamethasone, prednisone (↓ saquinavir levels, ↑ interacting drug levels; monitor anticonvulsant levels); clarithromycin, erythromycin, telithromycin (↑ saquinavir and macrolide levels); grapefruit juice, itraconazole, ketoconazole (↑ saquinavir levels); sildenafil (↑ or ↓ sildenafil levels; do not exceed 25 mg in 48 hrs)

Adverse Effects: Anorexia, headache, anemia, leukopenia, hyperglycemia (including worsening diabetes, new-onset diabetes, DKA), ↑ cholesterol/triglycerides (evaluate risk for coronary disease/pancreatitis), ↑ SGOT/SGPT, hyperuricemia, fat redistribution, possible increased bleeding in hemophilia

HIV Resistance Potential: Low (triple therapy); high (mono/double drug therapy)
Allergic Potential: Low
Safety in Pregnancy: B
Comments: Possible antagonism with indinavir. Potential synergy with AZT, ddC, 3TC, and ritonavir. Increased GI absorption with soft-gel capsules; take with large meal. Effective antiretroviral therapy consists of at least 3 antiretrovirals (same/different class)
Cerebrospinal Fluid Penetration: < 1%

REFERENCES:
Cameron DW, Japour AJ, Xu Y, et al. Ritonavir and saquinavir combination therapy for the treatment of HIV infection. AIDS 13:213-224, 1999.
Hsu A, Granneman GR, Cao G, et al. Pharmacokinetic interactions between two human immunodeficiency virus protease inhibitors, ritonavir and saquinavir. Clin Pharmacol Ther 63:453-64, 1998.
Murphy RL, Brun S, Hicks C, et al. ABT-378/ritonavir

---

* Resume dosing for CrCl < 10 mL/min after supplemental dose. "Usual dose" assumes normal renal and hepatic function. CrCl = creatinine clearance; CVVH = continuous veno-venous hemofiltration; HD = hemodialysis; PD = peritoneal dialysis. See pp. 252-255 for definitions/explanations, p. 1 for abbreviations

plus stavudine and lamivudine for the treatment of antiretroviral-naive adults with HIV-1 infection: 48-week results. AIDS 15:F1-9, 2001.

Noble S, Faulds D. Saquinavir. A review of its pharmacology and clinical potential in the management of HIV infection. Drugs 52:93-112, 1996.

Perry CM, Noble S. Saquinavir soft-gel capsule formation: A review of its use in patients with HIV infection. Drugs 55;461-86, 1998.

Panel on Clinical Practices for Treatment of HIV Infection. Guidelines for the use of antiretroviral agents in HIV-infected adults and adolescents. Department of Health and Human Services. April 23, 2001. www.hivatis.org

Vella S, Floridia M. Saquinavir: Clinical pharmacology and efficacy. Clin Pharmacokinet 34:189-201, 1998.

Sparfloxacin (Zagam)

Drug Class: Fluoroquinolone
Usual Dose: 200 mg (PO) q24h after a 400 mg (PO) loading dose
Pharmacokinetic Parameters:
Peak serum level: 1.4 mcg/mL
Bioavailability: 92%
Excreted unchanged: 60%
Serum half-life (normal/ESRD): 20 hrs/no data
Plasma protein binding: 45%
Volume of distribution (V_d): 3.9 L/kg
Primary Mode of Elimination: Hepatic
Dosage Adjustments:

CrCl ~ 40–60 mL/min	No change
CrCl ~ 10–30 mL/min	No change
CrCl < 10 mL/min	200 mg (PO) q48h (maintenance dose)
Post–HD dose	None
Post–PD dose	None
Post–CVVH dose	None
Moderate hepatic insufficiency	No change
Severe hepatic insufficiency	No information

Drug Interactions: No data
Adverse Effects: Drug fever/rash,

phototoxicity. May ↑ QT_c; avoid with other medications that prolong the QT_c interval and in patients with cardiac arrhythmias/heart block.
Resistance Potential: Low
Allergic Potential: Low
Safety in Pregnancy: C
Comments: Patients should be shielded from sunlight during and for 1 week after therapy. Concurrent administration of magnesium/aluminum containing antacids decreases sparfloxacin absorption by ~ 50%; take 2 hours before or 4 hours after antacids. Use another quinolone

REFERENCES:

Cunha BA. Sparfloxacin: A review of its microbiology, pharmacokinetics and clinical application. Adv Ther 14:348-56, 1997.

Goa KL, Bryson HM, Markham A. Sparfloxacin: A review of its antibacterial activity, pharmacokinetic properties, clinical efficacy, and tolerability in lower respiratory tract infections. Drugs 53:700-25, 1997.

Martin SJ, Meyer JM, Chuck SK, et al. Levofloxacin and Sparfloxacin: New quinolones antibiotics. Ann Pharmacother 32:320-36, 1998.

Stein GE, Havlichek DH. Sparfloxacin: Potential clinical and economic impact in the treatment of respiratory infections. Pharmacotherapy 17:1139-47, 1997.

Spectinomycin (Spectam, Trobicin)

Drug Class: Aminocyclitol
Usual Dose: 2 gm (IM) x 1 dose
Pharmacokinetic Parameters:
Peak serum level: 100 mcg/mL
Bioavailability: Not applicable
Excreted unchanged: 80%
Serum half-life (normal/ESRD): 1.6/16 hrs
Plasma protein binding: 20%
Volume of distribution (V_d): 0.25 L/kg
Primary Mode of Elimination: Renal
Dosage Adjustments:

CrCl ~ 40–60 mL/min	No change
CrCl ~ 10–30 mL/min	No change
CrCl < 10 mL/min	No change
Post–HD dose	None

---

* Resume dosing for CrCl < 10 mL/min after supplemental dose. "Usual dose" assumes normal renal and hepatic function. CrCl = creatinine clearance; CVVH = continuous veno-venous hemofiltration; HD = hemodialysis; PD = peritoneal dialysis. See pp. 252-255 for definitions/explanations, p. 1 for abbreviations

Post–PD dose	None
Post–CVVH dose	None
Moderate hepatic insufficiency	No change
Severe hepatic insufficiency	No change

Drug Interactions: None
Adverse Effects: Local pain at injection site
Resistance Potential: Low
Allergic Potential: Low
Safety in Pregnancy: B
Comments: Ineffective in pharyngeal GC (poor penetration into secretions)
Cerebrospinal Fluid Penetration: < 10%

REFERENCES:
Fiumara NJ. The treatment of gonococcal proctitis: An evaluation of 173 patients treated with 4 gm of spectinomycin. JAMA 239:735-7, 1978.
Holloway WJ. Spectinomycin. Med Clin North Am 66:169-173, 1995.
McCormack WM, Finland M. Spectinomycin. Ann Intern Med 84:712-16, 1976.

Stavudine (Zerit) d4t

Drug Class: Antiretroviral NRTI (nucleoside reverse transcriptase inhibitor)
Usual Dose: ≥ 60 kg: 40 mg (PO) q12h; < 60 kg: 30 mg (PO) q12h
Pharmacokinetic Parameters:
Peak serum level: 42 mcg/mL
Bioavailability: 86%
Excreted unchanged: 40%
Serum half-life (normal/ESRD): 1.0/5.5 hrs
Plasma protein binding: 0%
Volume of distribution (V_d): 0.5 L/kg
Primary Mode of Elimination: Renal
Dosage Adjustments: ≥ 60 kg / [≤ 60 kg]

CrCl ~ 40–60 mL/min	40 mg (PO) q12h [30 mg (PO) q12h]
CrCl ~ 10–30 mL/min	20 mg (PO) q24h [15 mg (PO) q24h]
CrCl < 10 mL/min	20 mg (PO) q12h [15 mg (PO) q24h]

Post–HD dose*	20 mg (PO) [15 mg (PO)]
Post–PD dose	No information
Post–CVVH dose*	20 mg (PO) [15 mg (PO)]
Moderate hepatic insufficiency	No change
Severe hepatic insufficiency	No change

Drug Interactions: Dapsone, INH, other neurotoxic agents (↑ risk of peripheral neuropathy)
Adverse Effects: Drug fever/rash, nausea, vomiting, GI upset, diarrhea, headache, insomnia, dose dependent peripheral neuropathy, myalgias, pancreatitis, ↑ SGOT/SGPT, thrombocytopenia, leukopenia, lactic acidosis with hepatic steatosis (rare, but potentially life-threatening toxicity with use of NRTIs)
HIV Resistance Potential: Low (triple therapy); high (mono/double drug therapy)
Allergic Potential: Low
Safety in Pregnancy: C
Comments: Pancreatitis may be severe/fatal. Avoid coadministration with AZT or ddC. Decrease dose in patients with peripheral neuropathy to 20 mg (PO) q12h. Pregnant women may be at increased risk for lactic acidosis/liver damage when stavudine is used with didanosine (ddI)
Effective antiretroviral therapy consists of at least 3 antiretrovirals (same/different classes)
Cerebrospinal Fluid Penetration: 30%

REFERENCES:
Dudley MN, Graham KK, Kaul S, et al. Pharmacokinetics of stavudine in patients with AIDS and AIDS-related complex. J Infect Dis 166:480-5, 1992.
Lea AP, Faulds D. Stavudine: A review of its pharmacodynamic and pharmacokinetic properties and clinical potential in HIV infection. Drugs 51:846-64, 1996.
Miller KD, Cameron M, Wood LV, et al. Lactic acidosis and hepatic steatosis associated with use of stavudine: Report of four cases. Ann Intern Med. 133:192-196, 2000.

---

* Resume dosing for CrCl < 10 mL/min after supplemental dose. "Usual dose" assumes normal renal and hepatic function. CrCl = creatinine clearance; CVVH = continuous veno-venous hemofiltration; HD = hemodialysis; PD = peritoneal dialysis. See pp. 252-255 for definitions/explanations, p. 1 for abbreviations

Murphy RL, Brun S, Hicks C, et al. ABT-378/ritonavir plus stavudine and lamivudine for the treatment of antiretroviral-naive adults with HIV-1 infection: 48-week results. AIDS 15:F1-9, 2001.

Panel on Clinical Practices for Treatment of HIV Infection. Guidelines for the use of antiretroviral agents in HIV-infected adults and adolescents. Department of Health and Human Services. April 23, 2001. www.hivatis.org

Streptomycin

Drug Class: Aminoglycoside
Usual Dose: 15 mg/kg (IM) q24h or 1 gm (IM) q24h (see comments)
Pharmacokinetic Parameters:
Peak serum level: 40 mcg/mL
Bioavailability: Not applicable
Excreted unchanged: 90%
Serum half-life (normal/ESRD): 2.5/100 hrs
Plasma protein binding: 35%
Volume of distribution (V_d): 0.26 L/kg
Primary Mode of Elimination: Renal
Dosage Adjustments:

CrCl ~ 40–60 mL/min	No change
CrCl ~ 10–30 mL/min	15 mg/kg (IM) q48h or 1 gm (IM) q48h
CrCl < 10 mL/min	15 mg/kg (IM) q72h or 1 gm (IM) q72h
Post–HD dose*	7.5 mg/kg (IM) or 500 mg (IM)
Post–PD dose*	3.75 mg/kg (IM) or 250 mg (IM)
Post–CVVH dose*	7.5 mg/kg (IM) or 500 mg (IM)
Moderate hepatic insufficiency	No change
Severe hepatic insufficiency	No change

Drug Interactions: Amphotericin B, cephalothin, cyclosporine, enflurane, methoxyflurane, NSAIDs, polymyxin B, radiographic contrast, vancomycin (↑ nephrotoxicity); cis-platinum (↑ nephrotoxicity, ↑ ototoxicity); loop diuretics (↑ ototoxicity); neuromuscular blocking agents (↑ apnea, prolonged paralysis); non-polarizing muscle relaxants (↑ apnea)
Adverse Effects: Most ototoxic aminoglycoside (usually vestibular ototoxicity); least nephrotoxic aminoglycoside
Resistance Potential: Low
Allergic Potential: Low
Safety in Pregnancy: D
Comments: May be given IV slowly over 1 hour. Dose for tularemia = 1 gm (IV/IM) q12h. Dose for plague = 2 gm (IV/IM) q12h. Dose for TB = 1 gm (IM) q24h 2-3x/week
Cerebrospinal Fluid Penetration: 20%

REFERENCES:
Davidson PT, Le HQ. Drug treatment of tuberculosis 1992. Drugs 43:651-73, 1992.

Kim-Sing A, Kays MB, Vivien EJ, et al. Intravenous streptomycin use in a patient infection with high-level gentamicin-resistant Streptococcus faecalis. Ann Pharmacother 27:712-4, 1993.

Morris JT, Cooper RH. Intravenous streptomycin: A useful route of administration. Clin Infect Dis 19:1150-1, 1994.

Van Scoy RE, Wilkowske CJ. Antituberculous agents. Mayo Clin Proc 67:179-87, 1992.

Telithromycin (Ketek)

Drug Class: Ketolide
Usual Dose: 800 mg (PO) q24h
Pharmacokinetic Parameters:
Peak serum level: 1.9 mcg/mL
Bioavailability: 57%
Excreted unchanged: 20%
Serum half-life (normal/ESRD): 9.8/11 hrs
Plasma protein binding: 65%
Volume of distribution (V_d): No data
Primary Mode of Elimination: Hepatic
Dosage Adjustments:

CrCl ~ 40–60 mL/min	No change
CrCl ~ 10–30 mL/min	No change
CrCl < 10 mL/min	No change
Post–HD dose	None
Post–PD dose	None

Post–CVVH dose	None
Moderate hepatic insufficiency	No change
Severe hepatic insufficiency	400 mg (PO) q24h

Drug Interactions: Carbamazepine (↑ carbamazepine levels, nausea, nystagmus, ataxia); amiodarone, procainamide, sotalol, astemizole, terfenadine, cisapride, pimozide (may ↑ QT interval, torsade de pointes); cyclosporine, digoxin, phenytoin, ritonavir (↑ interacting drug levels); efavirenz (↓ telithromycin levels); ergot derivatives (acute ergot toxicity); fluconazole, itraconazole, ketoconazole (↑ telithromycin levels, ↓ interacting drug levels); midazolam, triazolam (↑ interacting drug levels, sedation); statins (↑ risk of rhabdomyolysis); theophylline (additive nausea)
Adverse Effects: Nausea, diarrhea, dizziness, ↑ pulse rate (7-14 beats/min), ↑ SGOT/SGPT
Resistance Potential: Low
Allergic Potential: Low
Safety in Pregnancy: B
Comments: May take with or without food. Moitor potential hepatotoxicity with serial SGOTs/SGPTs

REFERENCES:
Bryskier A,. Ketolides-telithromycin, an example of a new class of antibacterial agents. Clin Microbiol Infect 6:661-9, 2000.
Felmingham D. Microbiological profile of telithromycin, the first ketolide antimicrobial. Clin Microbiol Infect 7:2-10, 2001.
Gustafsson I, Hjelm E, Cars O. In vitro pharmacodynamics of the new ketolides HMR 3004 and HMR 3647 (telithromycin) against Chalmydia pneumoniae. Antimicrob Agents Chemother 44:1846-7, 2000.

Terbinafine (Lamisil, Daskil)

Drug Class: Antifungal
Usual Dose: 250 mg (PO) q24h
Pharmacokinetic Parameters:
Peak serum level: 1 mcg/mL
Bioavailability: 80%

Excreted unchanged: 75%
Serum half-life (normal/ESRD): 24 hrs/no data
Plasma protein binding: 99%
Volume of distribution (V_d): 13.5 L/kg
Primary Mode of Elimination: Renal/hepatic
Dosage Adjustments:

CrCl ~ 40–60 mL/min	No change
CrCl ~ 10–30 mL/min	Avoid
CrCl < 10 mL/min	Avoid
Post–HD dose	Avoid
Post–PD dose	Avoid
Post–CVVH dose	Avoid
Moderate hepatic insufficiency	Avoid
Severe hepatic insufficiency	Avoid

Drug Interactions: Cimetidine (↓ terbinafine clearance, ↑ terbinafine levels); phenobarbital, rifampin (↑ terbinafine clearance, ↓ terbinafine levels)
Adverse Effects: Drug fever/rash, lymphopenia, leukopenia, ↑ SGOT/SGPT, visual disturbances, nausea, vomiting, GI upset
Resistance Potential: Low
Allergic Potential: Low
Safety in Pregnancy: B
Comments: May cause green vision and changes in the lens/retina
Cerebrospinal Fluid Penetration: < 10%

REFERENCES:
Abdel-Rahman SM, Nahata MC. Oral terbinafine: A new antifungal agent. Ann Pharmacother 31:445-56, 1997.
Amichai B, Grunwald MH. Adverse drug reactions of the new oral antifungal agents - terbinafine, fluconazole, and itraconazole. Int J Dermatol 37:410-5, 1998.
Gupta AK, Shear NH. Terbinafine: An update. J Am Acad Dermatol 37:979-88, 1997.
Trepanier EF, Amsden GW. Current issues in onychomycosis. Ann Pharmacother 32:204-14, 1998.

Tetracycline (various)

Drug Class: Tetracycline
Usual Dose: 500 mg (PO) q6h
Pharmacokinetic Parameters:
Peak serum level: 1.5 mcg/mL
Bioavailability: 60%
Excreted unchanged: 60%
Serum half-life (normal/ESRD): 8/108 hrs
Plasma protein binding: 60%
Volume of distribution (V_d): 0.7 L/kg
Primary Mode of Elimination: Renal
Dosage Adjustments:

CrCl ~ 40–60 mL/min	500 mg (PO) q8h
CrCl ~ 10–30 mL/min	500 mg (PO) q12h
CrCl < 10 mL/min	Avoid
Post–HD dose	Avoid
Post–PD dose	Avoid
Post–CVVH dose	Avoid
Moderate hepatic insufficiency	No change
Severe hepatic insufficiency	No change

Drug Interactions: Antacids, Al^{++}, Ca^{++}, Fe^{++}, Mg^{++}, Zn^{++}, multivitamins, sucralfate (↓ absorption of tetracycline); barbiturates, carbamazepine, phenytoin (↓ half-life of tetracycline); bicarbonate (↓ absorption and ↑ clearance of tetracycline); digoxin (↑ digoxin levels); insulin (↑ insulin effect); methoxyflurane (↑ nephrotoxicity)
Adverse Effects: Nausea, vomiting, GI upset, diarrhea, hepatotoxicity, vaginal candidiasis, photosensitizing reactions, benign intracranial hypertension (pseudotumor cerebri)
Resistance Potential: High (S. aureus, S. pneumoniae, N. gonorrhoeae)
Allergic Potential: Low
Safety in Pregnancy: D
Comments: Hepatotoxicity dose dependent (≥ 2 gm/day), especially in pregnancy/renal failure. Avoid prolonged sun exposure

Cerebrospinal Fluid Penetration:
Non-inflamed meninges = 5%
Inflamed meninges = 5%
Bile Penetration: 1000%

REFERENCES:
Cunha BA, Comer J, Jonas M. The tetracyclines. Med Clin North Am 66:293-302, 1982.
Pugliese A, Cunha BA. Tetraclyclines. Int J Urogyn 5:221-7, 1994.
Smilack JD, Wilson WE, Cocerill Fr 3rd. Tetracycline, chloramphenicol, erythromycin, clindamycin, and metronidazole. Mayo Clin Proc 66:1270-80, 1991.

Ticarcillin (Ticar)

Drug Class: Antipseudomonal penicillin
Usual Dose: 3 gm (IV) q6h
Pharmacokinetic Parameters:
Peak serum level: 300 mcg/mL
Bioavailability: Not applicable
Excreted unchanged: 85%
Serum half-life (normal/ESRD): 1/5 hrs
Plasma protein binding: 45%
Volume of distribution (V_d): 0.2 L/kg
Primary Mode of Elimination: Renal
Dosage Adjustments:

CrCl ~ 40–60 mL/min	3 gm (IV) q8h
CrCl ~ 10–30 mL/min	3 gm (IV) q12h
CrCl < 10 mL/min	3 gm (IV) q12h
Post–HD dose*	2 gm (IV)
Post–PD dose	None
Post–CVVH dose*	3 gm (IV)
Moderate hepatic insufficiency	No change
Severe hepatic insufficiency	No change

Drug Interactions: Aminoglycosides (inactivation of ticarcillin in renal failure); warfarin (↑ INR); oral contraceptives (↓ oral contraceptive effect); cefoxitin (↓ ticarcillin effect)
Adverse Effects: Drug fever/rash; E. multiforme/Stevens–Johnson syndrome,

---
* Resume dosing for CrCl < 10 mL/min after supplemental dose. "Usual dose" assumes normal renal and hepatic function. CrCl = creatinine clearance; CVVH = continuous veno-venous hemofiltration; HD = hemodialysis; PD = peritoneal dialysis. See pp. 252-255 for definitions/explanations, p. 1 for abbreviations

anaphylactic reactions (hypotension, laryngospasm, bronchospasm), hives, serum sickness. Dose-dependent inhibition of platelet aggregation is minimal/absent (usual dose is less than carbenicillin)

Resistance Potential: Low
Allergic Potential: High
Safety in Pregnancy: B
Comments: Administer 1 hour before or after aminoglycoside. Na^+ content = 5.2 mEq/g. Meningeal dose = usual dose
Cerebrospinal Fluid Penetration:
Non-inflamed meninges = 1%
Inflamed meninges = 30%

REFERENCES:

Donowitz GR, Mandell GL. Beta-lactam antibiotics. N Engl J Med 318:419-26 and 318:490-500, 1993.
Tan JS, File TM, Jr. Antipseudomonal penicillins. Med Clin North Am 79:679-93, 1995.
Wright AJ. The penicillins. Mayo Clin Proc 74:290-307, 1999.

Ticarcillin/clavulanate (Timentin)

Drug Class: Antipseudomonal penicillin
Usual Dose: 3.1 gm (IV) q6h
Pharmacokinetic Parameters:
Peak serum level: 300 mcg/mL
Bioavailability: Not applicable
Excreted unchanged: 85/45%
Serum half-life (normal/ESRD): [1/5]/[1/2] hrs
Plasma protein binding: 45/30%
Volume of distribution (V_d): 0.2/0.3 L/kg
Primary Mode of Elimination: Renal
Dosage Adjustments:

CrCl ~ 40–60 mL/min	No change
CrCl ~ 10–30 mL/min	3.1 gm (IV) q8h
CrCl < 10 mL/min	2 gm (IV) q12h
Post–HD dose*	3.1 gm (IV)
Post–PD dose*	3.1 gm (IV)
Post–CVVH dose*	3.1 gm (IV)

Moderate hepatic insufficiency	No change
Severe hepatic insufficiency	No change

Drug Interactions: Aminoglycosides (↓ aminoglycoside levels); methotrexate (↑ methotrexate levels); vecuronium (↑ vecuronium effect)
Adverse Effects: Drug fever/rash, E. multiforme/Stevens–Johnson syndrome, anaphylactic reactions (hypotension, laryngospasm, bronchospasm), hives, serum sickness
Resistance Potential: Low
Allergic Potential: High
Safety in Pregnancy: B
Comments: 20% of clavulanate removed by dialysis. Na^+ content = 4.75 mEq/g. K^+ content = 0.15 mEq/g
Cerebrospinal Fluid Penetration: < 10%

REFERENCES:

Donowitz GR, Mandell GL. Beta-lactam antibiotics. N Engl J Med 318:419-26 and 318:490-500, 1993.
Itokazu GS, Danziger LH. Ampicillin-sulbactam and ticarcillin-clavulanic acid: A comparison of their in vitro activity and review of their clinical efficacy. Pharmacotherapy 11:382-414, 1991.
Wright AJ. The penicillins. Mayo Clin Proc 74:290-307, 1999.

TMP–SMX (Bactrim, Septra)

Drug Class: Folate antagonist/sulfonamide
Usual Dose: 2.5-5 mg/kg (IV/PO) q6h
Pharmacokinetic Parameters:
Peak serum level: 2-8/40-80 mcg/mL
Bioavailability: 98%
Excreted unchanged: 50/70%
Serum half-life (normal/ESRD): 2-8/40-80 hrs
Plasma protein binding: 70%
Volume of distribution (V_d): 1.8/0.3 L/kg
Primary Mode of Elimination: Renal
Dosage Adjustments:

CrCl ~ 40–60 mL/min	1.25-2.5 mg/kg (IV/PO) q6h

---

* Resume dosing for CrCl < 10 mL/min after supplemental dose. "Usual dose" assumes normal renal and hepatic function. CrCl = creatinine clearance; CVVH = continuous veno-venous hemofiltration; HD = hemodialysis; PD = peritoneal dialysis. See pp. 252-255 for definitions/explanations, p. 1 for abbreviations

CrCl ~ 10–30 mL/min	0.625-1.25 mg/kg (IV/PO) q6h
CrCl < 10 mL/min	Avoid
Post–HD dose	Avoid
Post–PD dose	Avoid
Post–CVVH dose	Avoid
Moderate hepatic insufficiency	No change
Severe hepatic insufficiency	No change

Drug Interactions: *TMP component:*
Azathioprine (leukopenia); amantadine,
dapsone, digoxin, methotrexate, phenytoin,
rifampin, zidovudine (↑ interacting drug levels,
nystagmus with phenytoin); diuretics (↑ serum
K^+ with K^+-sparing diuretics, ↓ serum Na^+ with
thiazide diuretics); warfarin (↑ INR, bleeding).
SMX component: Cyclosporine (↓ cyclosporine
levels); phenytoin (↑ phenytoin levels,
nystagmus, ataxia); methotrexate (↑ antifolate
activity); sulfonylureas, thiopental (↑ interacting
drug effect); warfarin (↑ INR, bleeding)
Adverse Effects:
TMP: Folate deficiency
SMX: Leukopenia, thrombocytopenia, hemolytic
anemia ± G6PD deficiency, aplastic anemia, ↑
SGOT/SGPT, severe hypersensitivity reactions (E.
multiforme/Stevens–Johnson syndrome)
Resistance Potential: High (H. influenzae, S.
pneumoniae)
Allergic Potential: Very high (SMX); none
(TMP)
Safety in Pregnancy: X
Comments: Drug fever/rash increased in
HIV/AIDS. Excellent bioavailability (IV = PO).
1 SS tablet = 80 mg TMP + 400 mg SMX.
1 DS tablet = 160 mg TMP + 800 mg SMX.
1 SS tablet (PO) q6h = 10 mg/kg (IV) q24h.
1 DS tablet (PO) q6h = 20 mg/kg (IV) q24h.
Meningeal dose = 5 mg/kg (IV/PO) q6h
Cerebrospinal Fluid Penetration:
Non-inflamed meninges = 40%
Inflamed meninges = 40%
Bile Penetration: 100%

REFERENCES:
Cockerill FR, Edson RS. Trimethoprim-sulfamethoxazole.
  Mayo Clin Proc 66:1260-9, 1991.
El-Sadr W, Luskin-Hawk R, Yurik TM, et al. A
  randomized trial of daily and thrice weekly
  trimethoprim-sulfamethoxazole for the prevention of
  Pneumocystis carinii pneumonia in HIV infected
  individuals. Clin Infect Dis 29:775-83, 1999.
Giannakopoulos G, Johnson ES. TMP-SMX. Antibiotics
  for Clinicians 1:63-9, 1997.
Lundstrom TS, Sobel JD. Vancomycin, trimethoprim-
  sulfamethoxazole, and rifampin. Infect Dis Clin North
  Am 9:747-67, 1995.
Para MF, Dohn M, Frame P, et al, for the ACTG 268
  dapsoneStudy Team. Reduced toxicity with gradual
  initiation of trimethoprim-sulfamethoxazole as primary
  prophylaxis for Pneumocystis carinii pneumonia: AIDS
  Clinical Trials Group 268. J Acquire Immune Defic
  Syndr 24:337-43, 2000.
Smith LG, Sensakovic J. Trimethoprim-
  sulfamethoxazole. Med Clin North Am 66:143-56,
  1982.

Tobramycin (Nebcin)

Drug Class: Aminoglycoside
Usual Dose: 5 mg/kg (IV) q24h or 240 mg (IV)
q24h (preferred over q8h dosing)
Pharmacokinetic Parameters:
*Peak serum levels: 4-8 mcg/mL (q8h dosing);
  16-24 mcg/mL (q24h dosing)
Bioavailability: Not applicable
Excreted unchanged: 95%
Serum half-life (normal/ESRD): 2.5/56 hrs
Plasma protein binding: 10%
Volume of distribution (V_d): 0.24 L/kg*
Primary Mode of Elimination: Renal
Dosage Adjustments:

CrCl ~ 40–60 mL/min	2.5 mg/kg (IV) q24h or 120 mg (IV) q24h
CrCl ~ 10–30 mL/min	2.5 mg/kg (IV) q48h or 120 mg (IV) q48h
CrCl < 10 mL/min	1.25 mg/kg (IV) q48h or 60 mg (IV) q48h
Post–HD dose*	1.25 mg/kg (IV) or 80 mg (IV)
Post–PD dose*	0.6 mg/kg (IV) or 40 mg (IV)

---

* Resume dosing for CrCl < 10 mL/min after supplemental dose. "Usual dose" assumes normal renal and hepatic function. CrCl = creatinine clearance, CVVH = continuous veno-venous hemofiltration; HD = hemodialysis; PD = peritoneal dialysis. See pp. 252-255 for definitions/explanations, p. 1 for abbreviations

Post–CVVH dose*	1.42 mg/kg (IV) or 100 mg (IV)
Moderate hepatic insufficiency	No change
Severe hepatic insufficiency	No change

Drug Interactions: Amphotericin B, cyclosporine, enflurane, methoxyflurane, NSAIDs, polymyxin B, radiographic contrast, vancomycin (↑ nephrotoxicity); cis-platinum (↑ nephrotoxicity, ↑ ototoxicity); loop diuretics (↑ ototoxicity); neuromuscular blocking agents (↑ apnea, prolonged paralysis); non-polarizing muscle relaxants (↑ apnea)
Adverse Effects: Neuromuscular blockade with rapid infusion/absorption. Nephrotoxicity only with prolonged/extremely high serum trough levels; may cause reversible non–oliguric renal failure (ATN). Ototoxicity associated with prolonged/extremely high peak serum levels (usually irreversible): Cochlear toxicity (1/3 of ototoxicity) manifests as decreased high frequency hearing, but deafness is unusual. Vestibular toxicity (2/3 of ototoxicity) develops before ototoxicity, and typically manifests as tinnitus
Resistance Potential: High (P. aeruginosa)
Allergic Potential: Low
Safety in Pregnancy: C
Comments: Dose for synergy = 2.5 mg/kg (IV) q24h or 120 mg (IV) q24h. Single daily dosing greatly reduces nephrotoxic/ototoxic potential. Incompatible with solutions containing β–lactams, erythromycin, chloramphenicol, furosemide, sodium bicarbonate. IV infusion should be given slowly over 1 hour. May be given IM. Avoid intraperitoneal infusion due to risk of neuromuscular blockade. Avoid intratracheal/aerosolized intrapulmonary instillation, which predisposes to antibiotic resistance. V_d increases with edema/ascites, trauma, burns, cystic fibrosis; may require ↑ dose. V_d decreases with dehydration, obesity; may require ↓ dose. Renal cast counts are the best indicator of aminoglycoside nephrotoxicity, not serum creatinine. Dialysis removes ~ 1/3 of tobramycin from serum

Therapeutic Serum Concentrations:
Peak (q24h/q8h dosing) = 16-24/8-10 mcg/mL
Trough (q24h/q8h dosing) = 0/1-2 mcg/mL
Dose for synergy = 2.5 mg/kg (IV) q24h or 120 mg (IV) q24h
Intrathecal (IT) dose = 5 mg (IT) q24h
Cerebrospinal Fluid Penetration:
Non-inflamed meninges = 0%
Inflamed meninges = 20%
Bile Penetration: 30%

REFERENCES:
Begg EJ, Barclay ML. Aminoglycosides - 50 years on. Br J Clin Pharmacol 39:597-603, 1995.
Cunha BA. Aminoglycosides: Current role in antimicrobial therapy. Pharmacotherapy 8: 334-50, 1988.
Edson RS, Terrel CL. The aminoglycosides. Mayo Clin Proc 74:519-28, 1999.
Gilbert DN. Once-daily aminoglycoside therapy. Antimicrob Agents Chemother 35:399-405, 1991.
Hustinx WN, Hoepelman IM. Aminoglycoside dosage regimens: Is once a day enough? Clin Pharmacokinet 25:427-32, 1993.
Lortholary O, Tod M, Cohen Y, et al. Aminoglycosides. Med Clin North Am 79:761-87, 1995.
McCormack JP, Jewesson PJ. A critical reevaluation of the "therapeutic range" of aminoglycosides. Clin Infect Dis 14:320-39, 1992.

Trimethoprim (Proloprim, Trimpex)

Drug Class: Folate antagonist
Usual Dose: 100 mg (PO) q12h
Pharmacokinetic Parameters:
Peak serum level: 2-8 mcg/mL
Bioavailability: 98%
Excreted unchanged: 50%
Serum half-life (normal/ESRD): 12/24 hrs
Plasma protein binding: 70%
Volume of distribution (V_d): 1.8L/kg
Primary Mode of Elimination: Renal
Dosage Adjustments:

CrCl ~ 40–60 mL/min	No change
CrCl ~ 10–30 mL/min	100 mg (PO) q18h
CrCl < 10 mL/min	100 mg (PO) q24h
Post–HD dose	None

---

* Resume dosing for CrCl < 10 mL/min after supplemental dose. "Usual dose" assumes normal renal and hepatic function. CrCl = creatinine clearance; CVVH = continuous veno-venous hemofiltration; HD = hemodialysis; PD = peritoneal dialysis. See pp. 252-255 for definitions/explanations, p. 1 for abbreviations

Post–PD dose	None
Post–CVVH dose	None
Moderate hepatic insufficiency	No change
Severe hepatic insufficiency	No change

Drug Interactions: Azathioprine (leukopenia); amantadine, dapsone, digoxin, methotrexate, phenytoin, rifampin, zidovudine (↑ interacting drug levels, nystagmus with phenytoin); diuretics (↑ serum K^+ with K^+-sparing diuretics, ↓ serum Na^+ with thiazide diuretics); warfarin (↑ INR, bleeding)
Adverse Effects: Folate deficiency
Resistance Potential: No data
Allergic Potential: Low
Safety in Pregnancy: X
Comments: Useful in sulfa-allergic patients unable to take TMP-SMX.
Meningeal dose = 300 mg (PO) q6h
Cerebrospinal Fluid Penetration: 40%

REFERENCES:
Brogden RN, Carmine AA, Heel RC, et al. Trimethoprim: A review of its antibacterial activity, pharmacokinetics and therapeutic use in urinary tract infections. Drugs 23:405-30, 1982.
Friesen WT, Hekster YA, Vree TB. Trimethoprim: Clinical use and pharmacokinetics. Drug Intelligence & Clinical Pharmacy 15:325-30, 1981.
Neu HC. Trimethoprim alone for treatment of urinary tract infection. Rev Infect Dis 4:366-71, 1982.

Trimethoprim-Sulfamethoxazole, see TMP–SMX (Bactrim, Septra)

Trovafloxacin (Trovan)

Drug Class: Fluoroquinolone
Usual Dose: 300 mg (IV) q24h; 200 mg (PO) q24h
Pharmacokinetic Parameters:
Peak serum level: 3-6 (IV)/2-3 (PO) mcg/mL
Bioavailability: 86%
Excreted unchanged: 50%
Serum half-life (normal/ESRD): 11/11 hrs

Plasma protein binding: 76%
Volume of distribution (V_d): 1.3 L/kg
Primary Mode of Elimination: Hepatic
Dosage Adjustments:

CrCl ~ 40–60 mL/min	No change
CrCl ~ 10–30 mL/min	No change
CrCl < 10 mL/min	No change
Post–HD dose	None
Post–PD dose	None
Post–CVVH dose	None
Moderate hepatic insufficiency	150 mg (IV)/100 mg (PO) q24h
Severe hepatic insufficiency	Avoid

Drug Interactions: Al^{++}, Ca^{++}, Fe^{++}, Mg^{++}, Zn^{++} antacids, citrate/citric acid, dairy products (↓ absorption of trovafloxacin only if taken together); caffeine, theophylline (↑ interacting drug levels); NSAIDs (↑ risk of seizures), warfarin (↑ INR)
Adverse Effects: Drug fever/rash, GI upset, hepatic necrosis (may be fatal), seizures, mental confusion, encephalopathy, muscle contractions/spasticity, prolonged hypotension, local reaction/phlebitis IV, ↑ INR, pancreatitis, C. difficile diarrhea, non–C. difficile diarrhea
Resistance Potential: Low
Allergic Potential: High
Safety in Pregnancy: C
Comments: Give slowly over 2 hours to minimize hypotensive potential. Drug fevers more common than with other quinolones. Monitor for hepatotoxicity with daily SGOT/SGPTs. Monitor daily INRs. Avoid in patients with cirrhosis/liver disease, CNS/seizure disorders, or bleeding disorders. Use another quinolone
CNS Penetration: 23%

REFERENCES:
Cunha BA. Antimicrobial side effects. Med Clin North Am 85:149-85, 2001.
Cunha BA. Trovafloxacin adverse side effects. Antibiotics for Clinicians 2:137-9, 1998.

---

* Resume dosing for CrCl < 10 mL/min after supplemental dose. "Usual dose" assumes normal renal and hepatic function. CrCl = creatinine clearance; CVVH = continuous veno-venous hemofiltration; HD = hemodialysis; PD = peritoneal dialysis. See pp. 252-255 for definitions/explanations, p. 1 for abbreviations

Ernst ME, Ernst EJ, Klepser ME. Levofloxacin and trovafloxacin: The next generation of fluoroquinolones? Am J Health Syst Pharm 54:2569-84, 1997.

Garey KW, Amsden GW. Trovafloxacin: An overview. Pharmacology 19:21-34, 1999.

Haria M, Lamb HA. Trovafloxacin. Drugs 54:435-45, 1997.

Valacyclovir (Valtrex)

Drug Class: Antiviral (HSV, VZV)
Usual Dose: 500 mg (PO) q8h (HSV); 1 gm (PO) q8h (VZV) (see comments)
Pharmacokinetic Parameters:
Peak serum level: 4.5 mcg/mL
Bioavailability: 55%
Excreted unchanged: 1%
Serum half-life (normal/ESRD): 3/14 hrs
Plasma protein binding: 15%
Volume of distribution (V_d): 0.7 L/kg
Primary Mode of Elimination: Renal
Dosage Adjustments for HSV/VZV:

CrCl ~ 40–60 mL/min	250/500 mg (PO) q8h
CrCl ~ 10–30 mL/min	250/500 mg (PO) q12h
CrCl < 10 mL/min	250/500 mg (PO) q24h
Post–HD dose*	250/500 mg (PO)
Post–PD dose*	125/250 mg (PO)
Post–CVVH dose*	250/500 mg (PO)
Moderate hepatic insufficiency	No change
Severe hepatic insufficiency	No change

Drug Interactions: Cimetidine, probenecid (↑ acyclovir levels)
Adverse Effects: Headache, nausea, diarrhea, abdominal pain, weakness
Resistance Potential: Low
Allergic Potential: Low
Safety in Pregnancy: B
Comments: Converted to acyclovir in liver. Usual dose in adults:

Genital herpes (HSV-2):
  Prophylaxis = 1 gm (PO) q24h
  Episodic therapy for recurrences = 500mg (PO) q12h x 5 days
Shingles (VZV): 1 gm (PO) q8h x 7 days.
Meningeal dose = HSV dose
Cerebrospinal Fluid Penetration: 50%

REFERENCES:
Acost EP, Fletcher CV. Valacyclovir. Ann Pharmacotherapy 31:185-91, 1997.

Alrabiah FA, Sacks SL. New antiherpesvirus agents: Their targets and therapeutic potential. Drugs 52:17-32, 1996.

Geers TA, Isada CM. Update on antiviral therapy for genital herpes infection. Cleve Clinic J Med 67:567-73, 2000.

Perry CM, Faulds D. Valacyclovir: A review of its antiviral activity, pharmacokinetic properties, and therapeutic efficacy in herpesvirus infections. Drugs 52:754-72, 1996.

Valacyclovir. Med Lett Drugs Ther 38:3-4, 1996.

Valganciclovir (Valcyte)

Drug Class: Antiviral, Nucleoside inhibitor/analogue
Usual Dose: 900 mg (PO) q12h x 21 days (induction), then 900 mg (PO) q24h for life (maintenance)
Pharmacokinetic Parameters:
Peak serum level: 5.6 mcg/mL
Bioavailability: 59.4%
Excreted unchanged: 90%
Serum half-life (normal/ESRD): 4.1/67.5 hrs
Plasma protein binding: No data
Volume of distribution (V_d): 15.3 L/kg
Primary Mode of Elimination: Renal
Dosage Adjustments:

CrCl ~ 40–60 mL/min	450 mg (PO) q12h induction, then 450 mg (PO) q24h maintenance
CrCl ~ 10–40 mL/min	450 mg (PO) q48h induction, then 450 mg 2x/week maintenance
CrCl < 10 mL/min	Avoid

---

* Resume dosing for CrCl < 10 mL/min after supplemental dose. "Usual dose" assumes normal renal and hepatic function. CrCl = creatinine clearance; CVVH = continuous veno-venous hemofiltration; HD = hemodialysis; PD = peritoneal dialysis. See pp. 252-255 for definitions/explanations, p. 1 for abbreviations

Post–HD dose	No information
Post–PD dose	No information
Post–CVVH dose	No information
Moderate hepatic insufficiency	No change
Severe hepatic insufficiency	No change

Drug Interactions: Cytotoxic drugs (may produce additive toxicity: stomatitis, bone marrow depression, alopecia); imipenem (↑ risk of seizures); probenecid (↑ valganciclovir levels); zidovudine (↓ valganciclovir levels, ↑ zidovudine levels, possible neutropenia)
Adverse Effects: Drug fever/rash, diarrhea, nausea, vomiting, GI upset, leukopenia, anemia, thrombocytopenia, paresthesias/peripheral neuropathy, retinal detachment, aplastic anemia
Resistance Potential: Low
Allergic Potential: High
Safety in Pregnancy: C
Comments: Tablets should be taken with food. Valganciclovir is rapidly hydrolyzed to ganciclovir. Indicated for induction/maintenance therapy of CMV retinitis/infection. Not interchangeable on a tablet-to-tablet basis with oral ganciclovir. Much higher bioavailability than ganciclovir capsules; serum concentration equivalent to IV ganciclovir.
Meningeal dose = usual dose
Cerebrospinal Fluid Penetration: 70%

REFERENCES:

Jung D, Dorr A. Single-dose pharmacokinetics of valganciclovir in HIV and CMV seropositive subjects. J Clin Pharmacol 39:800-804, 1999.

Pescovitz MD, Rabkin J, Merion RM, et al. Valganciclovir results in improved oral absorption of ganciclovir in liver transplant recipients. Antimicrobial Agents Chemother 44:2811-15, 2000.

Martin D, Sierra-Madero J, Walmsley S, et al. Valganciclovir (VGCV) vs. IV ganciclovir (GVC) as induction therapy for newly diagnosed cytomegalovirus (CMV) retinitis: A randomized, controlled study. 7th Conference on retroviruses and opportunistic infections. San Francisco, CA (Abstract 231), 2000.

Vancomycin (Vancocin)

Drug Class: Glycopeptide
Usual Dose: 1 gm (IV) q12h (see comments)
Pharmacokinetic Parameters:
Peak serum level: 40 mcg/mL
Bioavailability: IV (not applicable)/PO (0%)
Excreted unchanged: 90%
Serum half-life (normal/ESRD): 6/230 hrs
Plasma protein binding: 10%
Volume of distribution (V_d): 0.7 L/kg
Primary Mode of Elimination: Renal
Dosage Adjustments:

CrCl ~ 40–60 mL/min	500 mg (IV) q12h
CrCl ~ 10–30 mL/min	500 mg (IV) q24h
CrCl < 10 mL/min	1 gm (IV) qweek
Post–HD dose	None
Post–PD dose	None
Post–CVVH dose*	1 gm (IV)
Moderate hepatic insufficiency	No change
Severe hepatic insufficiency	No change

Drug Interactions: Aminoglycosides, amphotericin B, polymyxin B (↑ nephrotoxicity)
Adverse Effects: "Red man/neck syndrome" with rapid IV infusion (histamine mediated), leukopenia, cardiac arrest, hypotension
Resistance Potential: Low
Allergic Potential: Low
Safety in Pregnancy: C
Comments: Not nephrotoxic. "Red man/neck syndrome" can be prevented/minimized by infusing IV vancomycin slowly over 1–2 hours. Intraperitoneal absorption = 40%. IV vancomycin use increases prevalence of VRE. For C. difficile diarrhea, use oral vancomycin 125 mg (PO) q6h. Vancomycin (IV/PO) ineffective for C. difficile colitis. Intrathecal (IT) dose = 20 mg (IT) in preservative free NaCl
Therapeutic Serum Concentrations:
Peak = 25-40 mcg/mL
Trough = 5-12 mcg/mL

---

* Resume dosing for CrCl < 10 mL/min after supplemental dose. "Usual dose" assumes normal renal and hepatic function. CrCl = creatinine clearance; CVVH = continuous veno-venous hemofiltration; HD = hemodialysis; PD = peritoneal dialysis. See pp. 252-255 for definitions/explanations, p. 1 for abbreviations

Potentially toxic peak levels: ≥ 80 mcg/mL
Cerebrospinal Fluid Penetration:
Non-inflamed meninges = 0%
Inflamed meninges = 25%
Bile Penetration: 50%

REFERENCES:
Cantu TG, Yamanaka-Yuen NA, Lietman PS. Serum vancomycin concentrations: Reappraisal of their clinical value. Clin Infect Dis 18:533-43, 1994.
Cunha BA. Vancomycin. Med Clin North Am 79:817-31, 1995.
Cunha BA, Deglin J, Chow M, et al. Pharmacokinetics of vancomycin in patients undergoing chronic hemodialysis. Rev Infect Dis 3:269-72, 1981.
French GL. Enterococci and vancomycin resistance. Clin Infect Dis 27:75-81, 1998.
Lacy MK, Tessier PR, Nicolau DP, et al. Comparison of vancomycin pharmacodynamics (1 gm every 12 or 25 h) against methicillin-resistant staphylococci. Intern J Antimicrob Agents 15:25-30, 2000.
Menzies D. Goel K, Cunha BA. Vancomycin. Antibiotics for Clinicians 2:97-9, 1998.
Wilheim MP. Vancomycin. Mayo Clin Proc 66:1165-70, 1991.

Voriconazole (Vfend)

Drug Class: Antifungal (2nd generation triazole)
Usual Dose: 400 mg (IV/PO) x 1 dose, then 200 mg (IV/PO) q12h
Pharmacokinetic Parameters:
Peak serum level: 4.8 mcg/mL
Bioavailability: 96%
Excreted unchanged: 5%
Serum half-life (normal/ESRD): 6/6 hrs
Plasma protein binding: 65%
Volume of distribution (V_d): 2 L/kg
Primary Mode of Elimination: Hepatic
Dosage Adjustments:

CrCl ~ 40–60 mL/min	No change
CrCl ~ 10–30 mL/min	No change
CrCl < 10 mL/min	No change
Post–HD dose	None
Post–PD dose	None
Post–CVVH dose	None

Moderate hepatic insufficiency	No change
Severe hepatic insufficiency	200 mg (IV/PO) q24h

Drug Interactions: Cyclosporine (↑ cyclosporine levels); phenytoin, rifampin, rifabutin (↓ voriconazole levels)
Adverse Effects: ↑ SGOT/SGPT, ↑ PT, skin rash, dose related visual disturbances (blurring vision, ↑ brightness)
Resistance Potential: Low
Allergic Potential: Low
Safety in Pregnancy: No data
Comments: Do not give voriconazole with rifampin, barbiturates, or carbamazepine. Voriconazole does not effect digoxin levels. Meningeal dose = usual dose
Cerebrospinal Fluid Penetration: 90%

REFERENCES:
Chandrasekar PH, Manavathu E. Voriconazole: A second-generation triazole. Drugs for Today 37:135-48, 2001.
McGinnis MR, Pasarell L, Sutton Da, et al. In vitro evaluation of voriconazole against some clinically important fungi. Antimicrob Agents Chemother 41:1832-4, 1997.
Sabo JA, Abdel-Rahman SM. Voriconazole: A new antifungal. Ann Pharmacotherapy 34:1032-43, 2000.

Zalcitabine (HIVID) ddC

Drug Class: Antiretroviral NRTI (nucleoside reverse transcriptase inhibitor)
Usual Dose: 0.75 mg (PO) q8h
Pharmacokinetic Parameters:
Peak serum level: 0.08 mcg/mL
Bioavailability: 85%
Excreted unchanged: 75%
Serum half-life (normal/ESRD): 1.2/10 hrs
Plasma protein binding: 0%
Volume of distribution (V_d): 0.54 L/kg
Primary Mode of Elimination: Renal
Dosage Adjustments:

CrCl ~ 40–60 mL/min	No change
CrCl ~ 10–30 mL/min	0.75 mg (PO) q12h

---

* Resume dosing for CrCl < 10 mL/min after supplemental dose. "Usual dose" assumes normal renal and hepatic function. CrCl = creatinine clearance; CVVH = continuous veno-venous hemofiltration; HD = hemodialysis; PD = peritoneal dialysis. See pp. 252-255 for definitions/explanations, p. 1 for abbreviations

CrCl < 10 mL/min	0.75 mg (PO) q24h
Post–HD dose	No information
Post–PD dose	No information
Post–CVVH dose	No information
Moderate hepatic insufficiency	No change
Severe hepatic insufficiency	No change

Drug Interactions: Cimetidine, probenecid, TMP-SMX (↑ zalcitabine levels); dapsone, didanosine, stavudine, INH, phenytoin, metronidazole, other neurotoxic agents or history of neuropathy (↑ risk of peripheral neuropathy); magnesium/aluminum containing antacids, metoclopramide (↓ bioavailability of zalcitabine); pentamidine IV, valproic acid, alcohol, other agents known to cause pancreatitis (↑ risk of pancreatitis)

Adverse Effects: Drug fever/rash, leukopenia, anemia, thrombocytopenia, hepatomegaly, hepatotoxicity/hepatic necrosis, peripheral neuropathy, pancreatitis, stomatitis, oral ulcers, dysphagia, arthritis, hyperglycemia, lipotrophy, wasting, lactic acidosis with hepatic steatosis (rare, but potentially life-threatening toxicity with use of NRTIs)

HIV Resistance Potential: Low (triple therapy); high (mono/double drug therapy)

Allergic Potential: High

Safety in Pregnancy: C

Comments: Foscarnet may increase toxicity. Do not use with stavudine, didanosine, or lamivudine to avoid additive toxicities. Food decreases absorption by 39%. Effective antiretroviral therapy consists of at least 3 antiretrovirals (same/different classes)

Cerebrospinal Fluid Penetration: 25%

REFERENCES:
Drugs for AIDS and associated infections. Med Lett Drug Ther 35:79-86, 1993.
HIV Trialists' Collaborative Group. Zidovudine, didanosine, and zalcitabine in the treatment of HIV infection: Meta-analyses of the randomised evidence. Lancet 353:2014-2025, 1999.

Panel on Clinical Practices for Treatment of HIV Infection. Guidelines for the use of antiretroviral agents in HIV-infected adults and adolescents. Department of Health and Human Services. April 23, 2001. www.hivatis.org
Shelton MJ, O'Donnell AM, Morse GD. Zalcitabine. Ann Pharmacotherapy 27:480-9, 1993.
Skowron G, Bozzette SA, Lim L, et al. Alternating and intermittent regimens of zidovudine and dideoxycytidine in patients with AIDS or AIDS-related complex. Ann Intern Med 118:321-30, 1993.

Zidovudine (Retrovir) ZDV Azidothymidine AZT

Drug Class: Antiretroviral NRTI (nucleoside reverse transcriptase inhibitor)

Usual Dose: 200 mg (PO) q8h or 300 mg (PO) q12h (see comments)

Pharmacokinetic Parameters:
Peak serum level: 1.2 mcg/mL
Bioavailability: 60%
Excreted unchanged: 16%
Serum half-life (normal/ESRD): 1.1/3 hrs
Plasma protein binding: 20%
Volume of distribution (V_d): 1.6 L/kg

Primary Mode of Elimination: Renal/hepatic

Dosage Adjustments:

CrCl ~ 40–60 mL/min	No change
CrCl ~ 10–30 mL/min	No change
CrCl < 10 mL/min	300 mg (PO) q24h
Post–HD dose*	300 mg (PO)
Post–PD dose	None
Post–CVVH dose*	300 mg (PO)
Moderate hepatic insufficiency	No change
Severe hepatic insufficiency	No change

Drug Interactions: Acetaminophen (↑ acetaminophen toxicity); atovaquone, fluconazole, lamivudine, methadone, probenecid, TMP-SMX, valproic acid (↑ zidovudine levels); cidofovir (↑ zidovudine levels, flu-like symptoms); clarithromycin, nelfinavir,

rifampin, rifabutin (↓ zidovudine levels);
dapsone, flucytosine, ganciclovir, interferon
alpha, bone marrow suppressive/cytotoxic
agents (↑ risk of hematologic toxicity);
indomethacin (↑ levels of zidovudine toxic
metabolite); phenytoin (↑ zidovudine levels, ↑ or
↓ phenytoin levels); ribavirin (↓ zidovudine
effect; avoid)
Adverse Effects: Nausea, vomiting, GI upset,
diarrhea, leukopenia, anemia, macrocytosis,
thrombocytopenia, headaches, ↑ SGOT/SGPT,
myalgias, insomnia, blue/black nail
discoloration, asthenia, lactic acidosis with
hepatic steatosis (rare, but potentially life-
threatening toxicity with use of NRTIs)
HIV Resistance Potential: Low (triple therapy);
high (mono/double drug therapy)
Allergic Potential: Low
Safety in Pregnancy: C
Comments: Synergistic with acyclovir, ddI, ddC,
alpha–interferon, or GM–CSF. Antagonized by
ganciclovir or ribavirin. Fat decreases GI
absorption. Also a component of Combivir and
Trizivir. Effective antiretroviral therapy consists of
at least 3 antiretrovirals (same/different classes).
Meningeal dose = usual dose
Cerebrospinal Fluid Penetration: 60%

REFERENCES:
Barry M, Mulcahy F, Merry C, et al. Pharmacokinetics and potential interactions amongst antiretroviral agents used to treat patients with HIV infection. Clin Pharmacol 36:289-304, 1999.
Been-Tiktak AM, Boucher CA, Brun-Vezinet F, et al. Efficacy and safety of combination therapy with delavirdine and zidovudine: A European/Australian phase II trial. Intern J Antimcrob Agents 11:13-21, 1999.
McDowell JA, Lou Y, Symonds WS, et al. Multiple-dose pharmacokinetics and pharmacodynamics of abacavir alone and in combination with zidovudine in human immunodeficiency virus-infected adults. Antimicrob Agents Chemother 44:2061-7, 2000.
Montaner JS, Reiss P, Cooper D, et al. A randomized, double-blind trial comparing combinations of nevirapine, didanosine, and zidovudine for HIV-infected patients: The INCAS trial. Italy, the Netherlands, Canada and Australia Study. J Am Med Assoc 279:930-937, 1998.
Panel on Clinical Practices for Treatment of HIV Infection. Guidelines for the use of antiretroviral agents in HIV-infected adults and adolescents. Department of Health and Human Services. April 23, 2001. www.hivatis.org
Simpson DM. Human immunodeficiency virus-associated dementia: A review of pathogenesis, prophylaxis, and treatment studies of zidovudine therapy. Clin Infect Dis 29:19-34, 1999.

ANTIMICROBIAL THERAPY AND INFECTIOUS DISEASE
REFERENCES AND SUGGESTED READINGS*

Amabile-Cuevas CF (ed). Antibiotic Resistance: From Molecular Basics to Therapeutic Options. R.G. Landes Company, Austin, 1996.

Ambrose P, Nightingale AT (eds). Principles of Pharmacodynamics. Marcel Dekker, Inc., New York, 2001.

Anderson RJ, Schrier RW (eds). Clinical Use of Drugs in Patients with Kidney and Liver Disease. W. B. Saunders Company, Philadelphia, 1981.

Armstrong D, Cohen J (eds). Infectious Diseases. Mosby, Philadelphia, 1999.

Bartlett JG, Gallant JE (eds). 2000-2001 Medical Management of HIV Infection. Port City Press, Baltimore, 2000.

Bennet WM, Aronoff GR, Golper TA, Morrison G, Brater DC, Singer I (eds). Drug Prescribing in Renal Failure, 2nd Edition. American College of Physicians, Philadelphia, 2000.

Brandstetter R, Cunha BA, Karetsky M (eds). The Pneumonias. Springer-Verlag, Berlin, 1993.

Chadwick DJ, Goode J (eds). Antibiotic Resistance: Origins, Evolution, Selection and Spread. John Wiley & Sons, New York, 1997.

Ciba Foundation Symposium 207. Antibiotic Resistance: Origins, Evolution, Selection and Spread. John Wiley & Sons, New York, 1997.

Conte Jr JE, Jacob LS, Polk Jr JC (eds). Antibiotic Prophylaxis in Surgery. J.B. Lippincott Company, Philadelphia, 1984.

Cook GC (ed). Manson's Tropical Diseases, 20th Edition. W.B. Saunders Company Ltd., London, 1996.

Cunha BA (ed). Medical Clinics of North America: Antimicrobial Therapy. W.B. Saunders Company, Philadelphia, 1982.

Cunha BA (ed). Medical Clinics of North America: Antimicrobial Therapy I. W.B. Saunders Company, Philadelphia, 1995.

Cunha BA (ed). Medical Clinics of North America: Antimicrobial Therapy II. W.B. Saunders Company, Philadelphia, 1995.

Cunha BA (ed). Infectious Disease in the Elderly. John Wright & Co., London, 1988.

Cunha BA (ed). Infectious Diseases in Critical Care Medicine. Marcel Dekker, New York, 1998.

Cunha BA (ed). Tick-Borne Infectious Diseases. Marcel Dekker, New York, 2000.

Cunha BA (ed). Medical Clinics of North America: Antimicrobial Therapy I. W.B. Saunders Company, Philadelphia, 2000.

Cunha BA (ed). Medical Clinics of North America: Antimicrobial Therapy II. W.B. Saunders Company, Philadelphia, 2001.

Dolin R, Masur H, Saag MS (eds). AIDS Therapy. Churchill Livingstone, New York, 1999.

Drugs for Parasitic Infections. Med Letter. March, 2000.

Gorbach SL, Bartlett JG, Blacklow NR (eds). Infectious Diseases, 2nd Edition. W.B. Saunders Company, Philadelphia, 1998.

Guerrant RL, Walker DH, Weller PF (eds). Tropical Infectious Disease: Principles, Pathogens & Practice. Churchill Livingstone, Philadelphia, 1999.

Ieada CM, Keaten, Jr, BL, Goldman MP, Gray LD, Aberg JA (eds). Infectious Diseases Handbook, 4th Edition. Lexi-Comp, Inc., Hudson, 2001.

Kaye D (ed). Infectious Disease Clinics of North America: Antibacterial Therapy: Pharmacodynamics, Pharmacology, New Agents. W.B. Saunders Company, Philadelphia, 1995.

Kaye D (ed). Infectious Disease Clinics of North America: Antibacterial Therapy: Pharmacodynamics, Pharmacology, New Agents. W.B. Saunders Company, Philadelphia, 2000.

Koneman EW, Allen SD, Janda WM, Schreckenberger PC, Winn Jr, WC (eds). Color Atlas and Textbook of Diagnostic Microbiology, 5th Edition. Lippincott-Raven Publishers, Philadelphia, 1997.

Kucers A, Crowe S, Grayson ML, Hoy J (eds). The Use of Antibiotics: A Clinical Review of Antibacterial, Antifungal, and Antiviral Drugs, 5th Edition. Butterworth-Heinemann, Oxford, 1997.

Lorian V (ed). Antibiotics in Laboratory Medicine, 4th Edition. Williams & Wilkens, Baltimore, 1996.

Mandell GL, Bennett JE, Dolin R (eds). Mandell, Douglas and Bennett's Principles and Practice of Infectious Disease, 5th Edition. Churchill Livingstone, Philadelphia, 2000.

Murray PR, Baron EJ, Pfaller MA, Tenover FC, Yolken RH (eds). Manual of Clinical Microbiology, 6th edition. ASM Press, Washington, D.C., 1995.

Neu HC (ed). Medical Clinics of North America: Update on Antibiotics I. W.B. Saunders Company, Philadelphia, 1987.

Neu HC (ed). Medical Clinics of North America: Update on Antibiotics II. W.B. Saunders Company, Philadelphia, 1988.

O'Grady F, Lambert HP, Finch RG, Greenwood D (eds). Antibiotic and Chemotherapy, 2nd Edition. Churchill Livingstone, New York, 1997.

Piscitelli SC, Rodvold KE (eds). Drug Interactions in Infectious Diseases. Humana Press, Totowa, 2001.

Pratt WB, Fekety R (eds). The Antimicrobial Drugs, 1st Edition. Oxford University Press, New York, 1986.

Ristuccia AM, Cunha BA (eds). Antimicrobial Therapy. Raven Press, New York, 1984.

* *See drug summaries (Chapter 7) for additional references*

Root RK (ed). Clinical Infectious Diseases: A Practical Approach. Oxford University Press, New York, 1999.

Schlossberg D (ed). Current Therapy of Infectious Disease, 2nd Edition. Mosby-Yearbook, St. Louis, 2001.

Scholar EM, Pratt WB (eds). The Antimicrobial Drugs, 2nd Edition. Oxford University Press, New York, 2000.

Strickland GT (ed). Hunter's Tropical Medicine and Emerging Infectious Diseases, 8th Edition. W.B. Saunders Company, Philadelphia, 2000.

Yoshikawa TT, Norman DC (eds). Antimicrobial Therapy in the Elderly. Marcel Dekker, New York, 1994.

Yu VL, Merigan, Jr. TC, Barriere SL (eds). Antimicrobial Therapy and Vaccines. Williams & Wilkens, Baltimore, 1999.

Zinner SH, Young LS, Acar JF, Ortiz-Neu C (eds). New Considerations for Macrolides, Azalides, Streptogramins, and Ketolides. Marcel Dekker, Inc., New York, 2000.

HIV INFECTION REFERENCES AND SUGGESTED READINGS

Ammassari A, Scoppettuolo G, Murri R, et al. Changing disease patterns in focal brain lesion-causing disorders in AIDS. J Acquir Immune Defic Syndr Hum Retroviral 18:365, 1998

Armstrong WS, Katz JT, Kazanjian PH. Human immunodeficiency virus-associated fever of unknown origin: a study of 70 patients in the United States and review. Clin Infect Dis 28:341, 1999

Barbut F, Meynard JL, Guiguet M, et al. Clostridium difficile-associated diarrhea in HIV-infected patients: Epidemiology and risk factors. J Acquir Immune Defic Syndr Hum Retroviral 16:176, 1997

Barreiro P, Soriano V, Blanco F, et al. Risks and benefits of replacing protease inhibitors by nevirapine in HIV-infected subjects under long-term successful triple combination therapy. AIDS 14:807-812, 2000.

Bartlett JG. Pneumonia in the patient with HIV infection. Infect Dis Clin North Am 12:807, 1998

Bartlett JG (ed). The Johns Hopkins Hospital Guide to Medical Care of Patients with HIV Infection, 9th edition, Lippincott Williams & Wilkins, Philadelphia, 2000

Bayard PJ, Berger TG, Jacobson MA. Drug hypersensitivity reactions and human immunodeficiency virus disease. J Acquir Immune Defic Syndr 5:1237, 1992

Bozzette SA, Finkelstein DM, Spector SA, et al. A randomized trial of three antipneumocystis agents in patients with advanced human immunodeficiency virus infection. NIAID AIDS Clinical Trials Group [see comments]. N Engl J Med 332:693, 1995

Bozzette SA, Sattler FR, Chiu J, et al. A controlled trial of early adjunctive treatment with corticosteroids for Pneumocystis carinii pneumonia in the acquired immunodeficiency syndrome. California Collaborative Treatment Group. N Engl J Med 323:1451, 1990

Brosgart CL, Louis TA, Hillman DW, et al. A randomized, placebo-controlled trial of the safety and efficacy of oral ganciclovir for prophylaxis of cytomegalovirus disease in HIV-infected individuals. AIDS 12:269-77, 1998.

Carr A, Marriott D, Field A, et al. Treatment of HIV-1-associated microsporidiosis and cryptosporidiosis with combination antiretroviral therapy. Lancet 351:256, 1998

Carr A, Samara K, Thorisdottir A, et al. Diagnosis, prediction, and natural course of HIV-1 protease-inhibitor associated lipodystrophy, hyperlipidaemia, and diabetes mellitus: a cohort study. Lancet 353:2093-2099, 1999.

Centers for Disease Control and Prevention. Notice to Readers: Updated guidelines for the use of rifabutin or rifampin for the treatment and prevention of tuberculosis among HIV-infected patients taking protease inhibitors or nonnucleoside reverse transcriptase inhibitors. MMWR 49:183-9, 2000.

Centers for Disease Control and Prevention. 1993 revised classification system for HIV infection and expanded surveillance case definition for AIDS among adolescents and adults. MMWR 41:1-19, 1992.

Chaisson RE, Keruly JC, Moore RD. Association of initial CD4 cell count and viral load with response to highly active antiretroviral therapy. J Am Med Assoc 284: 3128-3129, 2000.

Cinque P, Scarpellini P, Vago L, et al. Diagnosis of central nervous system complications in HIV-infected patients: Cerebrospinal fluid analysis by the polymerase chain reaction [editorial]. Aids 11:1, 1997

Cohen C, Hunt S, Sension M, et al. Phenotypic resistance testing significantly improves response to therapy: A randomized trial (VIRA3001). In: 7th Conference on Retrovirus and Opportunistic Infections. San Francisco: Abstract 237, 2000.

Cohn JA, McMeeking A, Cohen W, et al. Evaluation of the policy of empiric treatment of suspected Toxoplasma encephalitis in patients with the acquired immunodeficiency syndrome. Am J Med 86:521, 1989

Colson AE and Sax PE. Primary HIV-1 infection. In: UpToDate in Medicine (a CD-ROM textbook) 1998. Revised October, 1999

Cunha BA. Community-acquired pneumonia in patients with HIV. Drugs for Today 31:739, 1998

Cunha BA. Community-acquired pneumonia in HIV patients. Clinical Infectious Diseases 28:410, 1999

Cunha BA. Fever of unknown origin in HIV/AIDS patients. Drugs for Today 35:429, 1999

Currier JS, Williams PL, Koletar SL, et al. Discontinuation of Mycobacterium avium complex prophylaxis in patients with antiretroviral therapy-induced increases in CD4+ cell count. A randomized, double-blind, placebo-controlled trial. AIDS Clinical Trials Group 362 Study Team. Ann Intern Med 133:493, 2000

Deeks SG, Barbour JD, Martin JN, et al. Sustained CD4+ T cell response after virologic failure of protease inhibitor-based regimens in patients with human immunodeficiency virus infection. J Infect Dis 181:946, 2000

DeSimone JA, Pomerantz RJ, Babinchak TJ. Inflammatory reactions in HIV-1-infected persons after initiation of highly active antiretroviral therapy. Ann Intern Med 133:447, 2000

Detels R, Munoz A, McFarlane G, et al. Effectiveness of potent antiretroviral therapy on time to AIDS and death in men with known HIV infection duration. Multicenter AIDS Cohort Study Investigators. JAMA 280:1497, 1998

Durat J, Clevenbergh P, Halfon P, et al. Drug-resistance genotyping in HIV-1 therapy: the VIRADAPT randomized controlled trial. Lancet 353:2195-2199, 1999.

El-Sadr WM, Burman WJ, Grant LB, et al. Discontinuation of prophylaxis for mycobacterium avium complex disease in HIV-infected patients who have a response to antiretroviral therapy. N Engl J Med 342:1085-95, 2000.

Furrer H, Oparavil M, Bernasconi E, et al. Stopping primary prophylaxis in HIV-1 infected patients at high risk of toxoplasma encephalitis. Lancet 355:2217-8, 2000.

Gallant JE, Chaisson RE, Moore RD. The effect of adjunctive corticosteroids for the treatment of Pneumocystis carinii pneumonia on mortality and subsequent complications. Chest 114:1258, 1998

Garcia-Ordonez MA, Colmenero JD, Jimenez-Onate F, et al. Diagnostic usefulness of percutaneous liver biopsy in HIV-infected patients with fever of unknown origin. J Infect 38:94, 1999

Gildenberg PL, Gathe JC, Jr., Kim JH. Stereotactic biopsy of cerebral lesions in AIDS. Clin Infect Dis 30:491, 2000

Gorbach SL, Bartlett JG, Blackow, NR (eds). Infectious Diseases, 2nd edition. W.B. Saunders Co., Philadelphia, 1998

Graybill JR, Sobel J, Saag M, et al. Diagnosis and management of increased intracranial pressure in patients with AIDS and cryptococcal meningitis. The NIAID Mycoses Study Group and AIDS Cooperative Treatment Groups. Clin Infect Dis 30:47, 2000

Hardy WD, Feinberg J, Finkelstein DM, et al., for the AIDS Clinical Trials Group. A controlled trial of trimethoprim-sulfamethoxazole or aerosolized pentamidine for secondary prophylaxis of Pneumocystis carinii pneumonia in patients with the acquired immunodeficiency syndrome: AIDS Clinical Trials Group protocol 021. N Engl J Med 327:1842-8, 1992.

Havlir DV, Dube MP, Sattler FR, et al. Prophylaxis against disseminated Mycobacterium avium complex with weekly azithromycin, daily rifabutin, or both. N Engl J Med 335:392-8, 1996.

HIV Trialists' Collaborative Group. Zidovudine, didanosine, and zalcitabine in the treatment of HIV infection: Meta-analyses of the randomised evidence. Lancet 353:2014-2025, 1999.

Jacobson MA, Hahn SM, Gerberding JL, et al. Ciprofloxacin for Salmonella bacteremia in the acquired immunodeficiency syndrome (AIDS). Ann Intern Med 110:1027, 1989

Kourtis AP, Bulterys M, Nesheim SR, et al., Understanding the timing of HIV transmission from mother to infant. JAMA 285:709-712, 2001.

Ledergerber B, Egger M, Opravil M, et al. Clinical progression and virological failure on highly active antiretroviral therapy in HIV-1 patients: A prospective cohort study. Swiss HIV Cohort Study. Lancet 353:863, 1999

Leenders AC, Reiss P, Portegies P, et al. Liposomal amphotericin B (AmBisome) compared with amphotericin B both followed by oral fluconazole in the treatment of AIDS-associated cryptococcal meningitis. AIDS 11:1463, 1997

Lonergan JT, Behling C, Pfander H, et al. Hyperlactatemia and hepatic abnormalities in 10 human immunodeficiency virus-infected patients receiving nucleoside analogue combination regimens. Clin Infect Dis 31:162-166, 2000.

Lopez JC, Miro JM, Pena JM, Podzamczer D, and the GESIDA 04-98 Study Group. A randomized trial of the discontinuation of primary and secondary prophylaxis against Pneumocystis carinii pneumonia after HAART in patients with HIV Infection. N Engl J Med 344(3):159-167, 2001.

Maggi P, Larocca AM, Quarto M, et al. Effect of antiretroviral therapy on cryptosporidiosis and microsporidiosis in patients infected with human immunodeficiency virus type 1. Eur J Clin Microbiol Infect Dis 19:213, 2000

Manabe YC, Clark DP, Moore RD, et al. Cryptosporidiosis in patients with AIDS: Correlates of disease and survival. Clin Infect Dis 27:536, 1998

Martin DF, Kupperman BD, Wolitz RA, et al. Oral ganciclovir for patients with cytomegalovirus retinitis treated with a ganciclovir implant. N Engl J Med 340:1063-70, 1999.

Masur H, for the USPHS/IDSA Prevention of Opportunistic Infections Working Group: 2001 USPHS/IDSA guidelines for the prevention of opportunistic infections in persons infected with Human Immunodeficiency Virus. July, 2001, http://hivatis.org/trtgdlns.html#Opportunistic

Max B, Sherer R. Management of the adverse effects of antiretroviral therapy and medication adherence. Clin Infect Dis 30 Suppl 2:S96-S116, 2000.

Mendelson MH, Gurtman A, Szabo S, et al. Pseudomonas aeruginosa bacteremia in patients with AIDS. Clin Infect Dis 18:886, 1994

Montaner JS, Reiss P, Cooper D, et al. A randomized, double-blind trial comparing combinations of nevirapine, didanosine, and zidovudine for HIV-infected patients: the INCAS Trial. Italy, The Netherlands, Canada and Australia Study. J Am Med Assoc 279:930-937, 1998.

Murphy RL, Brun S, Hicks C, et al. ABT-378/ritonavir plus stavudine and lamivudine for the treatment of antiretroviral-naive adults with HIV-1 infection: 48-week results. AIDS 15:F1-9, 2001.

Palella FJ, Jr., Delaney KM, Moorman AC, et al. Declining morbidity and mortality among patients with advanced human immunodeficiency virus infection. HIV Outpatient Study Investigators. N Engl J Med 338:853-860, 1998.

Panel on Clinical Practices for Treatment of HIV Infection: Guidelines for the use of antiretroviral agents in HIV-infected adults and adolescents. Dept. of Health and Human Services. April 23, 2001, www.hivatis.org

Pierce M, Crampton S, Henry D, et al. A randomized trial of clarithromycin as prophylaxis against disseminated Mycobacterium avium complex infection in patients with advanced acquired immunodeficiency syndrome. N Engl J Med 335:384, 1996

Racoosin JA, Kessler CM. Bleeding episodes in HIV-positive patients taking HIV protease inhibitors: A case series. Haemophilia 5:266-269, 1999.

Saag MS, Graybill RJ, Larsen RA, et al. Practice guidelines for the management of cryptococcal disease. Infectious Diseases Society of America. Clin Infect Dis 30:710, 2000

Sax PE. Managing long-term complications of HIV care. Infectious Disease Special Edition 3:115-118, 2000

Sax PE. Opportunistic infections in HIV disease: Down but not out. Infectious Disease Clinics of North America 15:433-455, 2001

Schacker T, Collier AC, Hughes J, et al. Clinical and epidemiologic features of primary HIV infection. Ann Intern Med 125:257-264, 1996.

Schacker T, Zeh J, Hu HL, et al. Frequency of symptomatic and asymptomatic herpes simplex virus type 2 reactivations among human immunodeficiency virus-infected men. J Infect Dis 178:1616-22, 1998.

Schneider MME, Hoepelman AIM, Schattenkerk JKME, et al., and the Dutch AIDS Treatment Group. A controlled trial of aerosolized pentamidine or trimethoprim-sulfamethoxazole as primary prophylaxis against Pneumocystis carinii pneumonia in patients with human immunodeficiency virus infection. N Engl J Med 327:1836-41, 1992.

Sherman DS, Fish DN. Management of protease inhibitor-associated diarrhea. Clin Infect Dis 30:908, 2000

Smith NH, Cron S, Valdez LM, et al. Combination drug therapy for cryptosporidiosis in AIDS. J Infect Dis 178:900, 1998

Staszewski S, Morales-Ramirez J, Tashima KT, et al. Efavirenz plus zidovudine and lamivudine, efavirenz plus indinavir, and indinavir plus zidovudine and lamivudine in the treatment of HIV-1 Infection in adults. N Engl J Med 341:1865-1873, 1999.

Sterling TR, Vlahov D, Astemborski J, et al. Initial HIV-1 RNA level and progression to AIDS in women and men. N Engl J Med 344:720-725, 2001.

Tassie JM, Gasnault J, Bentata M, et al. Survival improvement of AIDS-related progressive multifocal leukoencephalopathy in the era of protease inhibitors. Clinical Epidemiology Group. French Hospital Database on HIV. AIDS 13:1881, 1999

U.S. Public Health Service Report: Updated U.S. Public Health Service guidelines for the management of occupational exposures to HBV, HCV, and HIV and recommendations for postexposure prophylaxis. MMWR 50(RR11):1-52, June 29, 2001. www.cdc.gov/mmwr/preview/mmwrhtml/rr5011a1.

Weber T. Cerebrospinal fluid analysis for the diagnosis of human immunodeficiency virus-related neurologic diseases. Semin Neurol 19:223, 1999

Weverling GJ, Mocroft A, Ledergerber B, et al. Discontinuation of Pneumocystis carinii pneumonia prophylaxis after start of highly active antiretroviral therapy in HIV-1 infection. EuroSIDA Study Group. Lancet 353:1293-1298, 1999.

INDEX

ANTIBIOTIC ESSENTIALS — ORDERING INFORMATION

Price (U.S. dollars)
1 - 9 copies:	$14.95 each
10 - 49 copies:	$13.95 each
50 - 100 copies:	$12.95 each
> 100 copies:	Call

Shipping
USA: UPS Ground delivery
1 - 3 copies:	add $5
4 - 10 copies:	add $7
10 - 49 copies:	add $10
50 - 100 copies:	add $15
> 100 copies:	Call

Call for Next Day, 2-day, or 3-day express delivery charges

Outside USA: Call, fax, or e-mail for delivery charges

Michigan residents: add 6%

4 Ways to Order:
By Internet:	www.physicianspress.com
By Phone:	(248) 616-3023
By Fax*:	(248) 616-3003
By Mail*:	Physicians' Press
	620 Cherry Street
	Royal Oak, Michigan 48073

*   Please print or type name, mailing address, credit card number and expiration date or purchase order number (if applicable), telephone number (important), fax number, and e-mail address. We accept VISA, MasterCard, and American Express

---

Visit our new website at www.physicianspress.com

- Antibiotic Essentials Updates
- Topical Reviews
- Self-Assessment Questions
- Clinical Pitfalls
- ECG Cases
- Bookstore

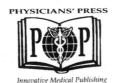

PHYSICIANS' PRESS

Innovative Medical Publishing